RADIOLOGY OF
Spinal Curvature

RADIOLOGY OF
Spinal Curvature

Arthur A. De Smet, M.D.

Associate Professor of Diagnostic Radiology;
Chief, Section of Skeletal Radiology,
The University of Kansas
College of Health Sciences and Hospital,
Kansas City, Kansas

with **290** *illustrations*

THE C. V. MOSBY COMPANY

ST. LOUIS • TORONTO • PRINCETON   1985

MOSBY

A TRADITION OF PUBLISHING EXCELLENCE

Editor: Carol Trumbold
Assistant editor: Anne Gunter
Editing supervisor: Peggy Fagen
Book design: Jeanne Genz
Cover design: Suzanne Oberholtzer
Production: Barbara Merritt, Billie Forshee, Ginny Douglas

Printed in the United States of America

The C.V. Mosby Company
11830 Westline Industrial Drive, St. Louis, Missouri 63146

Library of Congress Cataloging in Publication Data

De Smet, Arthur A.
  Radiology of spinal curvature.

  Bibliography: p.
  Includes index.
    1. Scoliosis—Diagnosis. 2. Spine—Radiography.
3. Scoliosis—Surgery. I. Title. [DNLM: 1. Spine—
radiography. 2. Scoliosis. 3. Kyphosis. 4. Lordosis.
5. Spondylolisthesis.   WE 735 D463r]
RD771.S3D47   1985   617'.3750757   84-22753
ISBN 0-8016-1264-0

AC/MV/MV 9 8 7 6 5 4 3 2 1   02/D/251

Contributors

Marc A. Asher, M.D.

Professor of Orthopedic Surgery,
The University of Kansas
College of Health Sciences and Hospital,
Kansas City, Kansas

Solomon Batnitzky, M.D.

Professor of Diagnostic Radiology,
Chief, Section of Neuroradiology,
The University of Kansas
College of Health Sciences and Hospital,
Kansas City, Kansas

Larry T. Cook, Ph.D.

Associate Professor of Diagnostic Radiology,
The University of Kansas
College of Health Sciences and Hospital,
Kansas City, Kansas

Hilton I. Price, M.D.

Associate Professor of Diagnostic Radiology,
The University of Kansas
College of Health Sciences and Hospital,
Kansas City, Kansas

*This book is dedicated
to my wife, Peg,
and my sons, Alan, Mark, and Brian.
Their importance to me and their love
provide the essential balance to the challenges
and pressures of my professional life.*

Preface

The idea to write this book was first stimulated by Dr. Donald Resnick of the University of California at San Diego and Mr. Samuel Harshberger of Mosby. They felt that there was a need for a textbook directed toward the radiologic evaluation of abnormal spinal curvature. Their comments reaffirmed my own experience as to the difficulty in achieving expertise in the radiology of spinal deformity. Although there are many excellent textbooks dealing with spinal deformity, their emphasis is on the complex clinical aspects of each condition. As a result, I had found it difficult to determine the role played by radiology from both these textbooks and related articles in the orthopedic literature. Because of the dedicated efforts of Dr. Marc Asher, our institution is a major referral center for spinal deformity problems. With this clinical stimulus and the invaluable assistance of Dr. Samuel J. Dwyer III, Dr. Larry Cook, and Mr. Mark Tarlton of our research section, I had already done considerable research in three-dimensional analysis of scoliosis. Therefore, because of this perceived need and a desire to increase my own knowledge, I enthusiastically agreed to make the considerable commitment of professional time that is required for a project of this kind.

My goal in writing this text was to provide a concise summary of the clinical and radiologic features of thoracic and lumbar spinal deformity for the general orthopedic surgeon and the diagnostic radiologist. With widespread school screening programs for scoliosis, both groups of physicians are becoming increasingly involved in the initial evaluation of patients with abnormal spinal curvature. I believe that both the radiologic and clinical aspects must be learned because of their strong interdependence. The general orthopedic surgeon will be familiar with many of the clinical concepts but may be unaware of the role of the radiographic evaluation in initial diagnosis and the monitoring of treatment. Similarly, the diagnostic radiologist has probably observed many of the described findings but his reports may not have detailed the important points because he was unaware of their clinical significance. I decided not to discuss abnormal curvature of the cervical spine in order to limit the length of the text and because abnormal cervical curvature does not share the rapid worsening with growth and the gravitational forces of trunkal weight that are so important in abnormal thoracic and lumbar curvature.

The first chapter includes a detailed discussion of the epidemiology, prognosis, and pathogenesis of idiopathic scoliosis. The following five chapters deal with the radiographic evaluation of scoliosis, both before and after orthosis or surgical treatment. Chapters seven through nine discuss the less common areas of secondary scoliosis, kyphosis, and lordosis. The last chapter discusses three-dimensional analysis of spinal curvature for both the specialist wishing to investigate this area and the non-research-oriented physician. A review of spinal curvature terminology is found in the Appendix. Although three-dimensional analysis will remain isolated to the academic centers, its use in research should increase. As further investigation is reported using these computer-assisted techniques, physicians will need background information to assess these results critically. Eight of the chapters end with a summary in which I have highlighted those features that I believe should be well known by all physicians evaluating patients with spinal curvature problems.

Although I have often seen extensive acknowledgments in other textbooks, I never previously fully appreciated how many individuals play a role in preparing and writing a major book. Although they are too numerous to mention individually, an important part is played by the technologists, secretarial staff, and file room personnel without whose day-to-day efforts I could not function professionally. I would like to thank Dr. Arch W. Templeton, Chairman of the Department of Diagnostic Radiology, for providing the excellent professional environment that has stimulated my research efforts.

With regard to this book itself, I would like to thank the following individuals for their efforts on my behalf. Our research clerk and department librarian, Mrs. Arlene Berridge, obtained, photocopied, and verified all of the reference material as well as tabulated much of the statistical data. One of our department secretaries, Mrs. Barbara Martin, cheerfully and willingly typed the entire manuscript, including its multiple revisions. Dr. Marc Asher and Mrs. Janice Orrick of the Section of Orthopedic Surgery provided many of the cases that were used for illustration and offered constructive criticism on the manuscript. From our department, Dr. Steven Fritz edited the radiation risk section and Dr. Solomon Batnitzky provided me with several illustrations. Although no longer associated with our institution, Dr. James Goin reviewed the entire manuscript for its clarity of presentation. The photography departments of this institution and Duke University Medical Center contributed their expertise in making the prints of scoliosis radiographs, which are so difficult to photographically reproduce. To all of these individuals, I owe a great debt of gratitude.

Arthur A. De Smet

Contents

Chapter One

An Overview of Idiopathic Scoliosis

*S*coliosis is a common deformity of the spine that has received considerable attention in the orthopedic literature but has been discussed only infrequently in the radiologic literature. This situation is unfortunate because scoliosis is both verified and quantified primarily by radiographic techniques. Interaction between orthopedists and radiologists can only improve evaluation of this complex condition. This text will emphasize idiopathic scoliosis because it is the most common and most thoroughly studied abnormality of spinal curvature. As such, it is an ideal prototype for understanding the principles of radiography of abnormal spinal curvature.

Scoliosis can be defined very simply as a lateral curvature of the spine. When a person is viewed from behind, the normal spine should be in a straight line. Any lateral deviation from that straight line is by definition a scoliosis. Although there are multiple causes of scoliosis,[78] 80% to 90% of the cases are idiopathic.[84] The terminology, patterns, epidemiology, and natural history of idiopathic scoliosis will be discussed as background for this important and common condition.

Terminology

The basis of all scientific study is the precise definition and measurement of the phenomenon under investigation. Evaluation of scoliosis research prior to the last two decades is handicapped by the lack of consistently defined and adequately detailed data for subsequent investigators to compare and validate earlier work. The Scoliosis Research Society was founded in 1966 to address this problem. The terminology committee of this society presented the first standardized list of terms relevant to scoliosis in 1978 and revised that list in 1981.[101] Because it is the only officially proposed terminology, the approved glossary will be used throughout this text and is presented in its entirety in the Appendix.

In order to describe fully a scoliotic curve, a number of descriptive terms must be used. The description of a scoliotic curve should routinely include etiology, age at presentation, curve direction, and curve level, for example, an idiopathic, adolescent, right thoracic scoliosis.

Age at Presentation

Idiopathic scoliosis is classified according to the age at which the scoliosis is first detected (with the realization that the age at presentation may not be the same time that the curve began). In most cases, the exact age that the scoliosis began is unknown, so the examiner can only guess at the age of onset. On the other hand, the age at presentation is known precisely. Curves should be differentiated according to patient age because of the differing prognosis and treatment options in the various age groups.

INFANTILE SCOLIOSIS

Infantile scoliosis refers to lateral spinal curvature beginning during the first 3 years of life. These patients are a distinctive subgroup of idiopathic scoliosis as emphasized by the fact that the condition is relatively rare (0.5%) in North America[93,107] but represents 9% to 13% of idiopathic scoliosis in Great Britain.[50,102] Also, unlike the other forms of scoliosis, there is frequent spontaneous resolution of infantile scoliosis in 28% to 92% of patients.* A recent fascinating study from Great Britain reported a decrease in infantile scoliosis from 41% of idiopathic scoliosis patients in 1970 down to 4% in 1981.[75] The author attributed the decrease to a change from positioning infants supine and tightly bundled to the current prone positioning without restrictive covers. This positioning difference may well have accounted for the frequency differences between North America and Great Britain.

These curves are single left thoracic 76% to 90% of the time and are one-and-one-half times more common in boys than in girls.† Untreated curves that do progress usually become very severe, exceeding a Cobb angle of 70 degrees.[53,102]

Unlike juvenile and adolescent scoliosis, prediction of subsequent progression is frequently possible by using the rib-vertebral angle of Mehta,[76] as described in Chapter Two. These patients also have associated congenital abnormalities including plagiocephaly (100%), mental retardation (13%), hip dislocation (3.5%), heart disease (2.5%), and inguinal hernia (7.4% of boys).[19,66,128] No incidence studies of spinal deformity have been performed in patients of this age, so the frequency of this condition is unknown.

JUVENILE SCOLIOSIS

These curves are defined as those first noted between 3 years of age and the onset of puberty. In its terminology, the Scoliosis Research Society did not give a definition for the onset of puberty, but it is commonly taken to mean thelarche (onset of breast development) in girls and pubarche (development of pubic hair) in boys. Since thelarche usually begins at age 10 years in girls and pubarche begins about age 12 years in boys,[5] the age range for juvenile scoliosis should be different for the two sexes. However, even recent studies[37,114] have used a range of 4 to 9 years of age to define juvenile scoliosis. Because the age range is similar to the physical development standards the distinction is not critical, but the inconsistency will hopefully be resolved in the future.

Juvenile scoliosis represents 12% to 16% of the cases of idiopathic scoliosis.[51,58,77,90] It affects both sexes equally and usually presents with a right thoracic pattern (41% to 48%) or a combined right thoracic and left lumbar

---

*See references 19, 50, 52, 53, 66, 75, 76, 113.
†See references 19, 50, 53, 66, 75, 113, 128.

pattern (22% to 32%).[37,114] Juvenile scoliosis is familial and commonly progressive, so it is more closely related to adolescent than infantile scoliosis. Undoubtedly some of the curves first detected during the rapid growth period of early adolescence are due to previously unrecognized juvenile scoliosis. Prognosis and treatment considerations are similar to those of adolescent scoliosis. This subgroup has been studied only infrequently, presumably because few children have physical examinations for spinal deformity at this age. Because population surveys of this age group have not been performed, the prevalence of juvenile scoliosis is unknown.

ADOLESCENT SCOLIOSIS

Adolescent scoliosis refers to those patients presenting with scoliosis at or after the onset of puberty but before completion of skeletal maturity. Most patients with idiopathic scoliosis present clinically during adolescence due to the rapid curve progression that occurs during accelerated growth. Skeletal maturity has not been defined in this context, but common usage has taken this to mean that skeletal growth has stopped. Adolescent scoliosis has been extensively studied and will be discussed in detail later in this chapter.

Curve Description

After specifying the age at presentation, each curve should be described by its direction and location. Supplementary terms such as *major* and *minor*, *primary* and *secondary*, and *structural* and *nonstructural* can also be used to describe other features of the curve.[42]

CURVE DIRECTION AND LOCATION

Curve direction is either right or left and denotes the direction in which the curve is convex, for instance, the common *right* thoracic scoliosis. Some physicians modify this terminology by adding the word *convexity* after the direction to emphasize how the direction is defined, but this addition is not necessary.

The curve location or level refers to the specific region of the spine that is curved and is defined by where the apex of the curve is located. The apex is the vertebra that is the most rotated or most deviated from the vertical axis. It is usually the most horizontal vertebra within the curve. After locating the apex, curve level is then defined as follows:

Cervical curve: apex between C1 and C6
Cervicothoracic curve: apex at C7 or T1
Thoracic curve: apex between T2 and T11
Thoracolumbar curve: apex at T12 or L1
Lumbar curve: apex between L2 and L4
Lumbosacral curve: apex between L5 and S1

SUPPLEMENTARY TERMS

Other terms can then be added to subcategorize the curves. The terms *structural* and *nonstructural* refer to the flexibility of the curve. A structural scoliosis is a lateral curvature of the spine that does not demonstrate normal segmental mobility on lateral bending or distraction. A structural scoliosis will not disappear on supine radiographs, when the patient bends toward the convexity of the scoliosis. A nonstructural scoliosis, such as that due to limb-length discrepancy, will correct completely with lateral bending.

A *major curve* is the largest curve in the scoliotic spine in contrast to the *minor* or smaller curves. Two curves of equal size in the same spine are termed a *double major* scoliosis. Since there is a well accepted standard deviation of 2.2 to 3.0 degrees[54,84] in measuring scoliosis, Willner recently defined *double major scoliosis* as consisting of two curves within 5 degrees of each other.[124]

A *primary* curve is the first structural curve to appear, with all other subsequent curves being *secondary* curves. This notation is seldom used because most patients are not seen until two curves are present, so radiographs are not available from the time when there was only one curve. Although the larger of two curves is usually the primary curve, a secondary curve can become larger than the primary, as has been illustrated by Moe.[78]

A *compensatory curve* develops above or below a structural curve to maintain body balance. A compensatory curve can become structural with time. Since it develops after a primary curve, every compensatory curve is by definition a secondary curve. The term *compensatory* is unnecessarily complicating because most secondary curves serve to restore balance.

If used only to indicate relative size, the terms *major* and *minor* are useful in emphasizing whether one curve is more deforming than the other. For instance, a patient with both thoracic and lumbar curves could have a double major thoracic and lumbar, a major thoracic and minor lumbar, or a minor thoracic and major lumbar curve pattern.

Therefore, it is suggested that each scoliotic spine be classified according to etiology, age at presentation, curve direction, and curve location. If two curves of different sizes are present, one should be labeled the major and the other the minor. If supine bending films are available, each curve segment can be classified as being structural or nonstructural.

Epidemiology
PREVALENCE

The frequency of scoliosis is not clear despite the fact that 39 studies have been reported.* The difficulty in interpreting these studies lies in lack of consistent epidemiologic techniques. The studies vary in their methods of case selection and criteria for defining a scoliotic curve. Almost all studies

---

*See references 1-4, 7, 9, 14, 15, 23, 27, 30, 31, 33, 39, 41, 44, 45, 49, 55, 68, 70, 71, 74, 82, 86-88, 92, 98, 104-106, 109, 110, 112, 118, 124, 125, 127.

have investigated prevalence (proportion of the population affected at a given time) rather than incidence (rate of occurrence of new cases).

Two methods of estimating the prevalence of scoliosis, tuberculosis (TB) screening chest radiographs[7,106,109] and retrospective analysis of referral center patients,[55] are less reliable than prospective screening. The TB screening chest radiographs are not optimally exposed for spine detail, and they evaluate only thoracic curves. Retrospective series from scoliosis referral centers are always biased in favor of more severe disease so that mild cases are not included in the studies, thereby giving a lower-than-actual prevalence.[63]

The most useful studies are those that screen large numbers of adolescent children without a case selection bias. A large number of studies have been reported in which a school nurse or physician performed a screening physical examination of a specific age group of children.* Unfortunately, many of these studies then reported a prevalence of scoliosis without obtaining a spinal radiograph or specifying whether or not the scoliosis was of a certain minimal magnitude. These studies have been summarized and are presented in Table 1-1. Although the popular forward bending test[70] was used by all the investigators as clinical evidence for possible scoliosis, there is considerable variation, with the reported prevalence varying from 0.07% to 8.5%. Either the different examiners had varying sensitivities for calling minimal asymmetries of the thorax abnormal or there might be population differences in the frequency of scoliosis. Even when the scoliosis is confirmed radiographically, there is considerable variation in the prevalence of small curves. If a 5 degree curvature is used as the minimal size for a scoliosis, the prevalence rate is still in a widely varying range from 1.2% to 16.0% (Table 1-2). The data in the original articles were carefully reviewed and frequently recalculated for Tables 1-2 through 1-8 to allow comparison between studies with consistent presentation of the data. With a minimum Cobb angle of 10 degrees for scoliosis as recommended by the Scoliosis Research Society, the prevalence is a more consistent 1.5% to 2.7% for ten studies, but five other studies have a range of 0.03% to 10.3% (Table 1-3). Only for the clinically more significant curves (over 20 degrees) is the prevalence a more consistent 0.3% to 0.6% (Table 1-4).

This variation in scoliosis prevalence might reflect differing methodologies but is more likely the result of different frequencies of scoliosis among population groups. Several small studies indicate that racial differences do exist, with a 0.5% prevalence for Lapps and 1.5% prevalence for non-Lapps in Norway,[109] a 2.5% prevalence for whites and a 0.03% prevalence for blacks in South Africa[104] and a 6.2% prevalence at one site (more than twice that at three other locations) in Greece.[111] In contrast, the large study of Shand and Eisberg[106] found no significant difference in the prevalence of scoliosis between whites and blacks. Since scoliosis has a definite familial tendency, it is not surprising that studies in different geographic regions give different frequencies of scoliosis.

---

*See references 2, 4, 9, 14, 23, 27, 30, 39, 41, 43-45, 49, 65, 68, 74, 82, 86, 92, 98, 104, 105, 110, 112, 115, 118, 125, 127.

TABLE 1-1
Scoliosis prevalence based on positive screening physicals

Authors	Year	Place	Age group (yr)	Number screened	Prevalence (%)
Cronis and Russell	1965	Delaware	6-18	68,301	0.07
Wynne-Davies	1968	Edinburg, U.K.	8-18	7,894	0.22
Baker and Zanyger	1970	Arizona	10-14	125	2.40
Grant et al.	1973	El Paso, Texas	5-18	6,058	0.83
Weiler	1974	Pennsylvania	12-14	8,096	2.80
Sells and May	1974	Seattle, Washington	12-15	3,096	1.60
Golomb and Taylor	1975	Sydney, Australia	10-15	3,299	8.50
Hensinger et al.	1975	Delaware	6-18	316,002	0.15
Flynn et al.	1977	Florida	13-15	38,710	1.80
Benson et al.	1977	Sacramento, California	10-14	7,815	1.50
Asher et al.	1980	Kansas	10-13	379,034	3.20
McCarthy et al.	1983	Little Rock, Arkansas	10-14	11,700	1.96

TABLE 1-2
Scoliosis prevalence: curves over 5 degrees

Authors	Year	Place	Age group (yr)	Number screened	Prevalence (%)
Brooks et al.	1975	California	12-14	3,492	13.6
Newman and Dewald	1977	Chicago, Illinois	14-18	861	16.0
Drennan et al.	1977	Denver, Colorado	11-12	15,904	3.4
Rogala et al.	1978	Montreal, Canada	12-14	26,947	4.5
Smyrnis et al.	1979	Athens, Greece	11-12	3,497	5.0
Goldberg et al.	1980	Dublin, Ireland	9-14	604	15.3
O'Brien	1980	Oswetry, England	11-14	903	3.3
Cooke et al.	1980	London, England	12-15	125	12.3
Willner	1982	Malmo, Sweden	7-16	17,181	2.8
Lonstein et al.	1982	Minnesota	10-14	1,393,553	1.2

TABLE 1-3
Scoliosis prevalence: curves over 10 degrees

Authors	Year	Place	Age group (yr)	Number screened	Prevalence (%)
Segil	1974	South Africa	White children	929	2.50
			African children	1,016	0.03
Brooks et al.	1975	California	12-14	3,492	5.90
Span and Makin	1976	Jerusalem, Israel	10-16	10,000	1.50
O'Brien	1977	Oswetry, England	11-14	869	2.00
Newman and Dewald	1977	Chicago, Illinois	14-18	861	10.30
Rogala et al.	1978	Montreal, Canada	12-14	26,947	2.10
Smyrnis et al.	1979	Athens, Greece	11-12	3,497	2.70
Dickson et al.	1980	Oxford, England	13-14	1,764	2.50
Goldberg et al.	1980	Dublin, Ireland	9-14	604	6.40
Smyrnis et al.	1980	Evia, Greece	10-15	9,382	6.20
		Lesvos, Greece	10-15	5,380	2.50
		Cnios, Greece	10-15	4,206	2.40
Gore et al.	1981	Wisconsin	10-14	8,393	2.00
Willner	1982	Malmo, Sweden	7-16	17,181	1.90

TABLE 1-4
Scoliosis prevalence: curves over 20 degrees

Authors	Year	Place	Age group (yr)	Number screened	Prevalence (%)
Brooks et al.	1975	California	12-14	3,492	0.4
Drennan et al.	1977	Denver, Colorado	11-12	15,904	0.5
Rogala et al.	1978	Montreal, Canada	12-14	26,947	0.3
Smyrnis et al.	1979	Athens, Greece	11-12	3,497	0.4
Torell et al.	1981	Goteborg, Sweden	<20	22,000	0.4
Gore et al.	1981	Wisconsin	10-14	8,393	0.4
Willner	1982	Malmo, Sweden	7-16	17,181	0.6

SEXUAL DIFFERENCES IN SCOLIOSIS PREVALENCE

Although most patients with idiopathic adolescent scoliosis requiring treatment are girls,[55] the relative frequency of scoliosis among boys and girls is not clear. Studies giving the results of screening by physical examination for a rib hump give a fairly consistent ratio of 1.5 to 2.0 girls to 1.0 boy.[2,71,105,118] However, studies giving distribution by Cobb angle are less consistent in pattern (Table 1-5). The ratio has varied from 1.2 to 3.6 girls per boy for curves over 5 degrees, from 1.6 to 5.3 girls per boy for curves over 10 degrees, and from 6.2 to 16.0 girls per boy for curves over 20 degrees. As a generalization of this data, however, it can certainly be concluded that scoliosis is more common in girls than boys, and the female predisposition is increased for larger curves. As a corollary, girls must have a higher propensity for scoliosis progression.

TABLE 1-5
Scoliosis prevalence by gender and curve size

Authors	Year	Place	Cobb angle (degrees)	Female prevalence (%)	Male prevalence (%)	Female/ male ratio
Brooks et al.	1975	California	>5	14.2	12.1	1.2
Newman and Dewald	1977	Chicago, Illinois	>5	21.4	10.1	2.1
Rogala et al.	1978	Montreal, Canada	>5	5.0	4.0	1.2
Smyrnis et al.	1979	Athens, Greece	>5	7.5	2.8	2.7
Willner	1982	Malmo, Sweden	>5	4.3	1.2	3.6
Newman and Dewald	1977	Chicago, Illinois	>10	14.7	5.6	2.6
Rogala et al.	1978	Montreal, Canada	>10	2.7	1.6	1.6
Smyrnis et al.	1979	Athens, Greece	>10	4.6	1.1	4.2
Gore et al.	1981	Wisconsin	>10	2.0	1.7	1.2
Willner	1982	Malmo, Sweden	>10	3.2	0.6	5.3
Rogala et al.	1978	Montreal, Canada	>20	0.5	0.08	6.2
Smyrnis et al.	1979	Athens, Greece	>20	0.8	0.05	16.0
Gore et al.	1981	Wisconsin	>20	0.5	0.1	5.0
Willner	1982	Malmo, Sweden	>20	1.1	0.14	7.9

CURVE PATTERNS

Although the informal impression at our institution is that right thoracic scoliosis is the most common pattern, the available literature is not consistent for any particular pattern (Table 1-6). Various authors have found the most common pattern to be the thoracic,[44,82,125] lumbar,[30] or thoracolumbar.[14,97,98] This inconsistency may reflect population genetic differences but just as likely stems from varying criteria for defining curve level. Brooks et al.[14] found a higher percentage of thoracolumbar curves (66.4%) than the other four investigators, but a curve was considered a thoracolumbar based on involvement of both thoracic and lumbar vertebrae rather than the currently accepted definition of the apex at the thoracolumbar junction. Willner[125] and Gore et al.[44] used the criteria of the Scoliosis Research Society and were the only authors to define their criteria. Their results parallel our empirical clinical experience, with thoracic curves (usually right convexity) being most common followed closely by thoracolumbar curves. Double major curves are the least common in all reported series.

TABLE 1-6
Curve patterns in adolescent scoliosis

Authors	Year	Thoracic (%)	Lumbar (%)	Thoracolumbar (%)	Double (%)	Cobb angle (degrees)
Brooks et al.	1975	8.2	13.3	66.4	11.6	>5
Newman and Dewald	1977	33.3	29.9	29.9	6.9	>5
Rogala et al.	1978	30.0	15.0	39.0	15.0	>5
Dickson et al.	1980	15.9	56.8	25.0	2.2	N.S.†
Gore et al.	1981	39.0 (32 R, 7 L)*	20.0 (2 R, 18 L)	27.0 (6 R, 21 L)	14.0	>10
Willner	1982	45.1 (37.5 R, 7.6 L)	12.0 (2.5 R, 9.5 L)	30.6 (11.6 R, 19.0 L)	12.9	>5

*R, Right convexity; L, left convexity as subdivisions of total percentage.
†N.S., Not stated

LIKELIHOOD OF PROGRESSION

The likelihood of curve progression in the still growing child is one of the most critical epidemiologic aspects of scoliosis. If the likelihood of small curve progression is low, then the expense and difficulties of brace treatment[77] cannot be justified. Only recently has the likelihood of curve progression been determined (Table 1-7). Analyzing the data by comparable curve sizes we find that the risk of progression is only 5.6% to 6.8% for all curves over 5 degrees, rises to 10.2% for curves over 10 degrees, and is as high as 46.2% to 78.8% for curves over 20 degrees (Table 1-7). The likelihood of progression at all curve sizes is much higher for girls than for boys.[69]

Analyses of progression by curve pattern have been more limited but appear most commonly for thoracic curves and less frequently for the other curve patterns (Table 1-8).

TABLE 1-7
Scoliosis progression by curve size

Authors	Year	Number followed	Curve size (degrees)	Sex	Progressive (%)
Brooks et al.	1975	134	>5	M/F	5.2
Rogala et al.	1978	603	>5	M/F	6.8
Rogala et al.	1978	603	>10	M/F	10.2
Smyrnis et al.	1979	112	7-16	M/F	22.6
Lonstein et al.	1981	727	5-29	M/F	23.2
Willner	1982	108	>19	M/F	46.2
Rogala et al.	1978	603	>20	M/F	78.8
Rogala et al.	1978	603	>10	M	3.8
				F	15.4
Smrynis et al.	1979	112	7-16	M	11.1
				F	27.6
Lonstein et al.	1981	727	5-29	M	13.1
				F	25.9
Willner	1982	108	>19	M	33.3
				F	47.2

TABLE 1-8
Scoliosis progression by curve location

Authors	Year	Curve location	Progression %
Smyrnis et al.	1979	R thoracic	77.8
		R thoracolumbar	25.0
		L thoracolumbar	7.1
		L lumbar	33.3
		Double	26.3
Dickson et al.	1980	Thoracic	38.0
		Thoracolumbar	18.0
		Lumbar	4.0

SCHOOL SCREENING

In the 1970s, many school screening programs were started[56,65,74,92,126] with enthusiastic endorsement by the American Academy of Orthopaedic Surgeons.[16] As a result, school screening for adolescent scoliosis is performed in many countries,[34] and at least 25% of the children are screened in 37 of the 50 states.[71] The rationale for beginning these programs was that early detection and treatment would prevent the significant cosmetic deformity, intractable back pain, and cardiopulmonary insufficiency that can result from undetected and untreated progressive scoliosis.

Recent studies have confirmed that these screening programs are valuable. In Minnesota, Kansas, and Sweden the screening programs have been associated with a reduction in the incidence of scoliosis surgery, a decrease in the average presenting size of scoliotic curves, and a decrease in the number of curves reaching 40 degrees.[2,71,115]

Natural History

Knowledge of the natural history of idiopathic scoliosis persisting into adulthood is important in determining the value of treatment. Scoliosis correction is indicated only if untreated scoliosis results in significant patient morbidity and mortality. The major reported complications of severe adult scoliosis are cardiopulmonary insufficiency, low back pain, and cosmetic deformity. An important related consideration is the likelihood of a moderate-sized curve progressing during adult life with resultant complications.

Although an early study based on an average of only 3 years of observation indicated that scoliosis did not progress after skeletal maturity,[94] many subsequent studies have shown that scoliosis can progress in adults.* Bjerkreim and Hassan[11] followed 70 patients for an average of 8½ years and found that progression averaged 3 degrees per year between ages 16 and 20 years and 1 degree per year after age 20. In a series of 20 patients with smaller curves, all less than 53 degrees, 40% of the curves increased a total of 5 to 10 degrees over a 7 to 17 year follow-up.[103] In two studies of the same patient population in Iowa at two different intervals, total curve progression was found to average 15 degrees for the first 24 years and 3.9 degrees for the next 10 years.[22,120] All investigators have found that thoracic curves and larger curves progress more frequently and severely than smaller curves at other levels. Significant progression is uncommon when the curve is less than 40 degrees at skeletal maturity.[119]

---

*See references 11, 22, 24, 57, 62, 95, 103, 120.

CARDIOPULMONARY COMPLICATIONS

Two large studies on the pulmonary function of patients with severe scoliosis have documented that the thoracic cage deformity results in reduced lung volume and decreased thoracic elasticity.[10,20] As a result of the restrictive lung disease, alveolar hypoventilation and pulmonary arterial hypertension develop with subsequent cor pulmonale. As the curve size increases, especially in thoracic curves, the patient's pulmonary function declines proportionately.[22,81,117,120] Even asymptomatic patients with curves in the 40 to 60 degree range have pulmonary function test findings of restrictive lung disease.[117]

Despite the well documented impaired cardiopulmonary status of severely scoliotic patients described above, the effect on mortality is not completely clear. In separate studies, Nachemson[79] and Nilsonne et al.[83] were each able to follow 90% of over 110 patients who had had documented scoliosis for over 38 and 50 years, respectively. Both studies found a mortality rate twice that of the normal population with cor pulmonale causing 60% to 80% of the deaths. Unfortunately, Nachemson's study included scoliosis of all causes, with paralytic and congenital scoliosis causing much of the increased mortality. The patients of Nilsonne et al. were thought on clinical grounds to have idiopathic scoliosis, but radiographs were not available to exclude other etiologies. Kolind-Sorensen[59] had somewhat comparable results in his series of 203 patients with idiopathic scoliosis over 40 degrees. He found that the mortality rate was normal for patients with scoliosis of 40 to 100 degrees but was twice as high for those with curves over 100 degrees. In a study of 762 scoliosis patients, Shneerson et al.[108] noted 43 deaths, with 58% of the deaths due to cardiorespiratory failure.

In contrast to the above studies, the patients in the series of reports from Iowa with serial radiographs available all had radiographically documented idiopathic scoliosis.[22,120] Despite the fact that these investigators documented significantly decreased pulmonary function in scoliotic patients, no increased mortality was found. The finding of no increased mortality has been questioned because only 54% and 60% of the patients could be located for follow-up.[78] Obviously, many of the patients who could not be located may have died, and thus there may have been a substantially increased mortality in this population.

In reviewing these studies, several important generalizations can be made: larger curves over 60 degrees, especially thoracic curves, frequently progress in adults and do cause increased mortality and morbidity due to the resultant restrictive lung disease.

LOW BACK PAIN

Although early studies reported that 90% to 100% of patients with lumbar curves had back pain,[51,83] subsequent studies have found a 30% to 60% incidence of back pain, which is similar to that of the general population.* Despite these latter studies, a debate still continues as to whether scoliotic patients have an increased incidence and severity of low back pain.[40,47] The source for this uncertainty lies in the high frequency of low back pain in the general population.

The degenerative changes in the older adult scoliotic lumbar spine can be quite impressive and are apparent proof for scoliosis causing low back pain due to the secondary degenerative disk disease.[13,36] However, one must be cautious in interpreting these findings and remember the high frequency of lumbar degenerative joint disease of the spine in nonscoliotic individuals. Whenever control series of a nonscoliotic population are compared to the scoliosis patients, the incidence of low back pain has been similar.†

In light of this evidence and the lower propensity for small lumbar curves to progress, it is believed that lumbar curves of less than 60 degrees need not be fused for the sole indication of preventing subsequent low back pain.[47] However, this conclusion does not negate the value of surgery for both scoliotic and nonscoliotic persons who have back pain due to lumbar degenerative joint disease.[60] Kostuik et al.[62] have shown that 83% of untreated patients with lumbar scoliosis and low back pain obtained significant pain relief with lumbar fusion. Although he evaluated mostly patients with thoracic and thoracolumbar scoliosis, Edgar[35] found that patients who had had spinal fusion were far less likely to have disabling back pain than patients with nonfused severe curves.

COSMETIC DEFORMITY

The unattractive physical appearance due to the "hunchback" deformity may well be the major complication of scoliosis in the view of most patients. Four separate studies have reported that the percentage of scoliotic patients who are unmarried can be twice as high as the unaffected population.[40,59,79,83] Many patients with severe scoliosis are embarrassed by their deformity, and a considerable number have psychologic disturbances.[8,12,40] Although the continuing Iowa study found no increase in the percentage of unmarried patients, 31% of the patients were unwilling to wear tight-fitting clothes or bathing suits because of the deformity.[22,90,120]

In the era prior to effective bracing, 92% of the spinal fusions performed for scoliosis were done for cosmetic reasons.[107] Because of the associated thoracic cage deformity, thoracic and thoracolumbar scoliosis is more likely than lumbar scoliosis to result in an unacceptable physical deformity.[12,51] Double major thoracic and lumbar curves usually result in a less detectable, balanced deformity.

---

*See references 12, 22, 60, 79-81, 120.
†See references 12, 22, 61, 79, 80, 120.

Pathogenesis

In 1941, a survey of 27 orthopedic surgeons revealed no consensus as to etiology of idiopathic scoliosis.[107] Favored theories at that time included endocrine or metabolic disturbance, muscle imbalance, vertebral growth disorder, postural or physiologic variation, and hereditary factors. Despite 40 years of subsequent research, the etiology is still unknown with data supporting many different theories.[48,91]

Family surveys have established a definite genetic component of scoliosis.[25,26,29,73,93] Among first-degree relatives (parents, siblings, and children) of a scoliotic patient, there is a 6.6% to 8.3% incidence of scoliosis with a polygenic pattern of inheritance.[28,38,127]

Differences in growth and development patterns between scoliotic and nonscoliotic individuals have recently been confirmed. Initially, there was conflicting data as to whether or not scoliotic patients are taller than their peers.[91] Recently it has been pointed out that after correction is made for the loss of height due to the scoliosis, scoliotic patients have longer spines and greater lower extremity lengths than those without scoliosis.* The greater height is probably due to the fact that adolescents with scoliosis have a longer duration of pubertal growth.[32,72,85,122,123] The relationship between this increased growth and subsequent development of scoliosis is unknown. Roaf[96] has proposed, based on his autopsy study of seven scoliotic spines, that overgrowth of the vertebral bodies compared to the posterior elements results in scoliosis. Further support for his theory has not been presented.

During the 1970s, exciting new investigations of the intervertebral disks suggested that collagen defects in the disks might cause scoliosis. Recent investigation, however, has revealed that collagen differences are minor[18] or may be secondary to the abnormal forces in the deformed spine.[6] Additional research suggests that defects in disk proteoglycans might contribute to the development of scoliosis.[91]

More recently, investigation has centered on neurologic causes of idiopathic scoliosis. Evidence is accumulating that aberrant neural responses in the paraspinal muscles play an important role in the pathogenesis of scoliosis progression.[46,67,89,116] This neurogenic dysfunction may arise from disturbance of the balance mechanism originating in the brainstem.[99,100,129]

---

*See references 17, 21, 64, 85, 121-123.

Summary

The enormous number of reported investigations and their conflicting results make it difficult to summarize clearly current knowledge about idiopathic scoliosis. Nevertheless, readers who are not specializing in this area need a concise overview. Although future research can invalidate any generalizations, the following outline represents my distillation of the "fundamentals" of idiopathic scoliosis.

1. Age at presentation
    a. Infantile: up to 3 years
    b. Juvenile: 4 to 9 years or onset of puberty
    c. Adolescent: 10 to 18 years or onset of skeletal maturity
2. Curve location and direction
    a. Thoracic: apex between T2 and T11
    b. Thoracolumbar: apex between T12 and L1
    c. Lumbar: apex between L2 and L4
    d. Double major: two curves within 5 degrees of each other
    e. Right or left: defined by the convexity
3. Epidemiology of idiopathic adolescent scoliosis
    a. Prevalence
        (1) Curves over 10 degrees—2% to 3%
        (2) Curves over 20 degrees—0.3% to 0.4%
    b. Gender patterns of prevalence
        (1) Female to male ratio—2.0 to 1.0 for curves >10 degrees
        (2) Female to male ratio = 6-8 to 1.0 for curves >20 degrees
    c. Distribution of curve patterns
        (1) Thoracic—40%
        (2) Thoracolumbar—30%
        (3) Lumbar—15%
        (4) Double major—15%
    d. Likelihood of progression:
        (1) >10 degrees, 10% to 20%
        (2) >20 degrees, 50% to 80%
    e. Progression more likely in girls and in patients with single major right thoracic scoliosis
4. Natural history
    a. Scoliosis can progress in adults
    b. Severe scoliosis results in restrictive lung disease and a two-fold increase in mortality
5. Pathogenesis: unknown with emphasis now on neuromuscular imbalance possibly arising from brainstem dysfunction

REFERENCES

1. Ascani, E., Giglio, G.C., and Salsano, V.: Scoliosis screening in Rome. In Zorab, P.A., and Siegler, D., editors: Scoliosis 1979, London, 1980, Academic Press, Inc.

2. Asher, M.A., Green, P., and Orrick, J.: A six-year report—spinal deformity screening in Kansas School Children, J. Kans. Med. Soc. **81**:568-571, 1980.

3. Avikainen, V.J., and Vaherto, H.: A high incidence of spinal curvature, Acta Orthop. Scand. **54**:267-273, 1983.

4. Baker, E.A., and Zangger, B.: School screening for idiopathic scoliosis, Am. J. Nurs. **70**:766-767, 1970.

5. Barnett, H.: Pediatrics, New York, 1968, Appleton-Century-Crofts.

6. Beard, H.K., Roberts, S., and O'Brien, J.P.: Immunofluorescent staining for collagen and proteoglycan in normal and scoliotic intervertebral discs, J. Bone Joint Surg. (Br.) **63**:529-534, 1981.

7. Bellyei, A., et al.: Prevalence of adolescent idiopathic scoliosis in Hungary, Acta Orthop. Scand. **48**:177-180, 1977.

8. Bengtsson, G., et al.: A psychological and psychiatric investigation of the adjustment of female scoliosis patients, Acta Psychiatr. Scand. **50**:50-59, 1974.

9. Benson, K.D., Wade, B., and Benson, D.R.: Results of school screening for scoliosis in the San Juan unified school district, Sacramento, California, J. Sch. Health **47**:483-484, 1977.

10. Bergofsky, E.H., Turino, G.M., and Fishman, A.P.: Cardiorespiratory failure in kyphoscoliosis, Medicine **38**:263-317, 1959.

11. Bjerkrem, I., and Hassan, I.: Progression in untreated idiopathic scoliosis after end of growth, Acta Orthop. Scand. **53**:897-900, 1982.

12. Bjure, J., and Nachemson, A.: Non-treated scoliosis, Clin. Orthop. **93**:44-52, 1973.

13. Briard, J.L., Jegou, D., and Cauchoix, J.: Adult lumbar scoliosis, Spine **4**:526-532, 1979.

14. Brooks, H.L., et al.: Scoliosis: a prospective epidemiological study, J. Bone Joint Surg. (Am.) **57**:968-972, 1975.

15. Brooks, L., et al.: The epidemiology of scoliosis—a prospective study, Orthop. Rev. **1**:17-23, 1972.

16. Brown, J., Bonnett, C., and Miller, M.J.: Scoliosis detection clinic, Orthop. Dig., March 1975, pp. 14-16.

17. Buric, M., and Momcilovic, B.: Growth pattern and skeletal age in school girls with idiopathic scoliosis, Clin. Orthop. **170**:238-242, 1982.

18. Bushell, G.R., et al.: The collagen of the intervertebral disc in adolescent idiopathic scoliosis, J. Bone Joint Surg. (Br.) **61**:501-508, 1979.

19. Ceballos T., et al.: Prognosis in infantile idiopathic scoliosis, J. Bone Joint Surg. (Am.) **62**:863-875, 1980.

20. Chapman, E.M., Dill, B.D., and Graybiel, A.: The decrease in functional capacity of the lungs and heart resulting from deformities of the chest: pulmonocardiac failure, Medicine **18**:167-202, 1939.

21. Clark, S., Harrison, A., and Zorab, P.A.: One year's study of growth and total hydroxyproline excretion in scoliotic children, Arch, Dis. Child **55**:467-470, 1980.

22. Collis, D.K., and Ponseti, I.V.: Long-term follow-up of patients with idiopathic scoliosis not treated surgically, J. Bone Joint Surg. (Am.) **51**:425-445, 1969.

23. Cooke, E.D., Carter, L.M., and Pilcher, M.F.: Identifying scoliosis in the adolescent with thermography, Clin. Orthop. **148**:172-176, 1980.

24. Coonrad, R.W., and Feierstein, M.S.: Progression of scoliosis in the adult, J. Bone Joint Surg. (Am.) **58**:156, 1976.

25. Cowell, H.R., Hall, J.N., and MacEwen, G.D.: Familial patterns in idiopathic scoliosis, J. Bone Joint Surg. (Am.) **51**:1236, 1969.

26. Cowell, H.R., Hall, J.N., and MacEwen, G.D.: Genetic aspects of idiopathic scoliois, Clin. Orthopaed. **86**:121-131, 1972.

27. Cronis, S., and Russell, A.Y.: Orthopedic screening of children in Delaware public schools, Dec. Med. J., April 1965, pp. 89-95.
28. Czeizel A., et al.: Genetics of adolescent idiopathic scoliosis, J. Med. Genet. 15:424-427, 1978.
29. De George, F.V., and Fisher, R.L.: Idiopathic scoliosis: genetic and environmental aspects, J. Med. Genet. 4:251-257, 1967.
30. Dickson, R.A., et al.: School screening for scoliosis: cohort study of clinical course, Br. Med. J. 265:1-7, 1980.
31. Drennan, J.C., Campbell, J.B., and Ridge, H.: Denver, a metropolitan public school scoliosis survey, Pediatrics 60:193-196, 1977.
32. Drummond, D.S., and Rogala, E.J.: Growth and maturation of adolescents with idiopathic scoliosis, Spine 5:507-511, 1980.
33. Drummond, D.S., Rogala, E., and Gurr, J.: Spinal deformity: natural history and the role of school screening, Orthop. Clin. North Am. 10:751-759, 1979.
34. Dwyer, A.F., et al.: School screening for scoliosis: our challenging responsibility, Aust. N.Z. J. Surg. 48:439-440, 1978.
35. Edgar, M.A.: Back pain assessment from a long-term follow-up of operated and unoperated patients with adolescent idiopathic scoliosis, Spine 4:519-520, 1979.
36. Epstein, J.A., Epstein, B.S., and Jones, M.D.: Symptomatic lumbar scoliosis with degenerative changes in the elderly, Spine 4:542-547, 1979.
37. Figueiredo, U.M., and James, J.I.P.: Juvenile idiopathic scoliosis, J. Bone Joint Surg. (Br.) 63:61-66, 1981.
38. Filho, N.A., and Thompson, M.W.: Genetic studies in scoliosis, J. Bone Joint Surg. (Am.) 53:199, 1971.
39. Flynn, J.C., Riddick M.F., and Keller, T.L.: Screening for scoliosis in Florida schools, J. Fla. Med. Assoc. 64:159-161, 1977.
40. Fowles, J.V., et al.: Untreated scoliosis in the adult, Clin. Orthop. 134:212-217, 1978.
41. Goldberg, C., et al.: Pilot study for a scoliosis screening project in south Dublin, Ir. Med. J. 73:265-268, 1980.
42. Goldstein, L.A., and Waugh, T.R.: Classification and terminology of scoliosis, Clin. Orthop. 93:10-22, 1973.
43. Golomb, M., and Taylor, T.K.F.: Screening adolescent school children for scoliosis, Med. J. Aust. 14:761-762, 1975.
44. Gore, D.R., et al.: Scoliosis screening: results of a community project, Pediatrics 67:196-200, 1981.
45. Grant, W.W., et al.: Health screening in school-age children, Am.J. Dis. Child. 125:520-522, 1973.
46. Haderspeck, K., and Schultz, A.: Progression of idiopathic scoliosis, Spine 6:447-455, 1981.
47. Hall, J., and Nachemson, A.: Debate: scoliosis, Spine 2:318-324, 1977.
48. Harrington, P.R.: The etiology of idiopathic scoliosis, Clin. Orthop. 126:17-25, 1977.
49. Hensinger, R., et al.: Orthopaedic screening of school-age children: review of a 10 year experience, Orthop. Rev. 4:23-28, 1975.
50. James, J.I.P.: Two curve patterns in idiopathic structural scoliosis, J. Bone Joint Surg. (Br.) 33:399-406, 1951.
51. James, J.I.P.: Idiopathic scoliosis, J. Bone Joint Surg. (Br.) 26:36-49, 1954.
52. James, J.I.P.: The management of infants with scoliosis, J. Bone Joint Surg. (Br.) 57:422-429, 1975.
53. James, J.I.P., Lloyd-Roberts, G.C., and Pilcher, M.F.: Infantile structural scoliosis, J. Bone Joint Surg. (Br.) 41:719-735, 1959.
54. Jeffries, B.F., et al.: Computerized measurement and analysis of scoliosis, Radiology 134:381-385, 1980.
55. Kane, W., and Moe, J.H.: A scoliosis-prevalence survey in Minnesota, Clin. Orthop. 69:216-218, 1970.

56. Kane, W.J., et al.: Scoliosis and school screening for spinal deformity, Am. Fam. Physician **17**:123-127, 1978.
57. Keim, H.A.: Scoliosis can progress in the adult, Orthop. Rev. **3**:23-28, 1974.
58. Keiser, R.P., and Shufflebarger, H.L.: The Milwaukee brace in idiopathic scoliosis, Clin. Orthop. **118**:19-24, 1976.
59. Kolind-Sorensen, V.: A follow-up study of patients with idiopathic scoliosis, Acta Orthop. Scand. **44**:98, 1973.
60. Kostuik, J.P.: Recent advances in the treatment of painful adult scoliosis, Clin. Orthop. **147**:238-252, 1980.
61. Kostuik, J.P., and Bentivoglio, J.: The incidence of low-back pain in adult scoliosis, Spine **6**:268-273, 1981.
62. Kostuik, J.P., Israel, J., and Hall, J.E.: Scoliosis surgery in adults, Clin. Orthop. **93**:225-234, 1973.
63. Leaver, J.M, Alvik, A., and Warren, M.D.: Prescriptive screening for adolescent idiopathic scoliosis: a review of the evidence, Int. J. Epidemiol. **11**:101-111, 1982.
64. Leong, J.C.Y., et al.: Linear growth in southern Chinese female patients with adolescent idiopathic scoliosis, Spine **7**:471-475, 1982.
65. Lezberg, S.: Screening for scoliosis, Phys. Ther. **54**:371-372, 1974.
66. Lloyd-Roberts, G.C., and Pilcher, M.F.: Structural idiopathic scoliosis in infancy, J. Bone Joint Surg. (Br.) **47**:520-523, 1965.
67. Lloyd-Roberts, G.C., et al.: Progression in idiopathic scoliosis, J. Bone Joint Surg. (Br.) **60**:451-460, 1978.
68. Lonstein, J.: Screening for spinal deformities in Minnesota schools, Clin. Orthop. **126**:33-42, 1977.
69. Lonstein, J., and Carlson, J.M.: Prognostication in idiopathic scoliosis, Orthop. Trans. **5**:22, 1981.
70. Lonstein, J., et al.: School screening for the early detection of spine deformities, Minn. Med., January 1976, pp. 51-57.
71. Lonstein, J., et al.: Voluntary school screening for scoliosis in Minnesota, J. Bone Joint Surg. (Am.) **64**:481-488, 1982.
72. Low, W.D., et al.: The development of southern Chinese girls with adolescent idiopathic scoliosis, Spine **3**:152-156, 1978.
73. MacEwen, G.D., and Cowell, H.R.: Familial incidence of idiopathic scoliosis and its implications in patient treatment, J. Bone Joint Surg. (Am.) **52**:405, 1970.
74. McCarthy, R.E., Morrissy, R.T., and Dwyer, A.P.: Scoliosis school screening in Arkansas, J. Ark. Med. Soc. **79**:315-317, 1983.
75. McMaster, M.J.: Infantile idiopathic scoliosis: can it be prevented?, J. Bone Joint Surg. (Br.) **65**:612-617, 1983.
76. Mehta, M.H.: The rib-vertebra angle in the early diagnosis between resolving and progressive infantile scoliosis, J. Bone Joint Surg. (Br.) **54**:230-243, 1972.
77. Moe, J.H., and Kettleson, D.N.: Idiopathic scoliosis: analysis of curve patterns and the preliminary results of Milwaukee-brace treatment in one hundred sixty-nine patients, J. Bone Joint Surg. (Am.) **52**:1509-1533, 1970.
78. Moe, J., et al.: Scoliosis and other spinal deformities, Philadelphia, 1978, W.B. Saunders, Co.
79. Nachemson, A.: A long term follow-up study of non-treated scoliosis, Acta Orthop. Scand. **39**:466-476, 1968.
80. Nachemson, A.: Adult scoliosis and back pain, Spine **4**:513-517, 1979.
81. Nachemson, A., and Elfstrom, G.: Intravital wireless telemetry of axial forces in Harrington distraction rods in patients with idiopathic scoliosis, J. Bone Joint Surg. (Am.) **53**:445-465, 1971.
82. Newman, D.C., and Dewald, R.L.: School screening for scoliosis, Ill. Med. J., January 1977, pp. 31-34.
83. Nilsonne, U., and Lundgren, K.D.: Long-term prognosis in idiopathic scoliosis, Acta Orthop. Scand. **39**:456-465, 1968.

84. Nordwall, A.: Studies in idiopathic scoliosis, Acta Orthop. Scand. (Suppl.) **150:** 73-101, 1973.
85. Nordwall, A., and Willner, S.: A study of skeletal age and height in girls with idiopathic scoliosis, Clin. Orthop. **110:**6-10, 1975.
86. O'Brien, J.P.: The incidence of scoliosis in Oswestry. In Zorab, P.A., and Siegler, D., editors: Scoliosis 1979, London, 1980, Academic Press, Inc.
87. O'Brien, J.P., and Akkerveeken, P.F.: School screening for scoliosis: results of a pilot study, Practitioner **219:**739-742, 1977.
88. Owen, R.: Current incidence of scoliosis in schoolchildren in the city of Liverpool. In Zorab, P.A., and Siegler, D., editors: Scoliosis 1979, London, 1980, Academic Press, Inc.
89. Pincott, J.R., and Taffs, L.F.: Experimental scoliosis in primates, J. Bone Joint Surg. (Br.) **64:**503-507, 1982.
90. Ponseti, I.V., and Friedman, B.: Prognosis in idiopathic scoliosis, J. Bone Joint Surg. (Am.) **32:**381-395, 1950.
91. Ponseti, I.V., et al.: Pathogenesis of scoliosis, Clin. Orthop. **120:**268-280, 1976.
92. Rapp, G.F.: Spinal screening for scoliosis, kyphosis and lordosis, J. Ind. State Med. Assoc. **71:**33-34, 1978.
93. Riseborough, F.J., and Wynne-Davies, R.: A genetic survey of idiopathic scoliosis in Boston, Massachusetts, J. Bone Joint Surg. (Am.) **55:**974-982, 1973.
94. Risser, J.C., and Ferguson, A.B.: Scoliosis: its prognosis, J. Bone Joint Surg. **18:**667-670, 1936.
95. Risser, J.C., Iqbal, Q.M., and Nagata, K.: Scoliosis after termination of vertebral growth, Ann. R. Coll. Surg. Engl. **59:**119-123, 1977.
96. Roaf, R.: Spinal deformities, London, 1977, Pitman Medical Publishing Co., Ltd.
97. Rogala, E.J., and Drummond, D.S.: Idiopathic scoliosis: a prospective study of the incidence and natural history based on a school screening of 26,947 children, J. Bone Joint Surg. (Br.) **59:**505, 1977.
98. Rogala E., Drummond, D.S., and Gurr, E.J.: Scoliosis: incidence and natural history, J. Bone Joint Surg. (Am.) **60:**173-176, 1978.
99. Sahlstrand, T.: An analysis of lateral predominance in adolescent idiopathic scoliosis with special reference to convexity of the curve, Spine **5:**512-518, 1980.
100. Sahlstrand, T., Ortengren, R., and Nachemson, A.: Postural equilibrium in adolescent idiopathic scoliosis, Acta Orthop. Scand. **49:**354-365, 1978.
101. Scoliosis Research Society: Scoliosis terminology, Orthop. Nursing, September/October 1982, pp. 38-40.
102. Scott, J.C., and Morgan, T.H.: The natural history and prognosis of infantile idiopathic scoliosis, J. Bone Joint Surg. (Br.) **37:**400-413, 1955.
103. Scott, M.M., and Piggott, H.: A short-term follow-up of patients with mild scoliosis, J. Bone Joint Surg. (Br.) **63:**523-525, 1981.
104. Segil, C.M.: The incidence of idiopathic scoliosis in the Bantu and white population groups in Johannesburg, J. Bone Joint Surg. (Br.) **56:**393, 1974.
105. Sells, C.J., and May, E.A.: Scoliosis screening in public schools, Am. J. Nurs. **74:**60-62, 1974.
106. Shands, Jr., A.R., and Eisberg, H.B.: The incidence of scoliosis in the state of Delaware, J. Bone Joint Surg. (Am.) **37:**1243-1249, 1955.
107. Shands, Jr., A.R., et al.: End-result study of the treatment of idiopathic scoliosis, J. Bone Joint Surg. **23:**963-977, 1941.
108. Shneerson, J.M., Sutton, G.C., and Zorab, P.A.: Causes of death, right ventricular hypertrophy, and congenital heart disease in scoliosis, Clin. Orthop. **135:**52-57, 1978.
109. Skogland, L.B., and Miller, J.A.A.: The incidence of scoliosis in northern Norway, Acta Orthop. Scand. **49:**635, 1978.
110. Smyrnis, P.N., et al.: School screening for scoliosis in Athens, J. Bone Joint Surg. (Br.) **61:**215-217, 1979.

111. Smyrnis, P.N., et al.: Incidence of scoliosis in the Greek islands. In Zorab, P.A., and Siegler, D., editors: Scoliosis 1979, London, 1980, Academic Press, Inc.

112. Span, Y., and Makin, M.: Incidence of scoliosis in school children in Jerusalem, J. Bone Joint Surg. (Br.) **58**:379, 1976.

113. Thompson, S.K., and Bentley, G.: Prognosis in infantile idiopathic scoliosis, J. Bone Joint Surg. (Br.) **62**:151-154, 1980.

114. Tolo, V.T., and Gillespie, R.: The characteristics of juvenile idiopathic scoliosis and results of its treatment, J. Bone Joint Surg. (Br.) **60**:181-188, 1978.

115. Torell, G., Nordwall, A, and Nachemson, A.: The changing pattern of scoliosis treatment due to effective screening, J. Bone Joint Surg. (Am.) **63**:337-341, 1981.

116. Trontelj, J.V., Pecak, F., and Dimitrijevic, M.R.: Segmental neurophysiological mechanisms in scoliosis, J. Bone Joint Surg. (Br.) **61**:310-313, 1979.

117. Weber, B., et al.: Pulmonary function in asymptomatic adolescents with idiopathic scoliosis, Am. Rev. Respir. Dis. **111**:389-397, 1975.

118. Weiler, D.R.: Scoliosis screening, J. Sch. Health **44**:563-565, 1974.

119. Weinstein, S.L., and Ponseti, I.V.: Curve progression in idiopathic scoliosis, J. Bone Joint Surg. (Am.) **65**:447-455, 1983.

120. Weinstein, S., Zavala, D.C., and Ponseti, I.V.: Idiopathic scoliosis: long-term follow-up and prognosis in untreated patients, J. Bone Joint Surg. (Am.) **63**:702-712, 1981.

121. Willner, S.: Growth in height of children with scoliosis, Acta Orthop. Scand. **45**:854-866, 1974.

122. Willner, S.: The proportion of legs to trunk in girls with idiopathic structural scoliosis, Acta Orthop. Scand. **46**:84-89, 1975.

123. Willner, S.: A study of height, weight and menarche in girls with idiopathic structural scoliosis, Acta Orthop. Scand. **46**:71-83, 1975.

124. Willner, S.: A comparative study of the efficiency of different types of school screening for scoliosis, Acta Orthop. Scand. **53**:769-774, 1982.

125. Willner, S., and Uden, A.: A prospective prevalence study of scoliosis in southern Sweden, Acta Orthop. Scand. **53**:233-237, 1982.

126. Winter, R.B., and Moe, J.H.: Orthotics for spinal deformity, Clin. Orthop. **102**:72-91, 1974.

127. Wynne-Davies, R.: Familial (idiopathic) scoliosis, J. Bone Joint Surg. (Br.) **50**:24-30, 1968.

128. Wynne-Davies, R.: Infantile idiopathic scoliosis, J. Bone Joint Surg. (Br.) **57**:138-141, 1975.

129. Yamamoto, H., et al.: An evaluation of brainstem function as a prognostication of early idiopathic scoliosis, J. Pediatr. Orthop. **2**:521-527, 1982.

Chapter Two

Radiographic Evaluation

*E*valuation of routine radiographs forms the foundation for the diagnosis and treatment of spinal deformity. Physicians obtaining scoliosis radiographs should be aware that radiography of the entire spine differs from conventional skeletal radiography. For most skeletal pathology, the films are collimated to a restricted area and image detail is optimized. For scoliosis radiographs, fine detail is not as critical because the alignment of the vertebrae is of prime concern. The specific radiographic techniques required for evaluation of spinal curvature are described in this chapter.

In addition to requiring special techniques, scoliosis radiographs are also evaluated in a distinctive manner. Although focal skeletal abnormalities are still searched for, proper evaluation of scoliosis films requires measurements of curvature, rotation, flexibility, and skeletal maturity that are not used elsewhere in the body. These measures will be discussed along with a detailed review of the potential risks from diagnostic radiographs. This latter topic is especially important. Because scoliotic patients undergoing treatment are usually children and adolescents, there is concern over the potential harm from repeated scoliosis radiographs in such young patients.

Radiographic Technique

The fundamental objective of spinal radiography is to assess spinal curvature in a reproducible manner with the patient in the upright position. Reproducibility is necessary so that changes in curvature on serial radiographs indicate curve progression rather than changes in technique. Spinal geometry is primarily evaluated with the patient in the upright position. The ability of the musculoskeletal forces to compensate for the effects of gravity determines the severity of an abnormal spinal curvature.

IMPORTANCE OF RADIOGRAPHS

Radiographs are essential for evaluation of spinal curvature abnormalities for five reasons. First, a clinically suspected abnormal curvature can be confirmed or disproved. School screening programs have shown that only 80% of children with the clinical signs of mild scoliosis actually have scoliosis on radiographic examination.[54] The remaining 20% have mild trunkal asymmetry, which is a well documented, normal variant.[15] Second, the etiology of the deformity can be determined with differentiation between the idiopathic and secondary forms. Third, the degree of deformity can be quantified to help decide on the initial clinical management. Fourth, the stability of the untreated deformity can be evaluated on serial examinations. Last, the results of treatment can be monitored. In selected cases, more specialized radiologic imaging procedures may be indicated. These procedures will be discussed in Chapter Three.

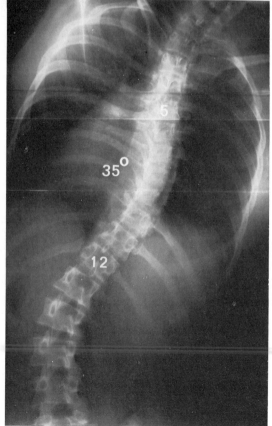

FIGURE 2-1
Idiopathic scoliosis in a 16-year-old girl.
Upright **(A)**, left bending **(B)**, and right
bending **(C)** supine radiographs show a
major right thoracic curve with a minor
left lumbar curve. The left lumbar curve
is more flexible, correcting 53.5% (100 ×
[43 degrees − 20 degrees]/43 degrees)
compared to 38.6% correction (100 × [57°
− 35°]/57°) for the thoracic curve.

RADIOGRAPHIC PROJECTIONS

Radiographic projections that can be used for the evaluation of scoliosis are the upright anteroposterior (AP), upright posteroanterior (PA), supine AP, and supine AP with left and right lateral bending (Fig. 2-1).[7,10,49,103] Because the scoliotic patient is evaluated clinically from behind, scoliosis radiographs are viewed similarly, with the patient's left to the viewer's left. This recommended convention will be used throughout this book. Additional material on techniques for scoliosis radiography has been presented by several authors.[7,10,58,69,100]

For most patients, only a single upright AP or PA film is necessary for the initial evaluation of scoliosis. The previous standard projection has been the AP, but recently multiple authors have recommended the use of the PA

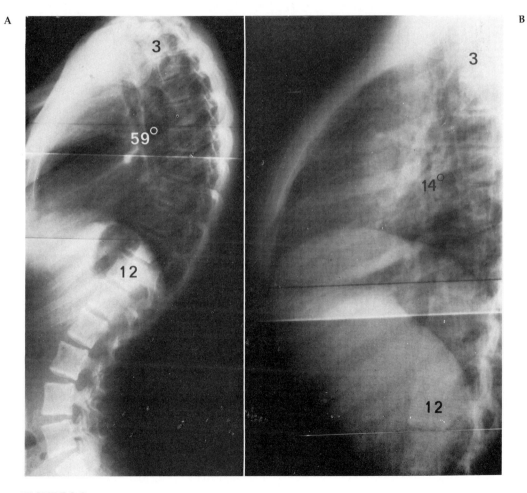

A

B

FIGURE 2-2
Postural thoracic hyperkyphosis in a 12-year-old girl.
A, Upright lateral radiograph—59 degrees hyperkyphosis.
B, Supine cross-table lateral film showing marked flexibility of the curve. Flexibility
$= 100 \times (59° − 14°)/59° = 76.3\%$.

projection to reduce breast irradiation.[3,4,39,43] The PA projection has been shown to reduce breast irradiation by 88% to 98%.[3,4,39] Supine and bending films are used to evaluate curve flexibility (Fig. 2-1) and to determine whether a curve is structural or nonstructural. Nonstructural curves are those that correct completely with bending toward the curve convexity. Supine and bending films are usually needed only in the evaluation of a patient prior to spinal instrumentation for scoliosis correction.[49]

Evaluation for sagittal plane deformity (abnormal kyphosis or abnormal lordosis) is done in the upright position with the lateral projection (Fig. 2-2, *A*). Kyphosis flexibility is determined using a cross-table lateral film with the patient lying supine on a bolster (Fig. 2-2, *B*). Lordosis flexibility is evaluated with a supine cross-table lateral film with the patient drawing his knees up against his chest. Spondylolisthesis stability is evaluated with upright flexion and extension lateral films of the lumbar spine (Fig. 2-3).

Supplementary views of specific regions of the spine are occasionally necessary. If congenital vertebral anomalies are suspected on the scoliosis films, routine films of the thoracic or lumbar spine are useful for better definition of the anomaly. Routine films of localized regions of the spine provide

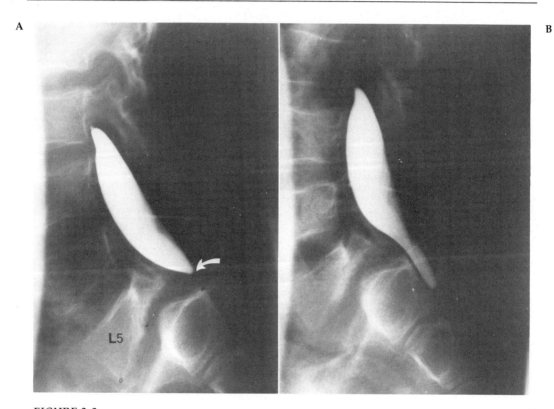

A

B

FIGURE 2-3
Grade 4 spondylolisthesis in a 10-year-old boy.
Upright films during myelography demonstrate forward motion of the fifth lumbar *(L5)* vertebra during flexion **(A)** with compression of the dural sac *(arrow)* compared to the extension film **(B).**

improved bony detail owing to the use of slower speed, higher resolution film-screen systems, and decreased scattered radiation with increased collimation.

The area of the lumbosacral junction needs special consideration. In patients with increased lumbar lordosis or increased sacral tilt, routine AP films of the lumbar spine may not adequately demonstrate the posterior elements

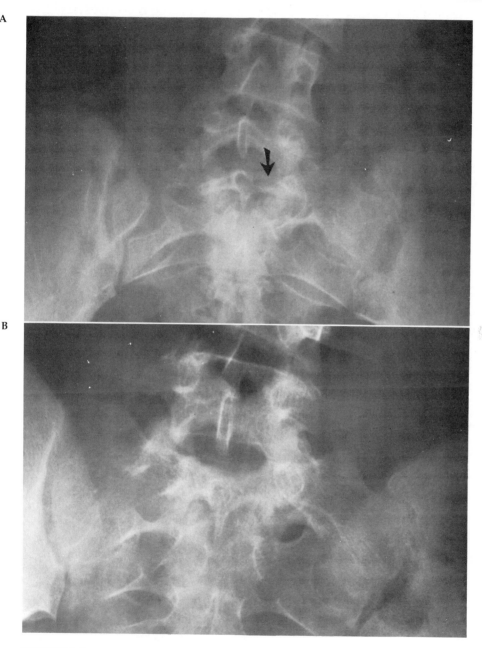

A

B

FIGURE 2-4
Routine AP film **(A)** shows questionable defect in posterior elements of upper sacrum *(arrow)*. Warner view **(B)** displays posterior elements en face and reveals intact posterior elements.

of the fifth lumbar vertebra or the upper sacrum. Although the incidence of spina bifida occulta is not increased in idiopathic scoliosis,[25] special views such as a Warner view with cephalad tilt of the x-ray tube will better define the posterior elements to detect if a congenital anomaly is present (Fig. 2-4).

TUBE, FILM, SCREEN, AND GRID SELECTION

A standard tube-to-film distance of 182.9 cm (6 feet) is used for all radiographs, including the upright and supine projections. If a shorter distance is used, the x-ray beam will not include the entire spine due to the anode heel effect. Since most ceiling mounted telescoping tube mounts will not raise to this distance, a second tube mounted on the overhead rails is needed for the supine films (Fig. 2-5). Using a smaller x-ray tube focal spot size such as 0.6 mm whenever possible will minimize geometric unsharpness of the image.

According to most authors, film size should be sufficient to include the entire thoracic and lumbar spine as well as the iliac crests.[7,10,103] Keim recommends that the top of the film include from the occiput down so that balance of the head relative to the trunk can be determined.[49] In small children, the standard 35 × 43 cm (14 × 17 inch) cassette is sufficiently long to include the

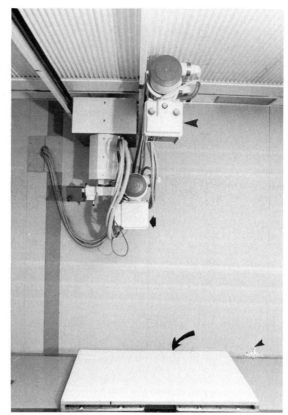

FIGURE 2-5
*Room layout for supine scoliosis
radiography.*
The standard tube on a telescoping mount *(arrow)* cannot be raised to a 182.9 cm tube-film distance so a second tube *(arrowhead)* is mounted on the overhead rails. The tube is centered to a movable grid-tunnel *(curved arrow)* for the film cassette. Controls for the overhead tube collimator and light are mounted on the table *(small arrowhead)*.

entire thoracic and lumbar spine. For older children and adults, a longer special cassette is needed. A 35 × 91 cm (14 × 36 inch) cassette is most commonly used.[7,10,103] These steel cassettes are cumbersome because of their weight and length. A modified 35 × 70 cm (14 × 28 inch) aluminum cassette is lighter and more convenient to use but is still long enough to include the entire thoracic and lumbar spine (Fig. 2-6).[29] This cassette weighs 4.4 kg and is 2.1 kg lighter than the 6.5 kg steel cassette. The shorter film length also saves on film costs.[29]

X-ray intensifying screens should contain the new rare-earth phosphors rather than the older calcium tungstate phosphors. The increased photon absorption and improved efficiency of photon to light conversion of high-speed rare-earth screens dramatically reduce patient radiation exposure. Although one group reported an average skin exposure of 1100 millirads for a single PA or AP scoliosis film,[62] average entrance skin exposure with modern techniques should be in the range of 20 to 65 millirads.[4,27,39,43,72] Failure to use high-speed rare-earth screens results in an increase in radiation exposure to 174 millirads.[66] The film should be selected to match the particular rare-earth phosphors present in the intensifying screens. The most common rare-earth phosphors, terbium-activated gadolinium oxysulfide and lanthanum oxy-

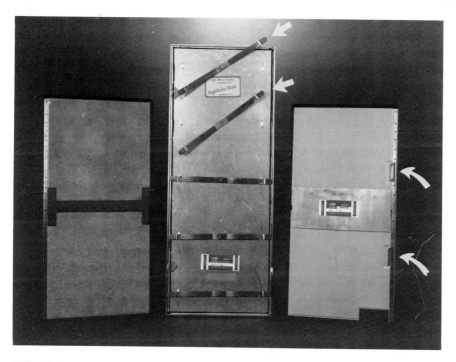

FIGURE 2-6
Scoliosis cassettes.
Comparison of 35 × 70 cm aluminum cassettes with longer, heavier steel cassette. Two latches *(curved arrows)* make opening and closing easier than the five locking straps *(arrows)*.
From De Smet, A.A., and Ritter, E.M.: Radiology **141**:249-250, 1981.

sulfide, emit light in the blue and green regions so the blue-sensitive films used with calcium tungstate screens are inappropriate with these rare-earth screens.[94] Standard contrast film is most often used, although a higher latitude film may be useful to minimize dark and light areas on the radiographs at the expense of vertebral edge definition.

Since patient thickness and density increase in the cephalocaudad direction, compensation is needed to provide uniform density of all the vertebrae on the radiographs. Without a compensation device, the upper thoracic spine must be overpenetrated to visualize adequately the lower lumbar spine. Aluminum wedge filters and lead-impregnated acrylic filters (Clear Pb filter, Victoreen Nuclear Associates, Carle Place, NY) can be used to reduce the x-ray tube output in the upper half of the spine[7,39,103] (Fig. 2-7). Solid aluminum filters are heavy and awkward to use. In addition, because the aluminum filter is opaque, the collimator localizer light cannot be used with the filter in place. Since the localizer light is needed to position the tube for each different projection, the aluminum filter must be removed and reinserted for each film. In addition to being lighter, an advantage of the acrylic filter is that it can be left on the collimator because it is transparent to light.

As an alternative to a tube filter, a gradient intensifying screen (Gradient Quanta III, Dupont, Wilmington, DE) can be used. This screen provides an 8:1 gradient from the high-speed end to the low-speed end.[76] The use of a gradient screen is simpler for the x-ray technologist but does not reduce patient radiation in the upper thorax as the gradient filters do. On the other hand, the gradient filter results in a lower contrast radiograph due to x-ray beam hardening and a less sharp image owing to scattered radiation from the filter.

Grid selection is also important. A focused grid of 8:1 ratio adequately reduces scattered radiation.[27] Higher ratio grids further reduce scatter but at the expense of increased radiation dose to the patient. Recently, it has been suggested that a patient-to-film air gap can be used instead of a grid to reduce scatter.[4,32] Unless the air gap is large, scatter reduction may be less than desired.[28]

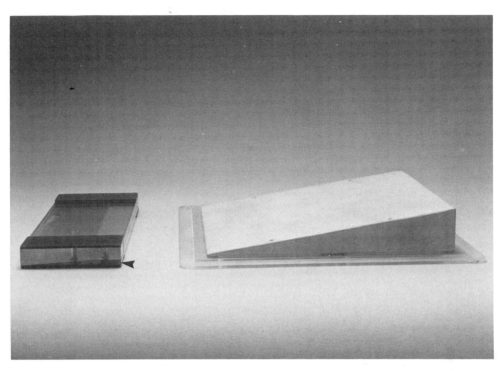

FIGURE 2-7
Gradient filters.
The acrylic filter *(left)* is transparent to light as well as smaller and lighter than the aluminum wedge filter *(right)*. The tapered lead-impregnated portion of the acrylic filter *(arrowhead)* is seen.

PATIENT RADIATION PROTECTION

The main methods for reducing patient irradiation have already been discussed and are (1) use of high-speed film-screen combinations, (2) proper selection of a grid, and (3) use of the PA projection to reduce breast radiation exposure. Proper collimation also reduces total body irradiation. On the PA (or AP) film, the superoinferior extent of the field can be from the lower cervical spine to the middle of the sacroiliac joints. The side-to-side extent should be no wider than the lateral spinal displacement unless the iliac crests must be visualized to assess skeletal maturity. Collimation for the lateral projection should be the same in the superoinferior direction. Side-to-side collimation should include from the posterior trunk skin surface to just inside the anterior chest wall. In this manner the breasts are not included in the primary x-ray beam except in patients with thoracic lordosis.

Gonadal shielding is provided by placing a lead waist apron at the level of the anterior superior iliac spine (Fig. 2-8). Placement of the apron at this level shields both the male and the female gonads from the primary beam and from off-focus radiation.[90]

If the AP position is used, breast shields have been advocated. These may consist of a lead stole or lead circles of varying sizes which are attached by Velcro strips to a light fabric vest.[72] The shields are useful in patients with small curves, but the apex of the curve may be obscured by the shields in patients with large thoracic curves. The use of the PA projection is simpler and as effective in reducing breast irradiation.

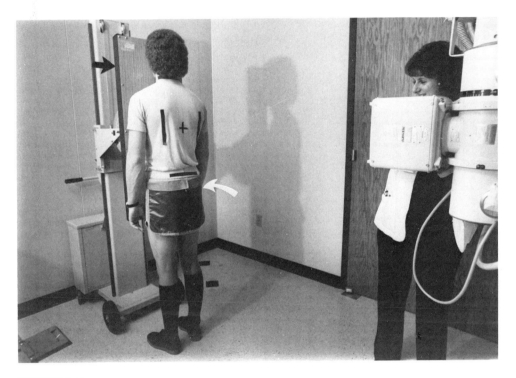

FIGURE 2-8
Positioning for PA radiograph.
Note height-adjustable cassette and grid holder *(arrow)* and lead apron in place
(curved arrow). Black tape on patient's shirt simulates desired beam collimation *(tape
strips)* and position of central ray *(crossed tape).*

PATIENT POSITIONING

The patient is instructed to stand normally erect with the arms at the sides for the PA and the AP projections (Fig. 2-8). The x-ray beam is centered in the sagittal midline of the patient and at a point halfway between the first thoracic and first sacral levels. All films are obtained with a nonforced end-inspiratory effort. The patient's shoes should be removed for upright films to eliminate the effects of shoe heels and lifts.

For the lateral projection, the patient's right side is placed against the cassette holder with the arms pulled slightly forward and holding on to a movable upright such as an intravenous bottle stand (Fig. 2-9). Raising the arms over the head should be avoided because it decreases the thoracic kyphosis and increases the lumbar lordosis. The x-ray beam is centered at a point halfway between the first thoracic and first sacral levels and 3 to 5 inches anterior to the posterior lumbar skin surface.

For the supine bending films, the patient bends maximally to one side and then to the opposite side (Fig. 2-10). The patient must be positioned toward one side of the film cassette to include the entire spine on the film. Usually this film can be collimated only 1 to 2 cm from each side to include the entire spine on the film. Top-to-bottom collimation is the same as for the routine AP or PA films. Recumbent bending films are best done with the patients supine because patients can bend easier on their backs than on their stomachs.

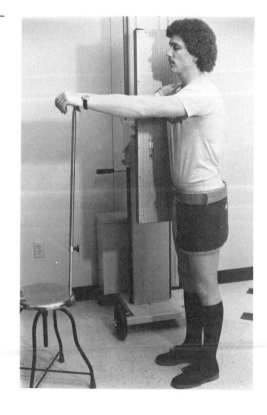

FIGURE 2-9
Patient positioning for lateral radiograph.
Lead apron is in place and arms are resting on adjustable stand.

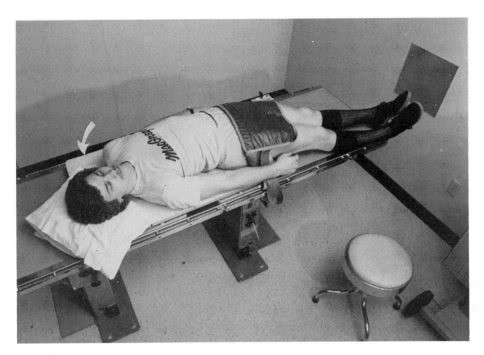

FIGURE 2-10
Supine bending positioning.
The patient bends maximally to one side while lying on the cassette grid tunnel
(curved arrow).

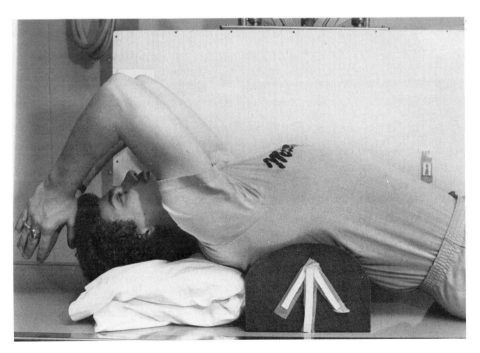

FIGURE 2-11
Cross-table lateral radiograph with the patient lying on a bolster to determine
kyphosis flexibility. Lead arrow records position of bolster on the radiograph.

Cross-table lateral films are performed with the patient recumbent to demonstrate curve flexibility. Correctibility of a thoracic kyphosis is determined by having the patient lie on a bolster pad placed beneath the palpable apex of the kyphosis (Fig. 2-11). The hands are placed together and drawn above the head. A radiopaque arrow on the bolster verifies its correct positioning.[7] Lumbar curve flexibility can be evaluated on a cross-table lateral film with the patient's knees drawn up to flatten the lumbar lordosis.

Evaluation of the Radiographs

The particular radiographs that are required will depend on the clinical situation. In most cases only a single upright AP or PA is needed for initial evaluation. A lateral film is indicated to exclude Scheuermann's disease or spondylolisthesis if there is a history of back pain or evidence of abnormal kyphosis or lordosis. Patients with Scheuermann's disease may have an associated scoliosis, but the scoliosis usually requires no treatment. Spondylolisthesis occurs in scoliotic patients at a frequency equal to or slightly greater than that of the general population.[36] Since the presence of low back pain may influence the decision as to treatment, it is important to know if the pain is due to spondylolisthesis rather than a lumbar scoliosis. A lateral film is also recommended prior to brace fitting, because the brace is designed differently for patients with thoracic hyperkyphosis or hypokyphosis.[101] Bending and cross-table lateral films are useful prior to surgery to estimate the degree of correction that can be achieved intraoperatively.[49]

CURVE EVALUATION

The first determination that needs to be made from the upright radiograph is whether an abnormal curvature exists. Scoliosis of less than 10 degree is clinically insignificant and further medical follow-up is seldom necessary. The parents of children with such small curves can be instructed in the forward bending test[53] to monitor change in the child's clinical appearance (Fig. 2-12). Curves of less than 10 degrees in a skeletally mature patient need no further evaluation.

The normal range for thoracic kyphosis as measured on lateral x-ray films has most commonly been stated to be 20 to 40 degrees.[12,58,71,77] One recent study extended the range to 20 to 50 degrees with an average of 37 degrees.[88] The upper limits of normal were also found to increase to 56 degrees in elderly adults.[37] Increased kyphosis is called hyperkyphosis, and decreased kyphosis is hypokyphosis. Occasionally the thoracic curve in a scoliotic patient may be markedly abnormal and be convex anteriorly resulting in thoracic lordosis.

The normal range of lumbar lordosis is less well-defined. Moe and co-authors recommend using a normal range of 40 to 60 degrees for lumbar lordosis but do not define their measurement levels.[58] Larger curves are hyperlordotic and smaller curves are hypolordotic. Propst-Proctor and Bleck studied 104 normal children and reported a normal range of 22 to 54 degrees for lumbar lordosis when measured from the first (L1) to the fifth (L5) lumbar vertebrae.[71] Stagnara et al. studied 100 young French adults and found a maximum range of 18 to 69 degrees from L1 to L5 and 32 to 82 degrees from L1 to the top of the sacrum.[88] At this institution, 20 to 50 degrees is used as the normal range for thoracic kyphosis, and 20 to 60 degrees is used for normal lumbar lordosis from L1 to L5.

If an abnormal curve is present, the next determination is whether the curve is idiopathic or secondary. Secondary scoliosis is discussed in Chapter Seven. Abnormal kyphosis and lordosis are discussed in Chapters Eight and Nine.

FIGURE 2-12
Forward bending test.
The patient is observed from behind after bending forward as if touching his toes. Any deviation of the spinous processes from the midline or the presence of a rib hump suggests scoliosis is present.

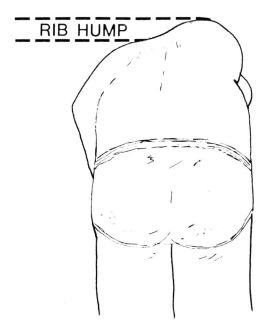

CURVE MEASUREMENT

Scoliosis, kyphosis, and lordosis are measured by the Cobb technique[50,55] as recommended by the Scoliosis Research Society. For this measurement, lines are drawn tangential to the superior endplate of the superior end vertebra and to the inferior endplate of the inferior end vertebrae (Fig. 2-13). The end vertebrae are those that are the most tilted from the horizontal. Perpendicular lines to these tangential lines construct the Cobb angle. Thoracic kyphosis and lumbar lordosis are measured in a similar fashion (Fig. 2-14). Because of the difficulty of visualizing the upper thoracic vertebrae, the superior end vertebra for thoracic kyphosis is usually at the third or fourth thoracic level. The Ferguson method can also be used to measure scoliosis (Fig. 2-15). The Ferguson method requires placement of a dot in the center of three vertebrae. Because the difficulty in identifying the exact center can cause considerable error in the measurement, use of the Ferguson method is not recommended.[49,50] Although it has been reported that the Cobb and Ferguson techniques do not give comparable scoliosis angles,[38,85] one study found no significant difference between the techniques in the average measured angles.[40] Another study found a linear correlation between the two measurements but reported that the Cobb angle was 1.38 times larger than the Ferguson angle for a given curve.[79] The Cobb method is the preferred one because it is easier to use, more reproducible, and is now accepted as the standard method.

There is a standard error of measurement of 2.2 to 3.0 degrees with the Cobb technique if the same end vertebrae are used for each measurement.[5,47,65,99] For this reason, if a curve measures within 5 degrees of a previous measurement on two serial films, the change is assumed to be due to measurement variation rather than a true change in the curve. If multiple observers pick the end vertebral bodies independently, the standard deviation of curve measurement is increased to 4.5 degrees owing to selection of different end vertebrae by the various observers.[67] As a result, the same end vertebrae must be used for serial measurements on a given patient. Although an early laboratory study[80] suggested that the PA projection would significantly change the Cobb angle when compared to AP films, a subsequent clinical study found only a minimal, clinically insignificant angle increase with the PA projection.[30]

Dawson et al. have recommended the use of an elaborate patient positioning device to minimize variations in patient positioning.[26] They found that with the use of the device, serial films on the same day gave Cobb measurements with a maximum difference of 6 degrees. In contrast, a comparison of free-standing and positioning device films gave a maximum difference of 17 degrees between the two techniques. The reason for this large difference may lie in the erectness of the patient's posture. In a study comparing PA and AP Cobb measurements, DeSmet et al. found that differences of more than 5 degrees on two films obtained in rapid sequence could be explained by differences in posture.[30] If the patient "slumps," a flexible curve becomes more prominent. With proper patient positioning, this slumping should occur infrequently. As a result, most centers have not felt it necessary to use a special positioning device.

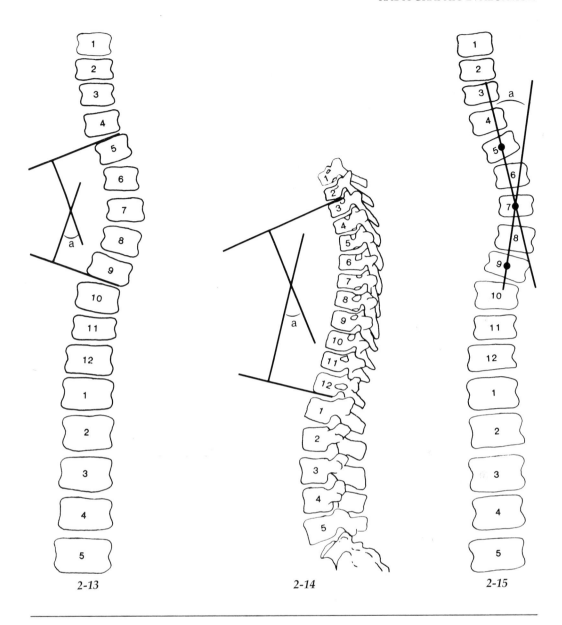

2-13

2-14

2-15

FIGURE 2-13
Cobb method.
The Cobb angle (*a*) is determined by lines drawn perpendicular to the tangents from the endplates of the most tilted superior (fifth thoracic) and inferior (ninth thoracic) vertebrae.

FIGURE 2-14
Cobb method for measurement of kyphosis.
Perpendicular lines from the tangents of the most tilted superior (third thoracic) and inferior (twelfth thoracic) vertebrae determine the thoracic kyphosis angle (*a*).

FIGURE 2-15
Ferguson measurement of scoliosis.
Dots are placed in the center of the apical and end vertebral bodies. Lines through these dots create the scoliosis angle (*a*).

Uniform positioning and technique are important but are not critical to ensure reliability of serial curve measurements. In an experimental study of two mounted scoliotic cadaver spines, a mean difference of 2.06 ± 1.09 degrees was found in the Cobb measurements for films made with changes of 10 degrees in spine rotation or 5 cm in x-ray tube centering.[85]

MEASUREMENT OF ROTATION

It has been shown both on anatomic specimens[78] and with computer modeling[81,82] that the spine rotates when scoliosis develops. The rigidity of the posterior ligaments and osseous elements requires that the tip of the spinous processes must rotate into the concavity of the curve. This rotation allows the posterior structures to remain the same length while the anterior elements elongate. The posterior elements function like the bowstring of an archery bow.

Although this rotation is well recognized, it has been difficult to measure accurately with new techniques still being proposed.[42] Initially, displacement of the spinous process from the midline was used to quantitate rotation,[20] but later investigation found this method to be unreliable owing to the acquired asymmetric development of the spinous processes of the scoliotic spine.[61] The most popular current method for measuring vertebral rotation is the method of Nash and Moe[61] or a modification of it.[65] In this technique, the displacement of the convex side pedicle is visually estimated[49] (Fig. 2-16) or measured on the film and expressed as a ratio with the vertebral body width (Fig. 2-17). Early investigators reported that on an AP radiograph the convex side pedicle

CONCAVE PEDICLE	ROTATION	CONVEX PEDICLE
Normal	0	Normal
Overlapping edge	1+	Slightly towards midline
Disappearing	2+	2/3's towards midline
Absent	3+	Midline
Absent	4+	Beyond midline

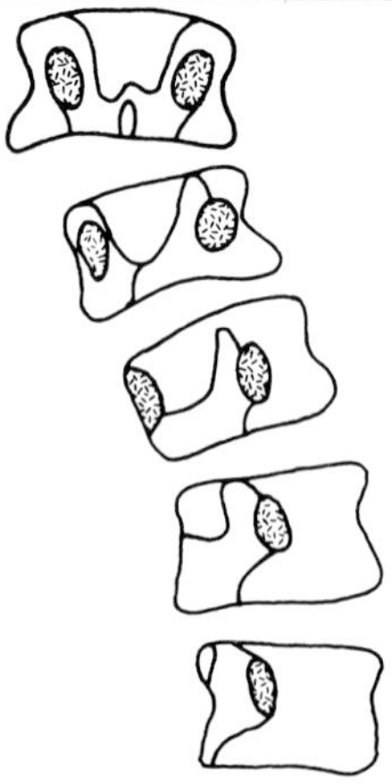

FIGURE 2-16
Nash and Moe grades.
Rotation is graded 0 to 4+, depending on changes in pedicle position.

migrated toward the midline in direct proportion to the degree of rotation.[61,65] More recent investigators could confirm this observation only when the specimen vertebrae did not have lateral or sagittal plane tilting.[6,31] Worse yet, it was also found that in certain circumstances a measured degree of pedicle displacement could have a 50% uncertainty in rotation measurement.[6] For example, a pedicle displacement measurement giving a calculated rotation of 30 degrees could actually represent rotation in a range from 15 to 45 degrees. This variation was due to variable vertebral morphology and tilting of the vertebrae. Thus, even in a specific patient, apparent changes in rotation after treatment might result from a change in vertebral tilt rather than a true change in rotation.

Mehta has stressed these problems with the Nash and Moe method and recommends determining rotation by the use of standard reference radiographs.[56] She has illustrated characteristic changes in the radiographic images of the pedicles, transverse processes, laminae, and spinous processes with rotation. By matching the illustrations with the visualized shape of the patient's apical vertebra, rotation can be determined to be 0, 15, 30, or 45 degrees. Unfortunately, in small to moderate curves the rotation is usually less than 30 degrees, so this quantitation is not very useful and has rarely been used in reported studies. In addition, no allowance is made for the image changes that occur with vertebral tilting.

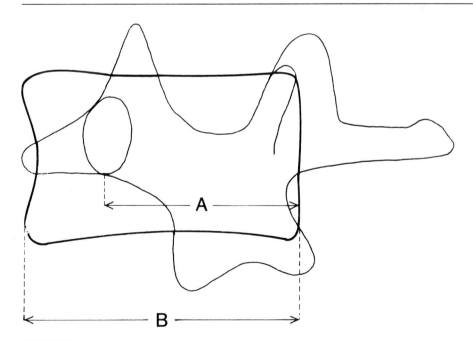

FIGURE 2-17
Quantitation of vertebral rotation.
The distance *(A)* from the midpoint of the convex pedicle to the concave vertebral margin divided by the vertebral body width *(B)* gives a ratio that decreases as rotation increases.

Recently, computed tomography (CT) has been used to measure vertebral rotation.[1,2] This technique provides a very accurate method for measuring rotation by clearly showing the axis of the vertebrae relative to the sagittal plane of the body. However, the significance of the data is uncertain because patients must be examined supine owing to the construction of CT scanners. Since curve magnitude frequently changes between the upright and supine positions, rotation should change also.

SKELETAL MATURITY

Determination of skeletal maturity is important in the management of patients with scoliosis because brace therapy is generally ineffective after cessation of skeletal growth, and curve progression is less frequent and less rapid after the growth spurt occurring during puberty. Skeletal maturity is most easily determined on the PA or AP scoliosis radiograph by the degree of ossification and fusion of the iliac crest apophysis. Risser had graded apophysis ossification from 0 to V, where *0* is the apophysis not yet ossified, *I* to *IV* the ossification progressing by quadrants, and *V* fusion of the apophysis (Fig. 2-18).[74] Progression from grades I to V usually occurs within a 2 year period.[16,89]

In Risser and Ferguson's original report, there was no progression of scoliosis in any patient with fused ilial apophyses (Risser V)[75]; however, the patients were followed for an average of 33 months only. Subsequently, numerous authors have noted that scoliosis may increase in severity after skeletal maturity.* However, the rate of progression is slow, and progression is more likely in curves greater than 40 degrees.

---

*See references 8, 21, 22, 48, 51, 83, 93, 98.

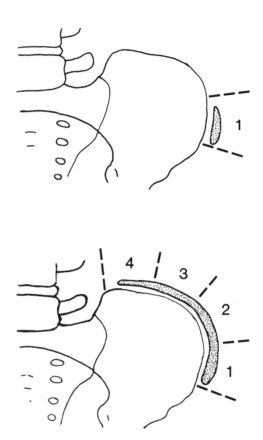

FIGURE 2-18
Iliac crest apophysis begins laterally (grade I) in the first quadrant *(upper figure)* and progresses medially to grade IV *(lower figure)* before fusion occurs (grade V).

Skeletal maturity can also be determined by the time of appearance and fusion of the vertebral ring apophyses (Fig. 2-19). These apophyses are difficult to visualize on AP or PA radiographs so they are more difficult to use for estimation of skeletal maturity than the iliac apophysis.[89] Fortunately, skeletal maturity determined by the Risser method correlates closely with the ring apophysis method.[93] Zaoussis and James reported that evaluation of skeletal maturity by the vertebral apophysis offered no advantage compared to the iliac apophysis method.[104] Others, however, believe that fusion of the vertebral ring apophyses is the most reliable indicator of the termination of spinal growth.[9]

CURVE FLEXIBILITY

Scoliosis curve flexibility is quantified by comparing the upright film with the supine bend film. The percentage of flexibility is defined as 100 times the difference between the upright Cobb curve measurement and the supine measurement with bend toward the curve convexity divided by the upright measurement (see Fig. 2-1). For example, a 40 degree right thoracic curve in the upright position that reduces to 30 degrees with right bending would have 25% flexibility ($100 \times [40° - 30°]/40°$). A curve with 0% flexibility would not change with bending and a curve with 100% flexibility would reduce to 0 degrees on the bending film. Kyphosis flexibility is quantified similarly by subtracting the Cobb angle on the lateral bolster film from the upright lateral measurement and dividing by the upright lateral measurement (see Fig. 2-2).

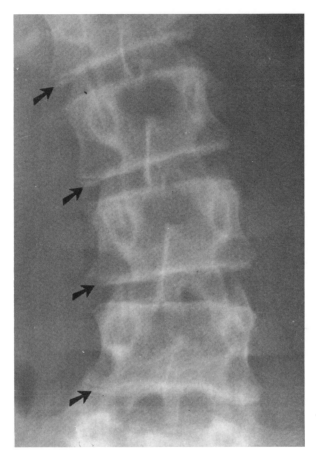

FIGURE 2-19
Unfused vertebral ring apophyses *(arrows)* in the lumbar spine indicating the
patient is not yet skeletally mature.

RIB-VERTEBRAL ANGLE

Measurement of the rib-vertebral angle has been recommended for use by Mehta as a predictor of which infantile scoliosis curves will progress and which will spontaneously resolve.[57] The rib-vertebral angle is measured by drawing a baseline tangentially across the inferior or superior endplate of the apical vertebra (Fig. 2-20). A line is then drawn perpendicular to this tangential line across the middle of the vertebra. Finally, a line is drawn from the midpoint of the head of each apical rib to the midpoint of the neck of the rib, just medial to the region where the neck widens into the shaft of the rib.[57] If the difference between these two angles is less than 20 degrees, the curve will probably resolve. If the difference is greater than 20 degrees, the curve will probably progress. On follow-up examination in 3 months, the angle difference will decrease in resolving curves and remain the same or increase in progressive curves. If the head of the convex rib overlaps the vertebral body, called phase II by Mehta, the curve will increase.[57] Two recent studies have confirmed Mehta's findings.[18,91]

Radiation Risk

An important issue today is the risk to the patient from exposure to diagnostic x-rays. This topic has been the subject of numerous editorials and reviews.* Several national and international agencies have issued reports and recommendations on ionizing radiation.[45,63,64,92] These reports should be studied by any physician wishing to review current knowledge regarding the potential hazards of diagnostic x-rays.

---

*See references 33, 41, 87, 95, 97, 102.

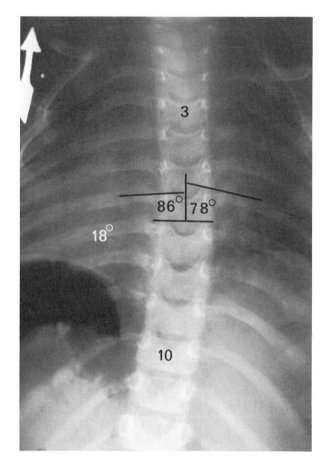

FIGURE 2-20
Rib-vertebral angle in infantile scoliosis.
At the apical vertebra lines are drawn through the middle of the head and neck of each rib up to a vertical line in the vertebral midline. The rib-vertebral angle difference of 8 degrees (86 to 78 degrees) correctly predicted spontaneous curve regression in this patient.

RADIATION MEASUREMENTS

Diagnostic x-rays are one form of radiated energy in the electromagnetic spectrum with wavelengths of 0.1 to 1.0 Å. Because of their unique energy level, x-rays are the most suitable form of electromagnetic radiation for evaluating the internal structure of the body. As x-rays pass through different body tissues, energy is absorbed by these tissues. To quantitate the energy in the x-ray beam, three basic measurements are used: the roentgen, the rad, and the rem. A *roentgen* (R) is a measure of *x-ray exposure* and is defined by the number of ionizations occurring in a volume of air. Exposure to 1 roentgen results in creation of ions equivalent to a charge of 2.58×10^{-4} coulombs per kilogram of air. The second measurement is the rad, which is a unit of *absorbed dose*. One *rad* is equal to the absorption of 100 ergs of energy in a gram of tissue. Because the size of the area irradiated and the kind of tissue irradiated will cause the total quantity of energy absorbed from a fixed x-ray exposure to vary, the rad is the most commonly used unit of measurement. The last commonly used measure is the rem. The rem is termed a measure of *dose equivalent* and takes into account the differing biologic effects of various forms of radiation. To determine the dose equivalent, the number of rads is multiplied by a quality factor which represents the relative hazard associated with the type of radiation in question. The quality factor for x-rays, gamma rays, and beta particles is one but is much higher for protons, neutrons, and alpha particles, which cause greater tissue damage.[19]

Therefore, for diagnostic x-rays, 1 rad of absorbed dose equals 1 rem absorbed by soft tissues. One roentgen of exposure to soft tissues results in 1.05 rad of energy absorbed. Thus the three measures are approximately equivalent for measuring soft tissue irradiation from diagnostic x-rays.

Recently, efforts have intensified to provide international standardization of units and measurements. Use of a system of units called the International System (SI) has been recommended.[35] These units are derived from the metric system. One roentgen has been defined as being equal to 2.58×10^{-4} coulombs per kilogram. Absorbed doses are measured in grays where 1 gray = 1 joule per kilogram = 100 rads. Dose equivalents are given in sieverts, where 1 sievert = 100 rems.

RADIOBIOLOGY

Damage to normal cells in the body from radiation exposure is a random phenomenon. Absorption of a given dose may or may not result in a harmful effect, although the higher the dose, the more likely the effect is to occur. Even if molecular changes do occur, they may be repaired by radiation repair mechanisms present in all normal mammalian cells.[87] If a small number of cells is killed, the functional reserve of the body will most likely limit the effect, and normal cell turnover will remove and replace the damaged cells. At very large doses, however, the functional reserve of the body may be insufficient to limit the immediate damage. Furthermore, killing of stem cell populations may limit or even prevent replacement of damaged cells. Acute radiation effects occur only at very high absorbed doses, with the effect depending on the whole body dose. Doses in the range of 200 to 1000 rads may result in death associated with bone marrow depression and loss of patency of small blood vessels. Doses from 1000 to 3000 rads will cause gastrointestinal tract mucosal exfoliation, while doses in excess of this quantity will cause prompt central nervous impairment resulting in rapid death. The median lethal dose for humans has been estimated at 250 to 450 rads.[17] Doses of this magnitude may occur during radiation therapy or result from nuclear energy accidents or nuclear weapons explosions but have little relevance to diagnostic radiology.

The more relevant aspect of radiobiology deals with the effect of low level exposure associated with most diagnostic examinations. Even at these low levels, damage may occur that is not repaired by the body. The list of possible effects from low level radiation exposure is lengthy, including cataracts, reduced fertility, damage to gonadal germ cells with long-term genetic effects, nonspecific life shortening, and the induction of neoplasm.[33] Exposure of developing embryos and fetuses during pregnancy may result in birth defects. However, each of these effects is highly unlikely, and, at low doses, the probability of any effect at all is very small. The exact dose-response relationship between radiation effects and low level exposure is controversial, but all authors agree that it is not significant unless the exposed population is very large. The frequency of each of the various effects with different dose levels has been ably summarized in a recent report by the National Research Council.[64]

CLINICAL STUDIES OF RADIATION EFFECTS

Exposure to repeated diagnostic x-rays at total absorbed doses of 100 to 500 rads is associated with an increased incidence of malignant neoplasms. The most frequent radiation-induced cancers are found in the female breast, the thyroid gland, and the hemopoietic tissues.[33] Many epidemiologic studies have found an increased incidence of neoplasm when these tissues received x-ray doses of over 100 rads.*

In light of these serious late effects of radiation, the concern over even the lower dosage of modern diagnostic x-rays is understandable. One investigator, using sophisticated statistical extrapolations, believes that he has shown an increased incidence of leukemia and heart disease from x-ray exposures as low as 1 roentgen.[13] However, clinical studies of patients and radiation workers subjected to x-ray exposures of less than 100 roentgens have failed to document any decrease in life span or increased incidence of neoplasm.[46,52,87] Early radiation workers were unaware of the harmful effects of x-rays, and many accumulated lifetime exposures of over 3000 roentgens.[96] With awareness of the risk of increased leukemia incidence and other life-shortening diseases, permissible doses for radiation workers have been established at a lifetime maximum of about 250 rems.[96] As a result of these changes, radiologists no longer have an increased incidence of neo-

*See references 11, 24, 44, 59, 60, 86.

51

plasm.[23,84,96] The data regarding the potential risk from prenatal diagnostic x-rays are highly controversial. While some clinical studies have found an increased incidence of birth defects and subsequent development of leukemia,[14] others question the validity of these studies.[68]

It is unlikely that epidemiologic studies will ever indicate a causal relationship between low level radiation and induced neoplasm because radiation-induced neoplasms cannot be distinguished from those occurring naturally.[34] If low level radiation induces neoplasm, the rate is so low compared to the normal rate of malignancy that a significant radiation-induced increase cannot be demonstrated.[97]

The potential for induced genetic defects in future generations has been of concern, but there is no evidence that low dose radiation to the testes or ovaries results in an increased incidence of genetic defects in future children.[70] Studies of Japanese A-bomb survivors who became pregnant between 1948 and 1953 found no increase in malformations, stillbirths, or neonatal deaths.[70] However, two expert committees have used laboratory test animals and high dose exposure human data to estimate the theoretical risk of low dose x-ray gonadal exposure. They estimated that for each rad of parental irradiation, there would be on the average 30[92] or between 5 and 75[64] genetic defects per million liveborn. This low figure should be compared to the spontaneous incidence of 107,000 genetic defects per million liveborn.[70]

IMPLICATIONS FOR SCOLIOSIS RADIOGRAPHY

In 1979, Nash et al.[62] reported that an adolescent girl having repeated scoliosis radiographs during bracing for scoliosis had a 110% increase in her risk of developing breast carcinoma because of the x-ray exposure. However, these authors reported an average skin exposure of 1129 milliroentgens for each AP film. Subsequently, multiple authors have reported that with modern techniques, skin exposure should average between 20 and 65 milliroentgens, a 17- to 56-fold reduction from that reported by Nash and Moe.[61] In addition, breast radiation can be decreased 88% to 98% from the entrance skin exposure by using the PA projection. The net effect is that the breast irradiation is reduced to 1 to 5 milliroentgens. The PA exposure also reduces x-ray irradiation of the thyroid 20-fold.[39] The net result is a theoretical but negligible increase in the incidence of breast or thyroid neoplasms. Because the bone marrow is still exposed with the PA projection, there is still a potential risk of induced leukemia. If one million people were exposed to 1 roentgen of whole body radiation, the number of radiation-induced leukemias has been theoretically calculated to range from 0.016 to 2.5. At a surface exposure of 20 to 65 milliroentgens, the theoretical increased rate of leukemia per scoliosis radiograph would be very small. In addition, since the whole body is not irradiated, the estimated rate would be even smaller. These conclusions are well documented in the recent thorough study of the risk of carcinogenesis from x-rays to scoliosis patients by Rao and Gregg.[73]

In conclusion, then, the risk from scoliosis radiography seems negligible when balanced against the complications of untreated scoliosis. Any risk can be made even smaller by using the PA projection, high-speed rare-earth screens, and good film collimation.

Summary

A. Radiographic technique
   1. 182.9 cm (6 foot) tube-to-film distance
   2. 0.6 mm focal spot x-ray tube
   3. Gradient compensation: wedge, gradient filter, or gradient screen
   4. 8:1 ratio grid
   5. Collimate from lower cervical spine to upper sacrum and side-to-side as much as possible
   6. 35 × 91 cm or 35 × 70 cm cassette
   7. High-speed rare-earth screen-film combination
B. Positioning
   1. PA upright—used routinely to reduce breast and thyroid exposure
   2. Lateral upright
      a. If back pain present or abnormal sagittal curve suspected
      b. Prior to bracing or surgery
   3. Supine bending
      a. To determine curve flexibility
      b. Prior to surgery to help determine the length of the fusion and achievable correction
   4. Cross-table lateral with bolster—prior to surgery for kyphosis flexibility
C. Evaluation
   1. Cobb angle for scoliosis, kyphosis, and lordosis—2 to 3 degrees standard error of measurement
      a. Normal thoracic kyphosis, 20 to 50 degrees
      b. Normal lumbar lordosis, 20 to 60 degrees
   2. Nash and Moe method for vertebral rotation—grades 0 to 4+
   3. Risser method for skeletal maturity—grades 0 to V
   4. Flexibility = 100 × (upright Cobb − supine bending Cobb)/upright Cobb
D. Radiation risk
   1. 1 rem = 1 rad ≃ 1 roentgen
   2. PA skin absorbed dose should be less than 100 millirads
   3. Harmful effects
      a. Future genetic damage—very low level risk, 5 to 75 birth defects per 1 million persons per rad exposure—unproven but estimated
      b. Somatic effects—not seen with low level exposure
      c. Induced neoplasm—not proven but estimated at one to six neoplasms per 1 million persons per rad exposure to specific organs (breast, thyroid, and bone marrow are most radiation sensitive)

REFERENCES

1. Aaro, S., and Dahlborn, M.: Estimation of vertebral rotation and the spinal and rib cage deformity in scoliosis by computer tomography, Spine **6**:460-467, 1981.
2. Aaro, S., and Dahlborn, M.: The longitudinal axis rotation of the apical vertebra, the vertebral, spinal, and rib cage deformity in idiopathic scoliosis studied by computer tomography, Spine **6**:567-572, 1981.
3. Andersen, P.E., Jr., Andersen, P.E., and van der Kooy, P.: Dose reduction in radiography of the spine in scoliosis, Acta Radiol. [Diagn.] (Stockh.) **23**:251-253, 1982.
4. Ardran, G.M., et al.: Assessment of scoliosis in children: low dose radiographic technique, Br. J. Radiol. **53**:146-147, 1980.
5. Beekman, C.E., and Hall, V.: Variability of scoliosis measurement from spinal roentgenograms, Phys. Ther. **59**:764-765, 1979.
6. Benson, D.R., Schultz, A.B., and Dewald, R.L.: Roentgenographic evaluation of vertebral rotation, J. Bone Joint Surg. (Am.) **58**:1125-1129, 1976.
7. Binstadt, D.H., Lonstein, J.E., and Winter, R.B.: Radiographic evaluation of the scoliotic patient, Minn. Med. **61**:474-496, 1978.
8. Bjerkreim, I., and Hassan, I.: Progression in untreated idiopathic scoliosis after end of growth, Acta. Orthop. Scand. **53**:897-900, 1982.
9. Blount, W.P., and Mellencamp, D.D.: Scoliosis treatment: skeletal maturity evaluation, Minn. Med. **56**:382-390, 1973.
10. Board, R.F.: Radiography of the scoliotic spine, Radiol. Technol. **38**:219-224, 1967.
11. Boice, J.D., Jr., and Monson, R.R.: Breast cancer in women after repeated fluoroscopic examinations of the chest, J. Natl. Cancer Inst. **59**:823-830, 1977.
12. Bradford, D.S., et al.: Scheuermann's kyphosis and roundback deformity, J. Bone Joint Surg. (Am.) **56**:740-758, 1974.
13. Bross, I.D.J., Ball, M., and Falen, S.: A dosage response curve for the one rad range: adult risks from diagnostic radiation, AJPH **69**:130-136, 1979.
14. Bross, I.D.J., and Natarajan, N.: Genetic damage from diagnostic radiation, JAMA **237**:2399-2401, 1977.
15. Burwell, R.G., et al.: Standardised trunk asymmetry scores: a study of back contour in healthy schoolchildren, J. Bone Joint Surg. (Br.) **65**:452-463, 1983.
16. Calvo, I.J.: Observations on the growth of the female adolescent spine and its relation to scoliosis, Clin. Orthop. **10**:40-46, 1957.
17. Casarett, A.P.: Radiation biology, Englewood Cliffs, N.J., 1968, Prentice-Hall, Inc.
18. Ceballos T., et al.: Prognosis in infantile idiopathic scoliosis, J. Bone Joint Surg. (Am.) **62**:863-875, 1980.
19. Christensen, E.E., Curry, T.S., III, and Dowdey, J.E.: An introduction to the physics of diagnostic radiology, Philadelphia, 1978, Lea & Febiger.
20. Cobb, J.R.: Outline for the study of scoliosis. In Instructional course lectures. The American Academy of Orthopaedic Surgeons, Vol. 5, Ann Arbor, 1948, J.W. Edwards, pp. 261-275.
21. Collis, D.K., and Ponseti, I.V.: Long-term follow-up of patients with idiopathic scoliosis not treated surgically, J. Bone Joint Surg. (Am.) **51**:425-445, 1969.
22. Coonrad, R.W., and Feierstein, M.S.: Progression of scoliosis in the adult, J. Bone Joint Surg. (Am.) **58**:156, 1976.
23. Court Brown, W.M., and Doll, R.: Expectation of life and mortality from cancer among British radiologists, Br. Med. J. **26**:181-187, 1958.
24. Court Brown, W.M., and Doll, R.: Mortality from cancer and other causes after radiotherapy for ankylosing spondylitis, Br. Med. J. **2**:1327-1332, 1965.

25. Cowell, M.J., and Cowell, H.R.: The incidence of spina bifida occulta in idiopathic scoliosis, Clin. Orthop. **118:**16-18, 1976.

26. Dawson, E.G., Smith, R.K., and McNiece, G.M.: Radiographic evaluation of scoliosis, Clin. Orthop. **131:**151-155, 1978.

27. DeSmet, A.A., Fritz, S.L., and Asher, M.A.: A method for minimizing the radiation exposure from scoliosis radiographs, J. Bone Joint Surg. (Am.) **63:**156-158, 1981.

28. DeSmet, A.A., Fritz, S.L., and Asher, M.A.: Minimizing radiation exposure from scoliosis radiographs (reply), J. Bone Joint Surg. (Am.) **63:**1500, 1981.

29. DeSmet, A.A., and Ritter, E.M.: An improved film cassette for scoliosis radiography, Radiology **141:**249-250, 1981.

30. DeSmet, A.A., et al.: A clinical study of the differences between the scoliotic angles measured on posteroanterior and anteroposterior radiographs, J. Bone Joint Surg. (Am.) **64:**489-493, 1982.

31. DeSmet, A.A., et al.: Evaluation of radiographic landmarks for three-dimensional spinal analysis. In Jacobs, R.R., editor: Pathogenesis of idiopathic scoliosis, Chicago, 1984, Scoliosis Research Society, pp. 44-59.

32. Dickson, R.A.: Letter, J. Bone Joint Surg. (Am.) **63:**1500, 1981.

33. Fabrikant, J.I.: Estimation of risk of cancer induction in populations exposed to low-level radiation, Invest. Radiol. **17:**342-349, 1982.

34. Fabrikant, J.I.: The BEIR-III report: origin of the controversy, AJR **136:**209-214, 1981.

35. Figley, M.M.: Introduction of SI units, AJR **134:**208, 1980.

36. Fisk, J.R., Moe, J.H., and Winter, R.B.: Scoliosis, spondylolysis, and spondylolisthesis: their relationship as reviewed in 539 patients, Spine **3:**234-245, 1978.

37. Fon, G.T., Pitt, M.J., and Thies, A.C. Jr.: Thoracic kyphosis: range in normal subjects, AJR **134:**979-983, 1980.

38. George, K., and Rippstein, J.: A comparative study of the two popular methods of measuring scoliotic deformity of the spine, J. Bone Joint Surg. (Am.) **6:**809-818, 1961.

39. Gray, J.E., Hoffman, A.D., and Peterson, H.A.: Reduction of radiation exposure during radiography for scoliosis, J. Bone Joint Surg. (Am.) **65:**5-12, 1983.

40. Greenspan, A., et al.: Scoliotic index: a comparative evaluation of methods for the measurement of scoliosis, Bull. Hosp. Joint Dis. Orthop. Inst. **39:**117-125, 1978.

41. Gregg, E.C.: Radiation risks with diagnostic x-rays, Radiology **123:**447-453, 1977.

42. Gross, C., Gross, M., and Alexander, D.: Scoliotic spinal anthropometry, Bull. Hosp. Joint Dis. Orthop. Inst. **43:**84-91, 1983.

43. Hellstrom, G., Irstam, L., and Nachemson, A.: Reduction of radiation dose in radiologic examination of patients with scoliosis, Spine **8:**28-30, 1983.

44. Hempelmann, L.H., et al.: Neoplasms in persons treated with x-rays in infancy: fourth survey in 20 years, J. Natl. Cancer Inst. **55:**519-530, 1975.

45. ICRP Publication 26: Recommendations of the International Commission on Radiological Protection, New York, 1977, Pergamon Press.

46. Jablon, S., and Miller, R.W.: Army technologists: 29-year follow up for cause of death, Radiology **126:**677-679, 1978.

47. Jeffries, B.F., et al.: Computerized measurement and analysis of scoliosis, Radiology **134:**381-385, 1980.

48. Keim, H.A.: Scoliosis can progress in the adult, Orthop. Rev. **3:**23-28, 1974.

49. Keim, H.A.: Scoliosis, Clin. Symp. CIBA **30:**2-30, 1978.

50. Kittleson, A.C., and Lim, L.W.: Measurement of scoliosis, AJR **108:**775-777, 1970.

51. Kostuik, J.P., Israel, J., and Hall, J.E.: Scoliosis surgery in adults, Clin. Orthop. **93:**225-234, 1973.

52. Linos, A., et al.: Low-dose radiation and leukemia, N. Engl. J. Med. **302:**1101-1105, 1980.

53. Lonstein, J., et al.: School screening for the early detection of spine deformities, Minn. Med., January 1976, pp. 51-57.

54. Lonstein, J., et al.: Voluntary school screening for scoliosis in Minnesota, J. Bone Joint Surg. (Am.) **64:**481-488, 1982.

55. McAlister, W.H., and Shackelford, G.D.: Measurement of spinal curvatures, Radiol. Clin. North Am. **13:**113-121, 1975.

56. Mehta, M.H.: Radiographic estimation of vertebral rotation in scoliosis, J. Bone Joint Surg. (Br.) **55:**513-520, 1973.

57. Mehta, M.H.: The rib-vertebra angle in the early diagnosis between resolving and progressive infantile scoliosis, J. Bone Joint Surg. (Br.) **54:**230-243, 1972.

58. Moe, J., et al.: Scoliosis and other spinal deformities, Philadelphia, 1978, W.B. Saunders Co.

59. Mole, R.H.: The sensitivity of the human breast to cancer induction by ionizing radiation, Br. J. Radiol. **51:**401-405, 1978.

60. Myrden, J.A., and Hiltz, J.E.: Breast cancer following multiple fluoroscopies during artificial pneumothorax treatment of pulmonary tuberculosis, Can. Med. Assoc. J. **100:**1032-1034, 1969.

61. Nash, C.L., and Moe, J.H.: A study of vertebral rotation, J. Bone Joint Surg. (Am.) **51:**223-229, 1969.

62. Nash, C.L., et al.: Risks of exposure to x-rays in patients undergoing long-term treatment for scoliosis, J. Bone Joint Surg. (Am.) **61:**371-374, 1979.

63. National Council on Radiation Protection and Measurements: Influence of dose and its distribution in time and dose-response relationships for low-LET radiations. NCRP report No. 64, Washington, D.C., 1980, NCRP.

64. National Research Council, Committee on the Biological Effects Ionizing Radiations: The effects on populations of exposure to low levels of ionizing radiation, 1980 (BEIR III), Washington, D.C., 1980, National Academy Press.

65. Nordwall, A.: Studies in idiopathic scoliosis, Acta Orthop. Scand. (Suppl.) **150:**73-101, 1973.

66. Nottage, W.M., Waugh, T.R., and McMaster, W.C.: Radiation exposure during scoliosis screening radiography, Spine **6:**456-459, 1981.

67. Oda, M., et al.: The significance of roentgenographic measurement in scoliosis, J. Pediatr. Orthop. **2:**378-382, 1982.

68. Oppenheim, B.E.: Genetic damage from diagnostic radiation? JAMA **242:**1390-1393, 1979.

69. Ozonoff, M.B.: Pediatric orthopedic radiology, Philadelphia, 1979, W.B. Saunders Co.

70. Pizzarello, D.J., and Witcofski, R.L.: Medical radiation biology, Philadelphia, 1982, Lea & Febiger.

71. Propst-Proctor, S.L., and Bleck, E.E.: Radiographic determination of lordosis and kyphosis in normal and scoliotic children, J. Pediatr. Orthop. **3:**344-346, 1983.

72. Raia, T.J., and Kilfoyle, R.M.: Minimizing radiation exposure in scoliosis screening, Appl. Radiol., January/February 1982, pp. 45-55.

73. Rao, P.S., and Gregg, E.C.: A revised estimate of the risk of carcinogenesis from x-rays to scoliosis patients, Invest. Radiol. **19:**58-60, 1984.

74. Risser, J.C.: The iliac apophysis: an invaluable sign in the management of scoliosis, Clin. Orthop. **11:**111-119, 1958.

75. Risser, J.C., and Ferguson, A.B.: Scoliosis: its prognosis, J. Bone Joint Surg. (Am.) **18**:667-670, 1936.

76. Ritter, E.M., et al.: Use of a gradient intensifying screen for scoliosis radiography, Radiology **135**:230-232, 1980.

77. Roaf, R.: Vertebral growth and its mechanical control, J. Bone Joint Surg. (Br.) **42**:40-59, 1960.

78. Roaf, R.: The basic anatomy of scoliosis, J. Bone Joint Surg. (Br.) **48**:786-792, 1966.

79. Robinson, E.F., and Wade, W.D.: Statistical assessment of two methods of measuring scoliosis before treatment, Can. Med. Assoc. J. **129**:839-841, 1983.

80. Schock, C.C., Brenton, L., and Agarwal, K.K.: The effect of PA versus AP x-rays on the apparent scoliotic angle, Orthop. Trans. **4**:32, 1980.

81. Schultz, A.B.: A biomechanical view of scoliosis, Spine **1**:162-171, 1976.

82. Schultz, A.B., et al.: A study of geometrical relationships in scoliotic spines, J. Biomech. **5**:409-420, 1972.

83. Scott, M.M., and Piggott, H.: A short-term follow-up of patients with mild scoliosis, J. Bone Joint Surg. (Br.) **63**:523-525, 1981.

84. Seltser, R., and Sartwell, P.E.: The influence of occupational exposure to radiation on the mortality of American radiologists and other medical specialists, Am. J. Epidemiol. **81**:2-22, 1965.

85. Sevastikoglou, J.A., and Bergquist, E.: Evaluation of the reliability of radiological methods for registration of scoliosis, Acta Orthop. Scand. **40**:608-613, 1969.

86. Shore, R.E., et al.: Breast neoplasms in women treated with x-rays for acute postpartum mastitis, J. Natl. Cancer Inst. **59**:813-822, 1977.

87. Sinclair, W.K.: Effects of low-level radiation and comparative risk, Radiology **138**:1-9, 1981.

88. Stagnara, P., et al.: Reciprocal angulation of vertebral bodies in a sagittal plane: approach to references for the evaluation of kyphosis and lordosis, Spine **7**:335-342, 1982.

89. Terver, S., Kleinman, R., and Bleck, E.E.: Growth landmarks and the evolution of scoliosis: a review of pertinent studies on their usefulness, Dev. Med. Child Neurol. **22**:675-684, 1980.

90. Thomas, S.R., et al.: Characteristics of extrafocal radiation and its potential significance in pediatric radiology, Radiology **146**:793-799, 1983.

91. Thompson, S.K., and Bentley, G.: Prognosis in infantile idiopathic scoliosis, J. Bone Joint Surg. (Br.) **62**:151-154, 1980.

92. United Nations Scientific Committee on Effects of Atomic Radiation: Sources and effects of ionizing radiation. Report A/32/40 to the General Assembly, 32nd session. Annex 1, Radiation carcinogenesis in animals, New York, 1977, United Nations.

93. Urbaniak, J.R., Schaefer, W.W., and Stelling, F.H., III: Iliac apophyses: prognostic value in idiopathic scoliosis, Clin. Orthop. **116**:80-85, 1976.

94. Venema, H.W.: X-ray absorption, speed, and luminescent efficiency of rare earth and other intensifying screens, Radiology **130**:756-771, 1979.

95. Wagner, H.N.: Radiation: the risks and the benfits, AJR **140**:595-603, 1983.

96. Warren S., and Lombard, O.M.: New data on the effects of ionizing radiation on radiologists, Arch. Environ. Health **13**:415-421, 1966.

97. Webster, E.W.: On the question of cancer induction by small x-ray doses, AJR **137**:647-666, 1981.

98. Weinstein, S., Zavala, D.C., and Ponseti, I.V.: Idiopathic scoliosis: long-term follow-up and prognosis in untreated patients, J. Bone Joint Surg. (Am.) **63**:702-712, 1981.

99. Wilson, M.S., Stockwell, J., and Leedy, M.G.: Measurement of scoliosis by orthopedic surgeons and radiologists, Aviat. Space Environ. Med. **54:**69-71, 1983.

100. Winter, R.B.: Congenital deformities of the spine, New York, 1983, Thieme-Stratton Inc.

101. Winter, R.B., and Carlson, J.M.: Modern orthotics for spinal deformities, Clin. Orthop. **126:**74-86, 1977.

102. Youker, J.E., et al.: Dose reduction in diagnostic radiology, Diagn. Imaging, April 1981, pp. 22-24, 50.

103. Young, L.W., Oestreich, A.E., and Goldstein, L.A.: Roentgenology in scoliosis: contribution to evaluation and management, AJR **108:**778-795, 1970.

104. Zaoussis, A.L., and James, J.I.P.: The iliac apophysis and the evolution of curves in scoliosis, J. Bone Joint Surg. (Br.) **40:**442-453, 1958.

Chapter Three ———————

Special
——— Radiographic Studies

Solomon Batnitzky and Hilton I. Price

*T*he evaluation, diagnosis, and management of patients with spinal curvature deformities are based nearly completely on radiographic information. Radiographs of the spine are essential and are the most valuable diagnostic tool available to the clinician. The important information that radiographs of the spine provide in the evaluation of patients with spinal curvature abnormalities has been discussed in detail in Chapter Two.

For most patients, only plain spine films are necessary for the evaluation and management of abnormal spinal curvature. In selected cases, however, additional specialized radiographic imaging techniques may be necessary for more accurate diagnosis. The value, advantages, and limitations of each imaging technique will be discussed for specific clinical conditions.

These imaging techniques include:
1. Conventional tomography
2. Myelography
3. Computed tomography (CT)
4. Computed tomographic metrizamide myelography (CTMM)
5. Magnetic resonance (MR)

Special Techniques
CONVENTIONAL TOMOGRAPHY (body section radiography, laminagraphy, planigraphy, and stratigraphy)

This technique provides an image of any selected plane through the body while blurring out the images of structures that lie above or below that plane. In cases of abnormal spinal curvature, thin-section pluridirectional tomography is useful to demonstrate better and more accurately the true anatomy of the deformity in cases where the actual pathology is obscure on plain radiographs (Figs. 3-2 and 3-3). This information may be helpful and important in planning corrective surgery.

MYELOGRAPHY

Myelography refers to the radiographic visualization of the spinal subarachnoid space with a contrast agent. It should be stressed that it is not a routine investigation performed on all patients with spine deformities.

Indications include the following:
1. To diagnose the presence or absence of surgically treatable intraspinal lesions
2. To ascertain the exact level and extent of the lesion
3. To exclude multiple lesions
4. To exclude the possibility of an operable lesion when the clinical situation and other diagnostic tests are inconclusive and equivocal

Myelography may be undertaken using either negative or positive contrast agents.

Negative contrast agents. Gas myelography[3] involves replacing the spinal subarachnoid fluid with air or oxygen. They are the least irritating and least toxic of all the different contrast agents that have been and are being used for myelography. Gas myelography is an excellent neuroradiologic technique to differentiate solid from cystic lesions of the spinal cord (Fig. 3-7) and also to demonstrate atrophy of the spinal cord. However, it is a time consuming and uncomfortable procedure for the patient. It is technically a difficult procedure to perform and requires meticulous technique and sophisticated equipment to be successful. Gas myelography has been used extensively in Scandinavia. However, it has not gained wide acceptance in the United States. With the advent of metrizamide and CT myelography, its use will be further limited.

Positive contrast myelography. Iophendylate[4] has been used as a satisfactory and reliable myelographic contrast agent with a high degree of diagnostic accuracy for the past 40 years. Metrizamide[5,25,44] is a relatively new nonionic water-soluble contrast agent that was approved for clinical use by the Food and Drug Administration in 1978 and has rapidly won wide acceptance for use as a myelographic agent. It has largely replaced iophendylate whenever positive contrast myelography is required.[35] The reader is referred to standard texts for a more detailed review of the advantages and disadvantages of the various myelographic contrast agents.[5]

Following a conventional metrizamide myelogram, spinal CT can be performed to provide additional information. (See below.)

COMPUTED TOMOGRAPHY (CT)

CT of the spine has added a new dimension to the diagnosis of lesions of the spine and its contents.[5,12,21] The new, high-resolution CT scanners provide exquisite demonstration of both the normal and pathologic anatomy of the spine and its contents. Unenhanced spinal CT is invaluable in demonstrating the bony, extradural, and paraspinal extent of tumors and other pathologic processes.

Consistent and reliable visualization of the intrathecal contents (cord, nerve roots, subarachnoid space), however, is difficult even with the new high-resolution scanners.

The use of metrizamide intrathecally provides additional information regarding the spinal contents and subarachnoid space.[1,11,37-39] This greatly extends the morphologic capabilities of spinal CT. One can perform a conventional metrizamide myelogram and follow this 4 to 6 hours later with a CT study of the suspected area of pathology. The 4 to 6 hour delay allows the metrizamide to become more dilute, as metrizamide in the concentration and dose used for myelography is far too dense for immediate CT scanning. Instead of performing a conventional metrizamide myelogram, one can inject a much smaller volume of a more dilute concentration of metrizamide intrathecally followed immediately by the CT scan. This has been termed *computed tomographic metrizamide myelography* (CTMM).

Pettersson et al.[37] in a retrospective study to assess the accuracy of metrizamide myelography in scoliosis showed that, in patients with severe scoliosis associated with dysraphic or segmentation anomalies or localized neurologic or radiologic abnormalities, CTMM is superior to metrizamide myelography and should be added to the latter or performed alone. In those cases, CTMM provided additional information that was essential for diagnosis and treatment. In idiopathic scoliosis with only vague neurologic disturbances, whole spine metrizamide myelography should always precede CTMM or be used alone. In less severe cases, the diagnostic accuracy of metrizamide myelography and CTMM is about the same.

Intraspinal neoplasms are best investigated by conventional myelography because of its ability to demonstrate multiple levels simultaneously. This may be followed by CT, which can complement myelography by providing additional information that might not be appreciated on conventional myelography.

MAGNETIC RESONANCE (MR)

MR imaging,[32] also known as *nuclear magentic resonance* (NMR), is a new imaging technique that is noninvasive and does not use ionizing radiation. This technique employs radiofrequency pulses in the presence of a magnetic field to generate high-quality medical images, which in many cases are more accurate and more specific than those provided by existing imaging techniques.[36,51] Due to the lack of bone artifacts with MR and to its ability to distinguish clearly white and gray matter and cerebrospinal fluid, MR has proved to be a more sensitive, superior, and less invasive method for diagnosing both acquired and congenital lesions of the spinal cord than CTMM and other radiologic techniques (Figs. 3-10 to 3-13, 3-19, and 3-28). Furthermore, the spine can be imaged directly in the transverse (axial), coronal, or sagittal planes. The patient does not require a lumbar puncture or hospital admission, and examination can be performed on an outpatient basis.

INDICATIONS

One or more of the preceding specialized imaging techniques may be necessary in patients with spinal curvature abnormalities when one of the following clinical conditions exists or cannot be excluded.
1. Congenital scoliosis with spinal dysraphism and segmentation anomalies
2. Idiopathic scoliosis with neurologic disturbances
3. Neurofibromatosis
4. Connective tissue disorders (the Marfan syndrome and the Ehlers-Danlos syndrome)
5. Spondylolisthesis

These conditions, with the exception of spondylolisthesis, are associated with a high incidence of intraspinal abnormalities, which will be discussed later in this chapter. The recognition of these spinal abnormalities is important in the scoliotic patient for two reasons[17]: first, there is a significant risk of inducing a neurologic deficit during surgical correction of the scoliosis in the presence of an untreated intraspinal abnormality and, second, to avoid the problems created by a solid spinal fusion covering an occult lesion that may manifest neurologically and require surgical treatment years later.

Once the diagnosis of an intraspinal abnormality has been made, the management of the intraspinal lesion takes precedence over the surgical correction of the scoliosis.[17,37]

Specialized Imaging of Pathologic States
SPINAL DYSRAPHISM AND MYELODYSPLASIA

Spinal dysraphism[19] represents a widespread spectrum of vertebral aberrations that may or may not be associated with congenital disorders of the formation of the spinal cord and nerves (myelodysplasia). All grades of this anomaly may be encountered, ranging from the most benign and least significant, spinal bifida occulta, to the most severe, the meningomyelocele. The incidence of scoliosis in spinal dysraphism is very common.[35,48] In patients with congenital scoliosis the incidence of intraspinal abnormalities is significant.

Congenital intraspinal anomalies associated with spinal dysraphism and myelodysplasia include diastematomyelia, syringohydromyelia, tight filum terminale syndrome, congenital tumors such as lipomas and teratomas, and embryonic malformations such as dermoids, epidermoids, and neurenteric cysts. All these entities and lesions overlap each other substantially, and more than one lesion or abnormality can be present in a patient.

Gillespie et al.[17] routinely obtain preoperative myelography on all patients with congenital scoliosis. In many instances, these lesions may be truly occult and the patient can present to the surgeon because of scoliosis with no significant neurological deficit. The diagnosis of these lesions is therefore of the utmost importance.

Diastematomyelia. Diastematomyelia is an uncommon congenital anomaly of the spine. It is a form of spinal dysraphism that is characterized by partial or complete sagittal clefting of one or more segments of the spinal cord without regard to the presence or absence of a bone spur or other fibro-osseous abnormality.[35]

The clinical features and symptoms in diastematomyelia are not specific and do not differ from those seen in the other forms of spinal dysraphism. In many cases diastematomyelia may be asymptomatic, being diagnosed on routine scoliosis surveys.

In diastematomyelia, the incidence of scoliosis is as high as 81%,[50] with an even higher incidence of other vertebral abnormalities.[22,50] In Gillespie's series of 31 cases of intraspinal anomalies in patients with congenital scoliosis, diastematomyelia accounted for 17 cases.[17] According to Hilal et al.[22] the incidence and severity of scoliosis with diastematomyelia increase with the age of the patient. Overall, diastematomyelia occurs in nearly 5% of all cases of congenital scoliosis.[50]

Until the advent of CTMM, the radiologic investigation of diastematomyelia was directed toward demonstrating the bony spur and the associated midline filling defect in the contrast column on myelography (Figs. 3-1 and 3-2). A radiologically visible bony spur is noted in about one third of patients.

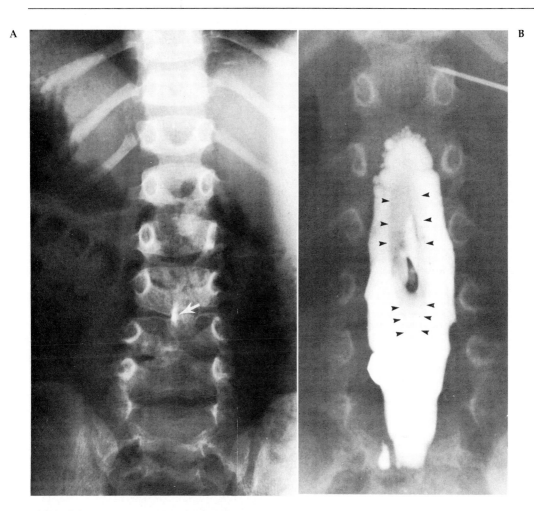

FIGURE 3-1
Diastematomyelia with tethered conus.
A, Lumbar spine radiograph reveals a bony spicule *(arrow)* at the L3-4 disk level. Spinal dysraphism is indicated by widening of the interpediculate distances from L2-S1 levels.
B, Myelography demonstrates splitting of the abnormally low-positioned conus medullaris *(arrowheads)* by the bony spur into a bifid conus that reunites to form a single filum terminale *(arrowheads)*.
From Batnitzky, S.: Intraspinal disorders. In Basic neuroradiology, St. Louis, 1983, Warren H. Green.

The spur can extend through the entire sagittal diameter of the canal or it might occupy only part of the canal. The spur can be attached to either the anterior or posterior canal walls or both. In about 5% to 6% of cases, the spurs are double, occurring at two different levels.[22,35]

Positive contrast myelography can demonstrate the split in the spinal cord. Myelography may reveal a midline filling defect in a contrast column that splits the contrast column into two columns at the level of the bony or fibrocartilaginous spur. The spur, especially if it is bony, may be seen within the filling defect. Myelography is also important to demonstrate the level of the conus in these patients, since diastematomyelia may be associated with a tethered conus. Air myelography is much less reliable in the evaluation of patients with diastematomyelia. Only rarely will myelography demonstrate the two hemicords and their extent in cases that do not have bony or fibrocartilaginous spurs.

CTMM has proved to be the definitive radiologic technique to diagnose and demonstrate diastematomyelia.[35,45] CTMM has demonstrated features of diastematomyelia that were previously not appreciated. A bony or fibrocarti-

FIGURE 3-2
Diastematomyelia.
AP tomogram demonstrates bony spur *(arrowhead)* at the L5 level in 2-year-old girl. The bony spur could not be appreciated on the plain lumbar radiographs. Lumbar scoliosis is also present.

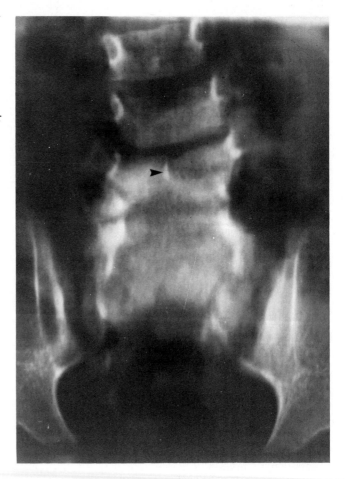

FIGURE 3-3
Extensive diastematomyelia without a
bony or fibrocartilaginous spur in a
12-year-old girl with asymptomatic
scoliosis.

A, Frontal digital radiograph of
thoracolumbar spine demonstrates
marked right convexity scoliosis.

B and **C,** AP tomograms of upper thoracic
area demonstrate some of the bony
abnormalities seen in diastematomyelia.
Multiple block vertebrae and widened
interpediculate distances are seen.
There is partial fusion of a midline
sagittal cleft of the T7 vertebral body
(arrows). Intersegmental fusion of the
pedicles and adjacent laminae on the
right side are identified. The right-sided
pedicles are linked by a discrete osseous
line—a congenital pedicular bar
(arrowheads).

Continued.

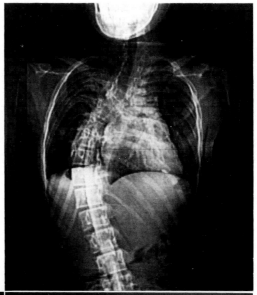

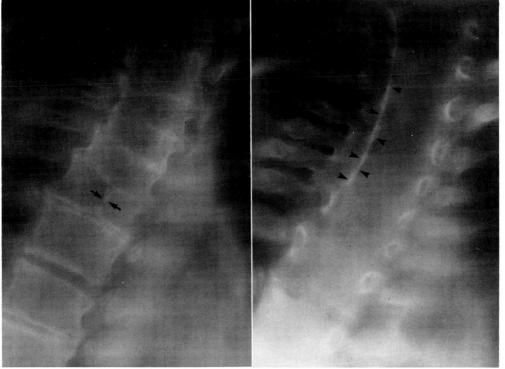

D

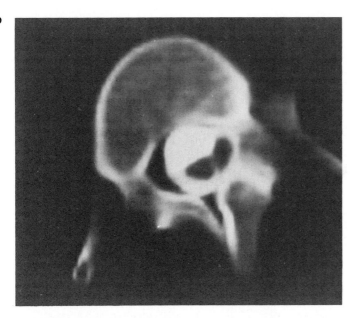

FIGURE 3-3, cont'd
D, CTMM at the T10 level shows two hemicords contained in a single dural and single arachnoid sheath. Both hemicords extended from C7 to L1. No bony or fibrocartilaginous spur was present.

laginous spur is a relatively uncommon finding in diastematomyelia (occurring in only about one third of cases). Furthermore, CTMM has demonstrated a split spinal cord within an unsplit dural sac in many cases, a finding that is difficult to appreciate on conventional myelography (Fig. 3-3).

Fifty percent of cases of diastematomyelia consist of two hemicords, which may or may not be equal in size, contained in a single arachnoid and a single dural tube with no fibrocartilaginous or osseous septum. The other 50% of cases have two hemicords, each with its own arachnoid and dural sheaths. The majority of the second group is associated with a sagittally oriented fibro-osseous septum (Fig. 3-4). Features of both general groups can be present in the same patient (Fig. 3-4).

Although CT may demonstrate the vertebral anomalies associated with diastematomyelia, plain films and conventional tomography of the spine are usually superior in revealing the full complexity of these anomalies[45] (Figs. 3-2 and 3-3).

Syringohydromyelia. Hydromyelia represents a persistence of the normal fetal condition in which the fourth ventricle communicates with the central canal of the neural tube. *Syringomyelia* refers to cavitation in the spinal cord, which may or may not communicate with the central canal. There has been much confusion with the use of these terms, as some authors have freely interchanged these terms. There is growing support to use the term *syringohydromyelia* to avoid confusion.[6,8,20]

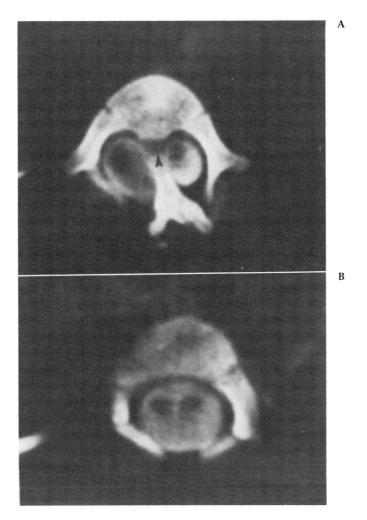

FIGURE 3-4
Diastematomyelia with bony spur in 2-year-old girl with abnormal gait and hypertrichosis.

A, CTMM in the upper lumbar area demonstrates large sagitally oriented bony spur extending across the spinal canal and splitting the cord and meninges into two asymmetric tubes, the right being greater than the left. Each hemicord is surrounded by its own subarachnoid space and dural sheath. Posteriorly the bony spur is attached to a bifid spinous process. Anteriorly a synchondrosis is present (the radiolucent junction between the anterior wall of the spinal canal and the bony spur) *(arrowhead).*

B, CTMM at a slightly higher level shows the two hemicords within a single dural sheath and surrounded by a single subarachnoid space.

Courtesy Thomas P. Naidich, MD, Chicago, Illinois.

Primary or congenital syringohydromyelia is frequently associated with congenital anomalies of the neural and spinal axis. Scoliosis is commonly an associated feature of syringohydromyelia.[6,8,31,49] Of those patients with symptoms of syringohydromyelia presenting before the age of 16 years, 87% will have scoliosis. Of those whose symptoms develop after the age of 16 years, the incidence of scoliosis is 48%.

Prior to the advent of CT, the definitive radiographic procedure to diagnose syringohydromyelia was myelography[8] (Figs. 3-5 and 3-6). It is necessary to perform both positive contrast myelography followed by a negative contrast study to make the diagnosis of syringohydromyelia using this technique (Fig. 3-7).

Myelography using either iophendylate or metrizamide will demonstrate a swollen cord in syringohydromyelia, the appearance of which is indistinguishable from an intramedullary tumor (Figs. 3-5 and 3-6). Air myelography can, at times, differentiate syringohydromyelia of the cord from an intramedullary tumor (Fig. 3-7). A swollen or expanded cervical cord demon-

FIGURE 3-5
Syringohydromyelia.
Frontal cervical myelogram in 45-year-old woman demonstrates marked swelling and enlargement of the cervical spinal cord, which is indistinguishable from any other intramedullary mass. Scoliosis of the upper thoracic spine is also present.

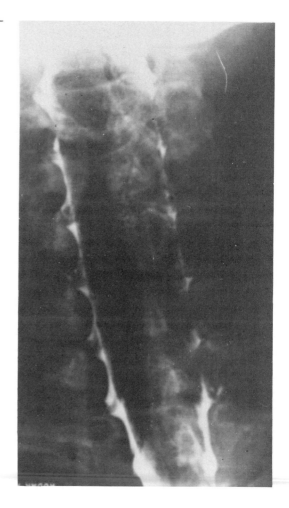

strated with positive contrast myelography in the head-down or horizontal positions will appear atrophied or collapsed on gas myelography in the upright position, since the fluid contents move caudad, collapsing the uppermost portion of the syringohydromyelic sac. This is known as the *collapsing cord* sign and is pathognomonic of syringohydromyelia.[5,8] It indicates a fluid-filled sac communicating with the fourth ventricle. No change in the appearance of the expanded cord will occur with changing position in the case of an intramedullary tumor. Syringohydromyelia may be localized to a few segments of the spinal cord (most commonly the cervical area) but may be extensive and involve the entire spinal cord (Fig. 3-6).

CT, especially CTMM, and more recently MR have revolutionized the radiologic diagnosis of syringohydromyelia.[8] Occasionally, one can see the cystic component of syringohydromyelia as a distinct area of decreased attenuation within the spinal cord on noncontrast CT scans[8] (Fig. 3-8). However, this is not a constant finding.

CTMM is a simple, safe, and accurate technique to demonstrate the in-

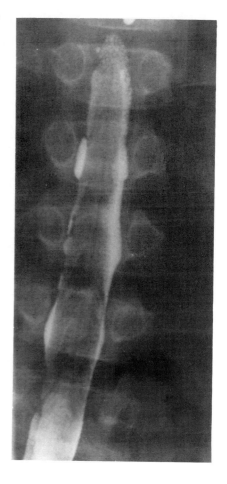

FIGURE 3-6
Syringohydromyelia with a tethered conus in
12-year-old boy.
Frontal myelogram of the lumbar region demonstrates extension of the intramedullary mass lesion (seen on the cervical thoracic study) into the lumbar region. A tethered conus is present with the cord ending at the level of L4. Note the thoracolumbar scoliosis.
From Batnitzky, S., et al.: RadioGraphics **3:**585-611, 1983.

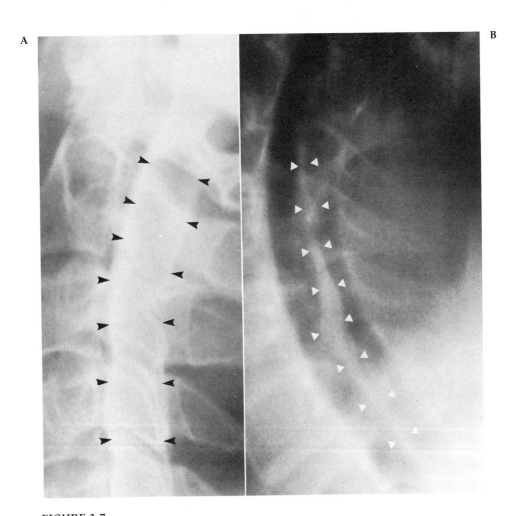

FIGURE 3-7
"Collapsing cord" sign in syringohydromyelia.
A, Lateral cervical myelogram in the head-down position demonstrates diffuse
widening of the spinal cord *(arrowheads)* with marked narrowing of the spinal
subarachnoid space.
B, Lateral air myelography in the same patient in the erect position demonstrates
collapse of the cervical cord *(arrowheads)* with a large subarachnoid space.
From Batnitzky, S.: Intraspinal disorders. In Basic neuroradiology, St. Louis, 1983, Warren H.
Green.

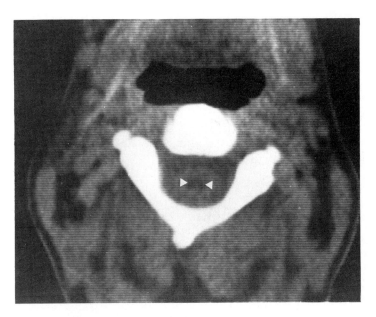

FIGURE 3-8
Syringohydromyelia.
Axial CT scan of the upper cervical area of a 42-year-old woman demonstrates a
syringohydromyelic cavity seen as an area of decreased attenuation *(arrowheads)*
within the spinal cord.
From Batnitzky, S., et al.: RadioGraphics **3:**585-611, 1983.

trathecal contents of the spine. It is a particularly useful and accurate technique in the diagnosis of syringohydromyelia. In many cases, CTMM will
demonstrate a swollen cord indistinguishable from any other intramedullary
lesion (Figs. 3-9, 3-10, and 3-13). It is important to note that in a significant
number of cases of syringohydromyelia the cord is actually normal in size or
even atrophic. This may explain why many patients in the past who had
proven syringohydromyelia at surgery or at autopsy had normal-appearing
myelograms.[8]

Changing from the supine to the lateral decubitus position may demonstrate a change in the shape and size of the cord (Fig. 3-9). The normal cord
does not change shape or size in the lateral decubitus position as seen on
CTMM.[8,38]

The demonstration of metrizamide in the syringohydromyelic cavity within the spinal cord is a pathognomonic finding[8,38] (Figs. 3-9, 3-15, and 3-16).
Delayed CT scans are often required to demonstrate filling of the cavity,
although in some instances it may fill soon after the intrathecal injection of
metrizamide. If a syrinx is suspected clinically and is not detected on the
initial scan a second scan 4 to 6 hours later, even a 24 hour–delayed scan,
should be obtained.

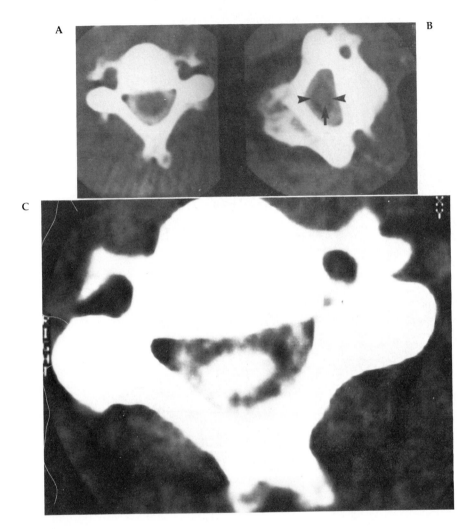

FIGURE 3-9

Syringohydromyelia, CT findings.

A, CTMM with the patient in the supine position shows widening of the cord and almost total obliteration of the subarachnoid space ventrally.

B, With the patient in the left lateral decubitus position, CTMM demonstrates that the sagittal diameter of the spinal cord has decreased in size *(arrowheads)*. The metrizamide can now be seen in the ventral subarachnoid space. Also note that the syrinx *(arrow)* is opacified by the metrizamide.

C, A delayed scan of the same patient after an interval of 4 hours shows increased opacification of the syringohydromyleic cavity.

From Batnitzky, S.: Intraspinal disorders. In Basic neuroradiology, St. Louis, 1983, Warren H. Green.

Preliminary experience using MR in evaluation of syringohydromyelia indicates that MR appears to be a method as sensitive but less invasive for the diagnosis and delineation of syringohydromyelia than other modalities, including CTMM[36,51] (Figs. 3-10 to 3-13). MR can distinguish relatively pure fluids like CSF from more heterogeneous fluid collections. This makes the differentiation between the cavities seen in syringohydromyelia and those seen with neoplastic cysts possible.

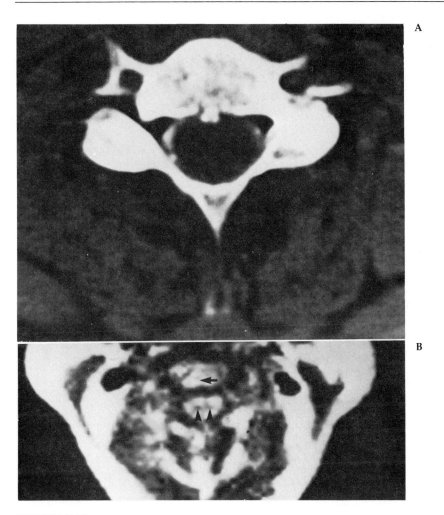

A

B

FIGURE 3-10
Syringohydromyelia.
A, CTMM demonstrates enlarged cervical spinal cord. Delayed scans at 4 and 24 hours did not demonstrate a syrinx.
B, Axial MR image demonstrates the syringohydromyelic cavity as a horizontal area of decreased signal intensity *(arrowheads)* within the spinal cord. Arrow points to the vertebral body.

Courtesy Andrew E. Yeates, MD, and Thomas H. Newton, MD, University of California at San Francisco.

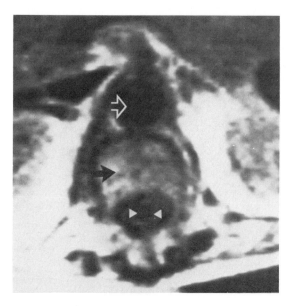

FIGURE 3-11
Syringohydromyelia.
Axial MR image demonstrates a syringohydromyelic cavity *(arrowheads)* in the lower thoracic region. Open arrow points to the aorta and closed arrow points to the vertebral body.

Courtesy Andrew E. Yeates, MD, and Thomas H. Newton, MD, The University of California at San Francisco.

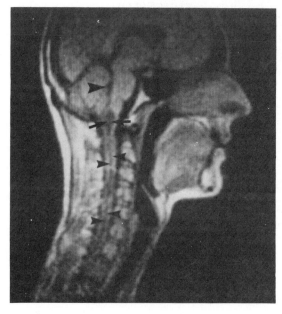

FIGURE 3-12
Syringohydromyelia.
Midsagittal MR image through the cervical spine and base of skull shows syringomyelia *(arrowheads)* and syringobulbia *(arrows)* in a 26-year-old man. The syringomyelia and syringobulbia communicate directly with the fourth ventricle *(large arrowhead)*

From Paushter, D.M., et al.: RadioGraphics **4**(Special edition):97-112, 1984.

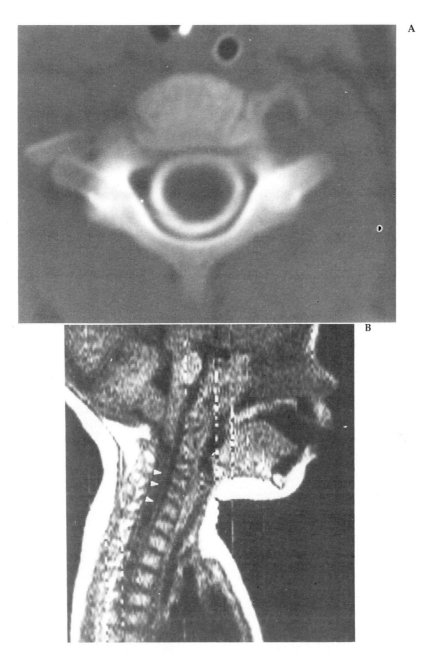

FIGURE 3-13
A 2½-year-old girl with syringohydromelia who presented with torticollis.
A, CTMM of midcervical region demonstrates large swollen cord and small
subarachnoid space.
B, Midsaggital MR image demonstrates a large syrinx *(arrowheads)* in the upper
cervical cord.

Courtesy Richard L. Gilmor, MD, Indianapolis, Indiana.

Tight filum terminale (tethered conus syndrome). The tight filum terminale syndrome refers to a complex of neurologic and orthopedic deformities associated with a short, thick filum terminale. The spinal cord is almost invariably low in position with the conus situated in the low lumbar or sacral canal.[15,19,24,35] The tight filum terminale syndrome may be far more common than generally appreciated. Congenital or acquired kyphoscoliosis is present in 25% of patients with a tight filum terminale, although scoliosis is only rarely the sole complaint.

Although myelography is still the radiographic examination of choice in a suspected tethered cord (Fig. 3-14), CTMM can be very useful and can provide information that is important in surgical planning. The size, position, and point of attachment of a spinal cord tethered to the dura are better shown on CTMM than metrizamide myelography.[24] Frequently associated abnor-

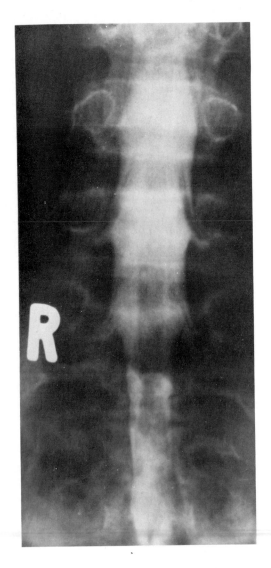

FIGURE 3-14
Tethered conus and diastematomyelia in 12-year-old boy.
Frontal myelogram of lumbosacral region demonstrates tethered conus extending into the sacrum up to the S3 level.

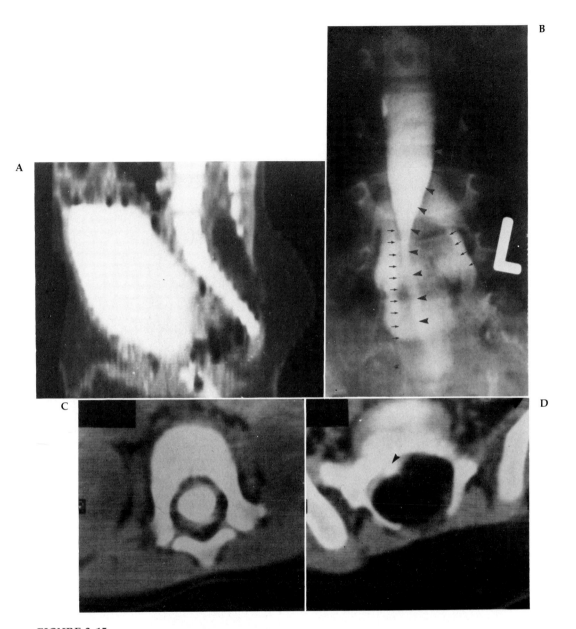

FIGURE 3-15
Lipomeningocele, tethered conus, and syringohydromyelia in 21-month-old boy.
A, Sagittal reformatted CT image of the lumbosacral region shows subcutaneous lumbosacral lipoma extending into the sacral canal up to the L5 level through a defect of the posterior elements of the sacrum.
B, At time of lumbar puncture for myelography, metrizamide was injected into the subarachnoid space and also inadvertently into the central canal. The central canal *(arrowheads)* is markedly dilated but tapers from L5 into the sacrum. The subarachnoid metrizamide *(arrows)* outlines the low tethered conus and lipoma, which cannot be differentiated from each other on the myelogram.
C, CTMM in the midlumbar region shows markedly dilated central canal filled with metrizamide.
D, CTMM at the S1 level shows the metrizamide-filled central canal within the low-lying conus *(arrowhead)*, which is displaced anteriorly and to the right by the large intrasacral lipoma.

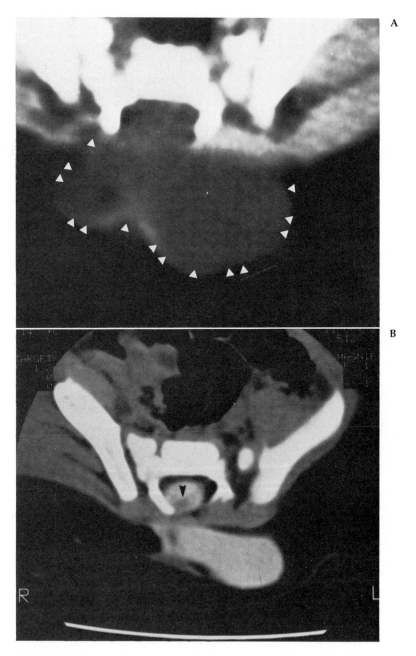

FIGURE 3-16
Lumbosacral meningocele, tethered conus, and syringohydromyelia in 5-day-old boy.
A, CT scan through the S1 level shows a large dorsally situated soft tissue mass
  (arrowheads) in the subcutaneous tissue. This soft tissue mass extends into the
  sacral canal through a large defect in the posterior neural arch.
B, CTMM at the level of S1 demonstrates a low-lying conus *(arrowhead),* which is
  situated posteriorly and slightly toward the right of the midline. Metrizamide
  has entered and filled the large meningocele.

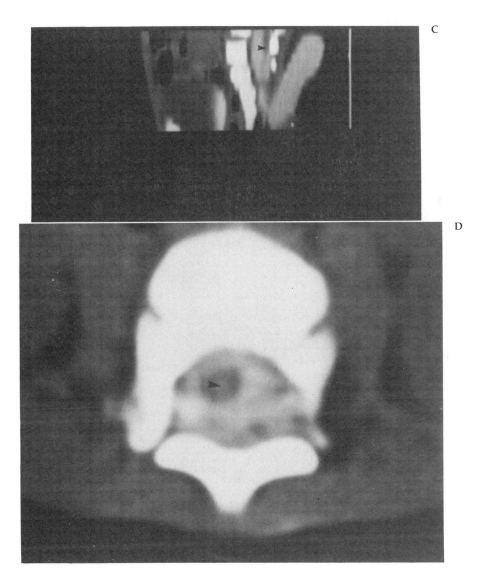

FIGURE 3-16, cont'd

C, Midsagittal reformatted CTMM image shows a low tethered conus *(arrowhead)* and the communication between the spinal subarachnoid space and the large meningocele.

D, Four hour–delayed CTMM at the level of L4 shows metrizamide within the central canal *(arrowhead)* of the tethered conus, confirming the additional diagnosis of syringohydromyelia.

malities such as syringohydromyelia, diastematomyelia, and lipomas of the filum terminale, which may not be evident on conventional myelography, will be demonstrated by CTMM (Figs. 3-15 and 3-16).

Congenital tumors and embryonic malformations. Congenital tumors such as lipomas and teratomas and embryonic malformations such as epidermoids, dermoids, and neurenteric cysts may be associated with spinal dysraphism and congenital scoliosis.[19,35]

Lipoma. The term *lipoma* is restricted to an abnormal, partially encapsulated mass of fat with an abnormally large amount of connective tissue, which has a definite connection to the spinal cord or leptomeninges.[13] The mere presence of fat does not constitute a lipoma. A high percentage of lipomas are associated with spinal dysraphism and its accompanying abnormalities[5,19,35] (Figs. 3-6 and 3-15).

Lipomas commonly involve the intradural extramedullary compartment but can occur in the extradural and intramedullary compartments. Lesions affecting the filum terminale are the most common.[13] In some cases the lipoma are impossible to separate from the cord radiologically and such differentiation can only be made at operation.

Metrizamide myelography followed by CTMM will demonstrate the location and extent of the lesion. On plain CT, as well as CTMM, lipomas have a characteristic low attenuation coefficient (-50 to -100 Hounsfield units).

Teratoma. Teratomas are true neoplasms containing disarranged tissues belonging to all three germinal layers at sites where these tissues do not normally occur.[16] An intraspinal teratoma can be extensive in location and size and many are cystic.[13,35] Though most teratomas are intradural-extramedullary in location, they can occur in the extradural and intramedullary compartments. From the radiologic point of view, they are indistinguishable from other intraspinal lesions.

Epidermoid and dermoid. Intraspinal epidermoids and dermoids are rare lesions accounting for 1% to 2% of all intraspinal tumors at all ages but representing 10% in patients below the age of 15 years.[35] They can be congenital or acquired in nature.[7,35] Congenital epidermoid and dermoid cysts arise from epithelial and dermal elements (including accessory organs such as hair follicles and sebaceous and sweat glands), respectively, that become sequestrated at the time of closure of the neural groove between the third and fifth weeks of embryonic life resulting in heterotopia of such elements. They are not true neoplasms but represent embryonic malformations.

Acquired or iatrogenic epidermoids or dermoids result from implantation of epithelial or dermal elements, respectively, into the spinal canal at the time of lumbar puncture performed with needles without stylets or with ill-fitting stylets.[7,35] Epidermoids and dermoids are identical from a radiologic point of view. They most commonly occur in the intradural extramedullary compartment (Fig. 3-17) but (rarely) also can be located in the intradural and intramedullary compartments.

Neurenteric cyst. Neurenteric cysts are rare lesions. They represent one of the spectrum of anomalies occurring in the split notocord syndrome.[19,35] These cysts are connected to the meninges through a midline defect in one or more vertebral bodies. Most neurenteric cysts arise in the lower cervical upper thoracic region, and the intraspinal component is usually situated ventral or ventrolateral to the spinal cord in the intradural extramedullary compartment. Myelography can demonstrate the characteristic appearance of multiple grapelike clusters in the intradural extramedullary compartment, although some cysts are unilocular and single. Typically, the presence of a posterior mediastinal mass can be seen on plain films and conventional tomography.

The appearance on CTMM is that of a ventral intradural extramedullary lesion with a paraspinal component, which can be quite large. The noncontrast CT appearance is similar to that of a duplication cyst. However, the presence of a vertebral abnormality points to the diagnosis of a neurenteric cyst.

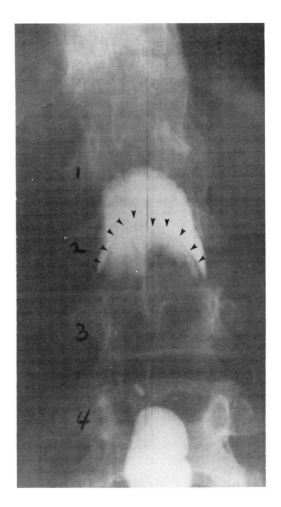

FIGURE 3-17
Congenital epidermoid in 30-year-old woman presented with asymptomatic scoliosis.
Frontal myelogram demonstrates the upper pole of an intradural lesion at the level of L2 *(arrowheads)*. There is flattening and erosion of the pedicles of L2 and L3. The lower pole of the tumor was situated at the inferior margin of L3.

IDIOPATHIC SCOLIOSIS WITH NEUROLOGIC DISTURBANCES

Although relatively uncommon, cases of so-called idiopathic scoliosis can complicate an intraspinal tumor. Scoliosis may be the earliest sign of disease of the spinal cord and nerves or the first sign sufficiently recognized to bring the patient to the physician (Figs. 3-17, 3-18, and 3-22). Scoliosis may be the dominant feature in patients with extensive intraspinal lesions. There have been reports in the literature of intramedullary ependymomas, astrocytomas, syringohydromyelia, arteriovenous malformation, arachnoiditis, and herniated disks that have presented with scoliosis.[2,9,10,34,37] Correct diagnosis is therefore of the utmost importance.

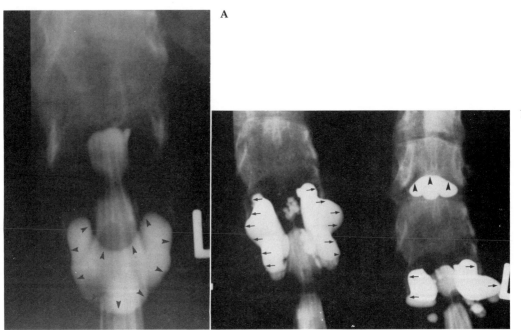

FIGURE 3-18
Large congenital extradural arachnoid cyst in 14-year-old boy who presented with thoracolumbar scoliosis.
A, Frontal myelogram shows lower portion of the cyst *(arrowheads)*. Note the thinning of the inner margins of the pedicles of T12, L1, and L2 with an increase in the interpediculate distance.
B, With the patient positioned head down, the lateral margins *(arrows)* and upper pole *(arrowheads)* of the cyst are demonstrated.
From Price, H.I., et al.: RadioGraphics **4**:283-313, 1984.

In patients presenting with idiopathic scoliosis, and whose neurologic examination reveals pathologic signs, metrizamide myelography followed by CTMM should be performed to exclude a possible cause for the scoliosis.[37] The exact role of MR imaging has yet to be determined. MR imaging may well become the definitive procedure in the evaluation of intraspinal disorders (Fig. 3-19).

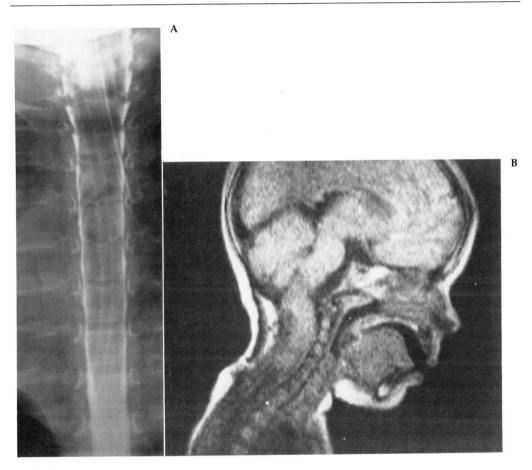

FIGURE 3-19
Astrocytoma of upper cervical cord in 4-year-old boy who presented with spastic paraparesis and torticollis.
A, Myelography of thoracocervical spine shows a large intramedullary lesion extending from the midthoracic region into the cervical area.
B, Midsagittal MR image of cervical spine and base of skull shows a markedly swollen upper cervical cord extending into the brainstem.
Courtesy Richard L. Gilmor, MD, Indianapolis, Indiana.

NEUROFIBROMATOSIS

Neurofibromatosis (von Recklinghausen's disease) is a hereditary hamartomatous disorder probably of neural crest origin involving not only neuroectoderm and mesoderm but also endoderm with the potential of appearing in any organ or system in the body.[23] It is transmitted as an autosomal dominant with markedly variable expressivity, but penetrance is virtually 100%.[40]

Abnormal curvature of the spine is the most common lesion in neurofibromatosis and has been reported in 10% to 41% of neurofibromatosis.[23,28] More than 80% of the scolioses occur before the age of 16 years, with the majority developing between 11 and 15 years. All types of scoliosis and kyphoscoliosis occur in patients with neurofibromatosis varying from mild, nonprogressive forms without vertebral dysplasia to grotesque forms with marked vertebral dysplasia and angulations.

Dural ectasia. Dural ectasia with enlargement of the spinal canal is a common finding in neurofibromatosis[23,27] (Figs. 3-20, 3-21, and 3-29). This ectasia,

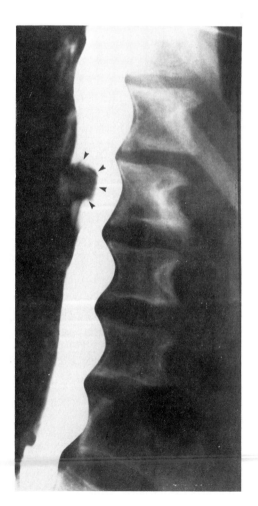

FIGURE 3-20
Widespread neurofibromatosis and right thoracolumbar scoliosis in a 13-year-old boy. Lateral myelogram shows the ectatic dural sac extending into the scalloped posterior margins at the lumbar vertebral bodies. The neurofibroma is also seen *(arrowheads),* which was clearly intradural on the AP film.

From Batnitzky, S.: Intraspinal disorders. In Basic neuroradiology, St. Louis, 1983, Warren H. Green.

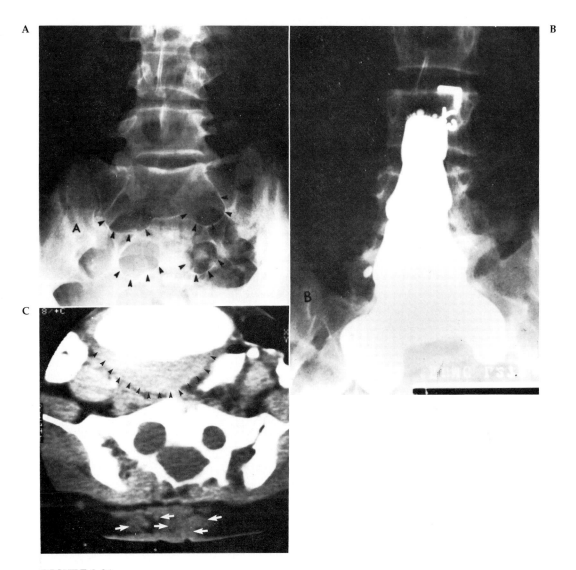

FIGURE 3-21
Dural ectasia with sacral lateral meningoceles in a 12-year-old girl with
neurofibromatosis.

A, Frontal roentgenogram of the sacrum shows marked enlargement of the sacral
  foramina *(arrowheads)* and widening of the interpediculate distance of L4 and L5.
B, Myelography reveals dural ectasia with the distal end of the dural sac widening
  into two large laterally situated meningoceles. These have also been termed
  sacral cysts.
C, CT of the sacrum at the S1 level demonstrates widening of the spinal canal
  together with marked sacral foraminal enlargement. Also note the large pelvic
  neurofibroma *(arrowheads)* involving the bladder wall. Multiple cutaneous
  neurofibromas *(arrows)* are also seen in the buttocks area.

A and B from Batnitzky, S.: Intraspinal disorders. In Basic neuroradiology, St. Louis, 1983,
Warren H. Green; C from Batnitzky, S., et al.: RadioGraphics **2**:500-528, 1982.

which probably results from mesodermal dysplasia of the meninges, may be localized to one or more segments but more commonly is diffuse. The thoracic and lumbar areas are the most common sites. It has been postulated that the basic abnormality is weakness of the dura, permitting transmission of the cerebrospinal fluid pulsations to the bone.[33] The dural ectasia over a period of years produces scalloping of the posterior margins of the vertebral bodies and erosion of the pedicles. Other connective tissue disorders such as the Ehlers-Danlos syndrome and the Marfan syndrome may also be associated with dural ectasia and the roentgenographic changes it produces.[18,27,33] According to Klatte et al.,[27] kyphoscoliosis in patients with neurofibromatosis is almost always associated with dural ectasia. They postulate that enlargement of the dural sac can erode the vertebrae to such a degree that normal stability is lost and kyphoscoliosis develops.

Neoplasms. Tumors of the central nervous system account for a major portion of the severe morbidity and increased mortality of neurofibromatosis. The combined frequency of such tumors is 5% to 10%. Patients with neurofibromatosis have an increased incidence of various intraspinal tumors.[30,42] These include schwannomas, neurofibromas, meningiomas, ependymomas, and astrocytomas.

Schwannomas and neurofibromas comprise two histologically similar but distinguishable types of tumors.[30] Schwannomas, also called *neurolemmomas* and *neurinomas,* arise from the cells of Schwann in the nerve sheath and occur not only in neurofibromatosis but frequently are solitary tumors in patients without the disorder. The dorsal nerve root is the primary site for the tumor.

Neurofibromas are a distinctive feature of neurofibromatosis and occur very rarely in any other setting. A neurofibroma is a complex structure histologically wherein all the cellular elements of the nerve—the Schwann cell, fibroblast and perineural cell—play a part in the tumor formation. Neurofibromas develop along mixed and autonomic nerve trunks and nerve endings.

Schwannoma is the most common solitary extramedullary spinal tumor in neurofibromatosis[30] (Figs. 3-22 and 3-23). On occasion, multiple tumors may be present. Neurofibromas frequently occur at multiple sites (Figs. 3-24 and 3-25). The thoracic and cauda equina regions are characteristic sites for multiple tumor involvement. Both schwannomas and neurofibromas are typically intradural tumors but can also occur in the extradural compartment in some cases. Both tumors can extend through the intervertebral foramen to present as a so-called *dumbbell* tumor, where one part of the tumor lies within the spinal canal (either in the intradural or extradural compartment) and the other part is extradural and extraspinal in location (Figs. 3-25 and 3-26).

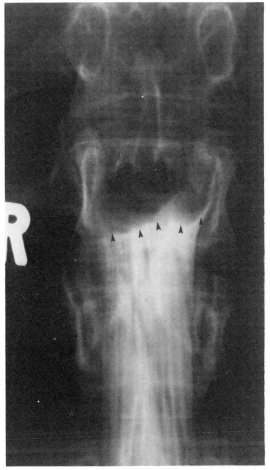

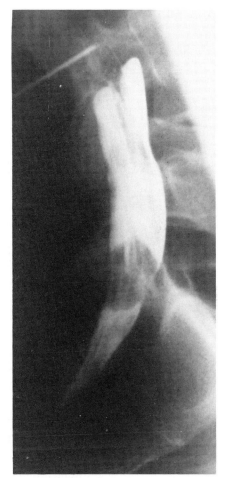

3-22   *3-23*

FIGURE 3-22
Intradural schwannoma.
Frontal myelogram in 42-year-old woman with a family history of
neurofibromatosis who presented with asymptomatic scoliosis demonstrates
complete block to the flow of the contrast material at the T12 level due to a
left-sided intradural schwannoma. The arrowheads point to the lower pole of the
tumor, which is lobulated.

FIGURE 3-23
Schwannoma.
Lateral myelogram demonstrates large intradural schwannoma at the L5-S1 level in
30-year-old man with multiple neurofibromatosis.

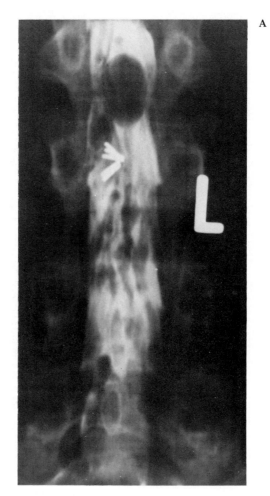

A

FIGURE 3-24
Multiple neurofibromas in a 36-year-old man with multiple neurofibromatosis.
A, Frontal myelogram of the lumbar area shows multiple intradural lesions of
varying size representing multiple neurofibromas.

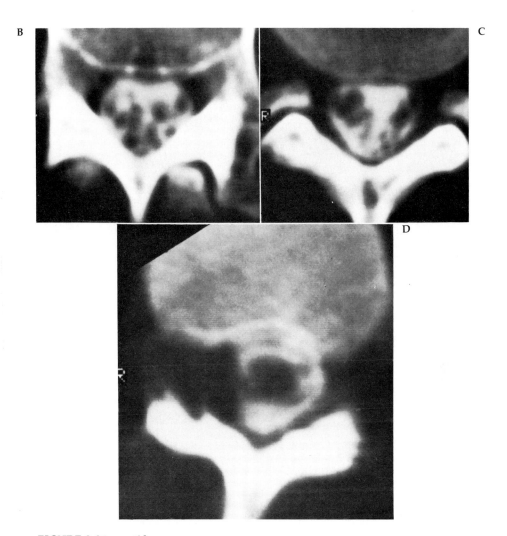

FIGURE 3-24, cont'd

B and **C,** CTMM at the L3 and L4 levels demonstrates the multiple neurofibromas of varying sizes seen as filling defects within the metrizamide column.

D, CTMM at the C5 level demonstrates an extradural defect on the right side due to a dumb-bell neurofibroma, which is enlarging the right intervertebral foramen and displacing the cord toward the left side.

A

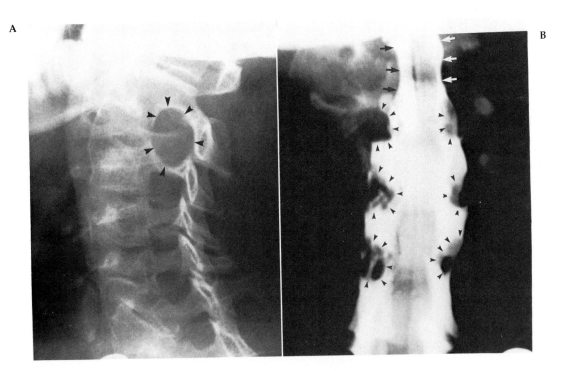

B

FIGURE 3-25
Bilateral dumb-bell neurofibromas.

A, Oblique view of the cervical spine showing marked enlargement of the left
intervertebral foramen at C2 *(arrowheads).* The other intravertebral foramina are
also enlarged but to a lesser extent. Identical findings were present in the right
intervertebral foramina.

B, Frontal cervical myelogram reveals displacement of the dural sac *(arrows)* away
from the bony spinal canal bilaterally by the extradural components of the
bilateral dumb-bell neurofibromas at C2. The nerve root sheaths *(arrowheads)* of
the rest of the cervical cord are enlarged bilaterally by surgically proven multiple
intradural neurofibromas.

From Batnitzky, S.: Intraspinal disorders. In Basic neuroradiology, St. Louis, 1983, Warren H.
Green.

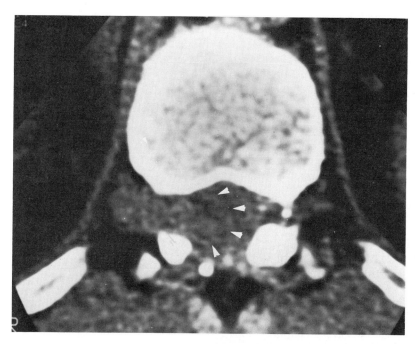

FIGURE 3-26
Dumb-bell schwannoma.
CT of T11 demonstrates a dumb-bell schwannoma *(arrowheads)* widening the right
intervertebral foramen and displacing the dural sac toward the left side. A
postlaminectomy defect and residual droplets of iophendylate are also noted.

Spinal meningiomas[30] arise from the ventral aspect of the spinal canal in
neurofibromatosis and tend to occur mostly in the thoracic region (Fig. 3-27).
Meningiomas, which can also be multiple, typically present in adulthood as
do schwannomas, although the latter tend to occur at an earlier age (average
age of diagnosis is 38 years versus 50 years).[46] Spinal root neurofibromas are
commonly found in children.[19] Meningiomas and schwannomas in non-
neurofibromatosis patients are more common in females than males.[12,30,43]
The sex ratio of both meningiomas and schwannomas in neurofibromatosis
patients has not been determined.

All three tumors can resemble each other radiologically. Schwannomas
and neurofibromas tend to be larger than meningiomas, and bone changes
are four times more frequent with schwannomas and neurofibromas than
meningiomas.[6] These bony changes consist of erosion of the pedicles, widening of the interpediculate distance, widening of the intervertebral foramen,
and scalloping of the posterior surface of the vertebral bodies (Figs. 3-20 to
3-22, 3-25, and 3-29).

Because of the multiplicity of lesions in neurofibromatosis, a survey of the entire spine is essential. This should be performed with conventional myelography because of its ability to demonstrate multiple levels simultaneously. This can be followed by CTMM at the level or levels of pathology to provide additional information that may not be appreciated on myelography. CT is particularly useful and, in fact, superior to myelography in demonstrating the extent and size of the extradural component of a dumbbell lesion (Fig. 3-26).

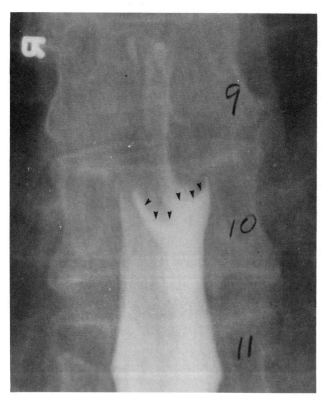

FIGURE 3-27
Thoracic meningioma in 36-year-old woman with neurofibromatosis.
Frontal thoracic myelogram with the patient in the head-down position demonstrates the lower pole of a left-sided intradural extramedullary tumor at the T10 level *(arrowheads).* The spinal cord is displaced to the contralateral side.

The intramedullary tumors of neurofibromatosis include ependymoma and less often astrocytoma[30] (Fig. 3-28). These tumors occur in adults but can (rarely) be seen in children. The ependymoma frequently occurs at multiple sites. A solitary tumor often involves the conus medullaris and the filum terminale, whereas multiple ependymomas can be seen at all levels of the neuraxis. Astrocytomas can exist separately or with ependymomas in the spinal cord. The cervical and thoracic cords are the most common sites.

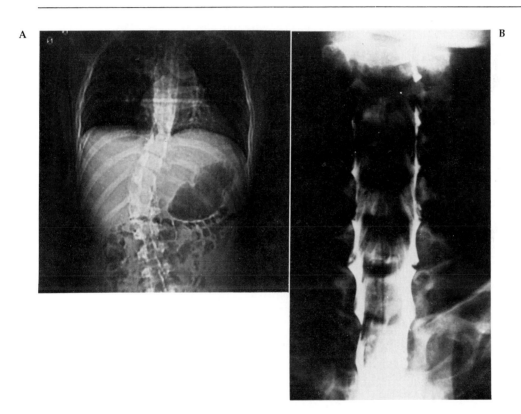

FIGURE 3-28
Intramedullary ependymoma extending into the posterior fossa in 16-year-old boy
with neurofibromatosis.

A, Frontal digital radiograph of thoracolumbar area shows right convexity
thoracolumbar scoliosis.

B, Frontal cervical myelogram demonstrates swelling and enlargement of the
cervical spinal cord. Lumbar and thoracic myelography demonstrated multiple
intradural extramedullary neurofibromas of varying sizes.

Continued.

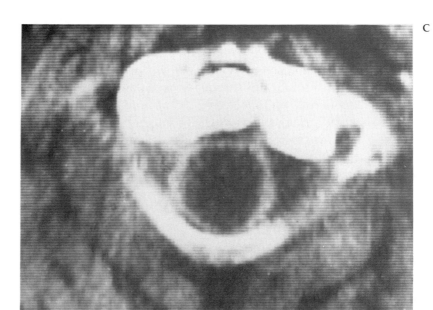

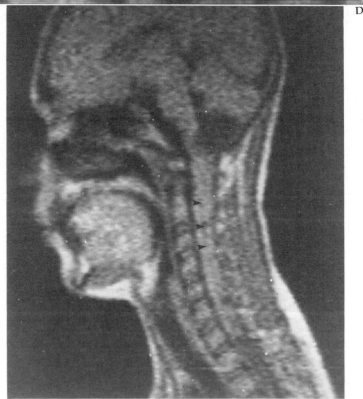

FIGURE 3-28, cont'd

C, CTMM at level of C2 shows a swollen spinal cord with a narrowed subarachnoid space. Delayed scans at 6, 12, and 24 hours did not demonstrate a syrinx.

D, Midsagittal MR image of the cervical spine and base of skull demonstrates an enlarged swollen spinal cord in the cervical area. Cystic areas *(arrowheads)* are noted within the swollen cord. A large cystic component is present in the posterior fossa. The cervical and posterior fossa lesion proved to be an ependymoma of the cord that was extending into the posterior fossa.

Lateral meningocele. Numerous developmental neural anomalies such as syringohydromyelia and lateral meningocele can occur in neurofibromatosis patients.[27,30,42] Lateral meningoceles are a manifestation of dural ectasia. Lateral saccular protrusions of dura—meningoceles—may extend through and enlarge the intervertebral foramen similar to that seen in a dumbbell neurofibroma or schwannoma (Figs. 3-21 and 3-29).

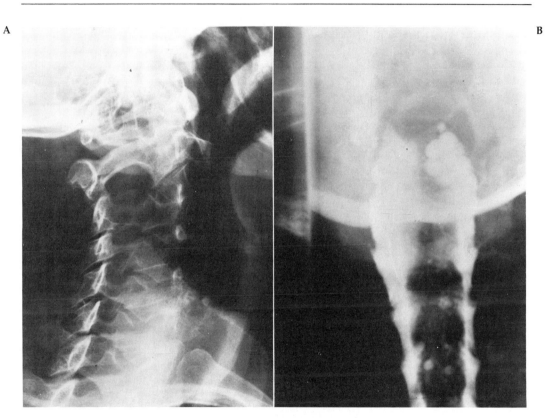

FIGURE 3-29
Lateral meningoceles in a 40-year-old woman with multiple neurofibromatosis and marked kyphoscoliosis.
A, Oblique view of cervical spine shows marked enlargement of the right C2-3 intervertebral foramen. The opposite oblique radiograph also showed enlargement of the C2-3 intervertebral foramen on the left side.
B, Frontal cervical myelogram demonstrates no abnormality. The lateral view (not shown) of the cervical myelogram revealed scalloping of the posterior margins of the cervical vertebrae due to dural ectasia.

Continued.

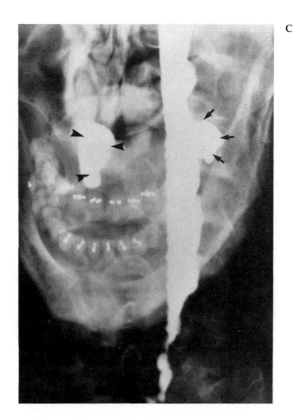

C

FIGURE 3-29, cont'd

C, With the patient in the left lateral decubitus position, contrast material fills a
lateral meningocele *(arrows)*, which is extending through and enlarging the C2-3
intervertebral foramen. The right C2-3 lateral meningocele *(arrowheads)* contains
residual contrast from the right lateral decubitus position which was obtained
first.

A

B

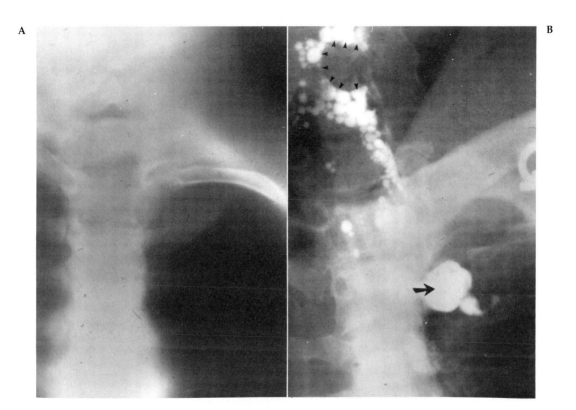

FIGURE 3-30
Lateral thoracic meningocele.
A, AP tomogram of left lung apex shows extrapleural soft tissue mass.
B, Myelography confirms the diagnosis of a lateral meningocele *(arrow).* Also note
the cervical intradural neurofibroma *(arrowheads).*

In the thoracic region, a lateral meningocele can produce a paraspinal mass (Fig. 3-30). Mediastinal neurofibromas are surprisingly rare. A posterior mediastinal mass in a patient with neurofibromatosis, particularly with kyphoscoliosis, is more likely to be a lateral meningocele than a neurofibroma. Lateral thoracic meningoceles are easily detected by CT. On axial images, the protrusion of the meninges through the enlarged intervertebral foramen can readily be detected (Fig. 3-31). However, at times differentiation from a schwannoma or neurofibroma may be difficult without the use of CTMM.

Lateral meningoceles at all levels have been reported in neurofibromatosis but characteristically occur in the thoracic region.[27] Lateral meningoceles are fairly specific to neurofibromatosis cases; 70% to 85% of the reported cases of lateral thoracic meningoceles have been associated with neurofibromatosis.[28,30,33,42]

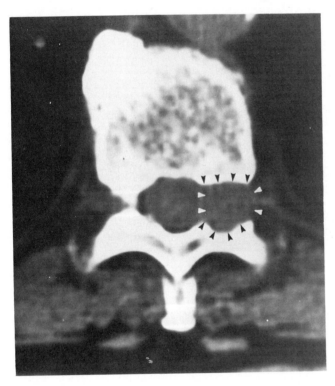

FIGURE 3-31
Lateral thoracic meningocele in a patient with neurofibromatosis.
Axial CT scan at the T9 level shows lateral thoracic meningocele *(arrowheads)* extending through widened left intervertebral foramen. The attenuation values within the soft tissue mass approximate those of cerebrospinal fluid.

CONNECTIVE TISSUE DISORDERS

The Marfan syndrome is a familial, multisystem disorder of connective tissue.[18] Kyphosis and scoliosis are frequent findings. The spinal canal enlarges in both the sagittal and coronal planes with posterior scalloping of the vertebral bodies. These changes can simulate an intraspinal tumor or neurofibromatosis. These bony changes, as in neurofibromatosis, are due to dural ectasia.[18,27,33] Apart from the dural ectasia no other known intraspinal abnormalities are part of this syndrome.

The Ehlers-Danlos syndrome is a familial disorder of connective tissue in which kyphoscoliosis is frequently present at the thoracolumbar junction.[18] Dural ectasia producing scalloping of the posterior vertebral bodies is also a feature of this syndrome.[18,27,33] This can mimic an intraspinal tumor. Subcutaneous calcifications with a predilection for the lower extremities is a characteristic feature of Ehlers-Danlos syndrome.

Homocystinuria, an inborn error of amino acid metabolism, may resemble the Marfan syndrome and the Ehlers-Danlos syndrome.[18] Mental retardation and osteoporosis are prominent features of this condition. In doubtful cases, the urine test for homocystinuria will establish the diagnosis.

SPONDYLOLISTHESIS

Spondylolisthesis refers to the displacement of one vertebral body on another. It is most frequently associated with a disruption in the pars interarticularis but can also occur with an intact pars. The fifth lumbar (L5)–first sacral (S1) level is most commonly involved when a pars defect is present. The defect can be unilateral but in the majority of cases is bilateral.[14] The L4-5 level is the most common site of degenerative spondylolisthesis with an intact pars.[14,26]

Plain radiographs of the lumbar spine adequately demonstrate the spinal malalignment. The presence of vertebral instability can be evaluated with lateral flexion and extension radiographs. The need for additional roentgenologic investigation depends on the patient's clinical symptoms and the anticipated treatment.

Conventional tomography is helpful in cases where the defect in the pars interarticularis is not well demonstrated on plain radiographs, and these can be obtained in the lateral and oblique projection.[14] The nature of the pars defect, associated callus formation, and secondary degenerative changes in the apophyseal joints may be clearly identified. Tomography is helpful in identifying bilateral defects.[14] Following surgical fusion of a spondylolisthesis, tomography is helpful in the evaluation of the bony graft and in excluding the presence of a pseudoarthrosis.

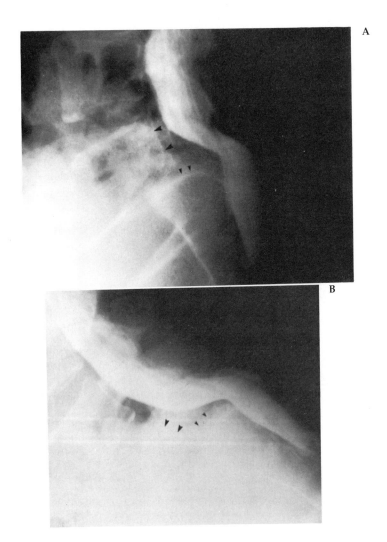

FIGURE 3-32
Spondylolisthesis.
A and B, Lateral extension and flexion views, respectively, of metrizamide
myelogram of a 27-year-old woman with low back pain, demonstrate a ventral
extradural defect at the L5-S1 level due to the spondylolisthesis. There is
increasing spondylolisthesis between the extension and flexion positions. The
large arrowheads point to the posterior margins of L5 and the small arrowheads
outline the superior surface of the sacrum.

Myelography. When the patient's clinical findings are suggestive of nerve root entrapment or spinal stenosis, metrizamide myelography can be extremely useful in identifying intraspinal abnormalities associated with or coincidental to the spondylolisthesis. Patients with neurologic defects in whom surgical fusion is to be performed should be evaluated preoperatively by myelography.[14]

Myelography is the most effective means of studying the dynamics of the spondylolisthesis (Fig. 3-32). Using stress views and films taken in the upright position, the true nature and severity of the lesion can be ascertained. In the performance of the lumbar portion of a myelogram, it is wise to avoid the level of abnormality as this can contribute to difficulties in both performing and interpreting the study. Usually a higher intervertebral level is selected, for example, L3-4 when the spondylolisthesis is at L5-S1.

The myelographic abnormalities in spondylolisthesis include a step-off deformity of the sac at the level of the defect (Fig. 3-32). This ventral defect can be accentuated if lateral flexion and extension studies are performed. In addition, a dorsal defect may be visible due to hypertrophic changes in the vertebral laminae and ligamentum flavum. These areas of encroachment can cause a variable degree of dural sac compression varying from partial to complete obstruction. Secondary degenerative changes in the apophyseal joints and disk may cause further spinal stenosis.

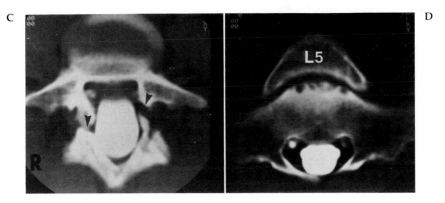

FIGURE 3-32, cont'd
C, CTMM at the L5-S1 level demonstrates the defects in the pars articularis bilaterally *(arrowheads).* The apparent enlargement of the sagittal diameter of the spinal canal at the level of the spondylolisthesis ("double canal" appearance) is due to geometric distortion of the canal from the increased lumbar lordosis.
D, Note the overriding of the vertebral bodies of L5 on S1.

Computed tomography (CT). High-resolution spinal CT is rapidly replacing the more invasive procedures as the primary radiologic investigation of patients with low back pain including patients with spondylolisthesis.

The presence of a pars defect is clearly identified on CT (Figs. 3-32 and 3-33). The transverse processes, pedicles, and superior facets move with the subluxed vertebral body and the laminae, dorsal spinous process, and inferior articular facets remain with the subjacent inferior vertebral segment.[47]

CT can identify the degree of spinal stenosis due to both bony and soft tissue changes. This may involve the central spinal canal diameter as well as the lateral recesses and intervertebral foramina. The axial CT scans tend to overestimate the degree of compression of the spinal canal by bulging or herniated disks in patients with spondylolisthesis.

The "double canal" appearance has been described in spondylolisthesis (Figs. 3-32 and 3-33). This is due to the vertebral body subluxation resulting in a geometric distortion of the canal from the increased lumbar lordosis with an apparent increase in the sagittal diameter of the canal at the level of the spondylolisthesis.[41] The CT gantry is usually unable to tilt sufficiently to produce scans parallel to the disk. Sagittal reconstructions are more helpful in the evaluation of the spinal canal diameter[41] (Figs. 3-32 and 3-33).

The vertical height of the intervertebral foramen is reduced due to the inferior positioning of the pedicle in the roof of the foramen. The orientation of the foramen is thus changed from a vertical to a horizontal plane. The diameter may be further compromised by lateral osteophyte formation. The perineural fat normally visible in the intervertebral foramen may be obliterated by the bulging intervertebral disk or the callus developing around the pars defect.

Degeneration of the disk at the level of the spondylolisthesis is not uncommonly found; however, the disk herniation, if present, occurs at the interspace above the pars defect.[41] Associated anomalies of the vertebral column, for instance, spina bifida occulta and hypoplastic facets, can be clearly identified on CT.[14]

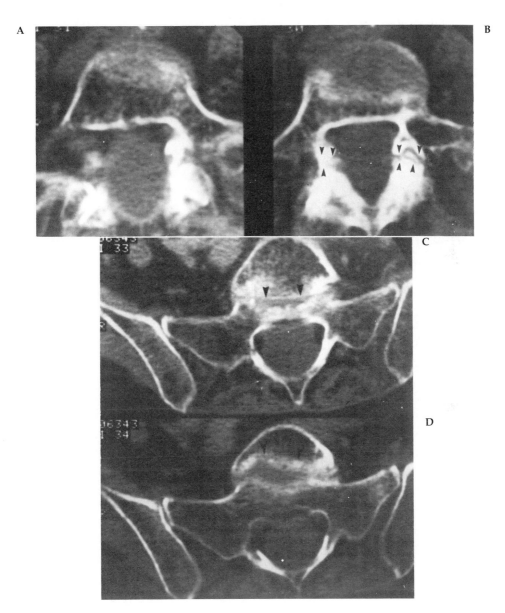

FIGURE 3-33
Spondylolisthesis in 66-year-old woman with low back pain.
A and B, CT without metrizamide shows the bilateral pars defects *(arrowheads)*
with marked sclerosis around the edges. The "double canal" appearance is also
present.
C and D, Overriding of the L5 *(arrowheads)* and the S1 vertebral bodies is seen
with marked sclerosis of the edges due to bony ebernation.

Severe degenerative disease involving the apophyseal joints can result in secondary spondylolisthesis with an intact pars interarticularis[26,41] (Fig. 3-34). This results in severe spinal stenosis as the lamina moves forward across the spinal canal.[41]

The severe degenerative disease at the apophyseal joints and intervertebral disk are clearly visualized on CT as are the changes of spinal stenosis. The overriding of the articular facets can be identified without a defect in the pars interarticularis. The presence of a vacuum phenomenon at the apophyseal joint suggests the preservation of the neural arch.[29]

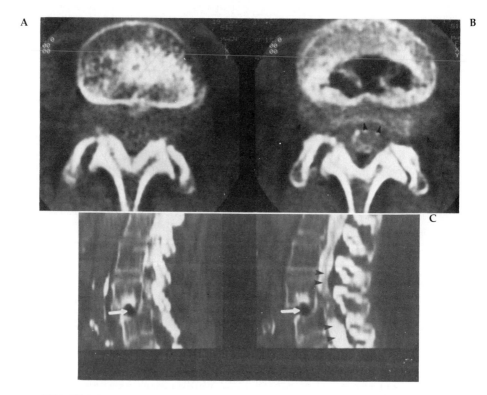

FIGURE 3-34
Degenerative spondylolisthesis in 62-year-old woman.
A and B, CTMM shows nearly total occlusion of the subarachnoid space at the L4-5 level due to degenerative spondylolisthesis. Bilateral subluxation of the apophyseal joints and bulging of the intervertebral disk *(arrowheads)* contribute to the near-total extradural obstruction. Note the vacuum disk phenomen in B.
C, Sagittal reformatted image of CTMM shows metrizamide *(arrowheads)* above and below the level of obstruction. Also note the vacuum disk *(arrow)*.

REFERENCES

1. Arni, H., et al.: Metrizamide spinal computer tomography following myelography, Comput. Tomogr. **4**:17-125, 1980.
2. Banna, M., and Gryspeerdt, G.L.: Intraspinal tumors in children (excluding dysraphism), Clin. Radiol. **22**:17-32, 1971.
3. Batnitzky, S.: Negative contrast myelographic agents. In Miller, R.E., and Skukas, J., editors: Radiographic contrast agents, Baltimore, 1977, University Park Press.
4. Batnitzky, S.: Positive contrast myelography: water-soluble iodinated organic agents. In Miller, R.E., and Skukas, J., editors: Radiographic contrast agents, Baltimore, 1977, University Park Press, pp. 419-427.
5. Batnitzky, S.: Intraspinal disorders. In Sarwar, M., Azar Kia, B., and Batnitzky, S., editors: Basic neuroradiology, St. Louis, 1983, Warren H. Green, pp. 758-838.
6. Batnitzky, S., et al.: Meningomyelocele and syringohydromyelia, Radiology **120**:351-357, 1976.
7. Batnitzky, S., et al.: Iatrogenic intraspinal epidermoid tumors, JAMA **237**:148-150, 1977.
8. Batnitzky, S., et al.: The radiology of syringohydromyelia, RadioGraphics **3**:585-611, 1983.
9. Boldrey, E., et al.: Scoliosis as a manifestation of disease of the cervicothoracic portion of the spinal cord, Arch. Neurol. Psychiatr. **61**:528-544, 1949.
10. Burrows, E.H., and Leeds, N.E.: Neuroradiology, New York, 1981, Churchill Livingstone, pp. 488-529.
11. Di Chiro, G., and Schellinger, D.: Computed tomography of spinal cord after lumbar intrathecal introduction of Metrizamide (computer-assisted myelography), Radiology **120**:101-104, 1976.
12. Dorwart, R.H., LaMasters, D.L., and Watanabe, T.J.: Tumors. In Newton, T.H., and Potts, D.G., editors: Computed tomography of the spine and spinal cord, San Anselmo, Calif., 1983, Clavadel Press, pp. 115-147.
13. Emery, J.L., and Lendon, R.G.: Lipomas of the cauda equina and other fatty tumors related to neurospinal dysraphism, Dev. Med. Child Neurol. **11**(Suppl. 20):62-70, 1969.
14. Epstein, B.S.: The spine—a radiological text and atlas, Philadelphia, 1976, Lea & Febiger, pp. 585-607.
15. Fitz, C.R., and Harwood-Nash, D.C.: The tethered conus, AJR **125**:515-523, 1975.
16. Friede, R.L.: Developmental neuropathology, New York, 1975, Springer-Verlag, pp. 266-271.
17. Gillespie, R., et al.: Intraspinal anomalies in congenital scoliosis, Clin. Orthop. **93**:103-109, 1973.
18. Goldman, A.B.: Collagen diseases, epiphyseal dysplasias and related conditions. In Resnick, D., and Niwayana, G., editors: Diagnosis of bone and joint disorders, Philadelphia, 1981, W.B. Saunders Co., pp. 2492-2545.
19. Harwood-Nash, D.C.: Neuroradiology in infants and children, St. Louis, 1976, The C.V. Mosby Co., pp. 1072-1227.
20. Harwood-Nash, D.C., and Fitz, C.R.: Myelography and syringohydromyelia in infancy and childhood, Radiology **113**:661-669, 1974.
21. Haughton, V.M., and Williams, A.L.: Computed tomography of the spine, Postgrad. Radiol. **2**:35-60, 1982.
22. Hilal, S.K., Martin, D., and Pollack, E.: Diastematomyelia in children, Radiology **112**:609-621, 1974.
23. Holt, J.F.: Neurofibromatosis in children, AJR **130**:615-639, 1978.
24. Kaplan, J.O., and Quencer, R.M.: The occult tethered conus syndrome in the adult, Radiology **137**:387-391, 1980.
25. Kieffer, S.A., et al.: Contrast agents for myelography: clinical and radiological evaluation of amipaque and pantopaque, Radiology **129**:695-705, 1978.
26. Kirkaldi-Willis, W.H., et al.: Pathological anatomy of lumbar spondylosis and

stenosis correlated with the CT scan. In Post, M.J.D., editor: Radiographic evaluation of the spine, New York, 1980, Masson Publishing Co., pp. 34-55.

27. Klatte, E.C., Franken, E.A., and Smith, J.A.: The radiographic spectrum in neurofibromatosis, Semin. Roentgenol. **11**:17-33, 1976.

28. Leeds, N.E., and Jacobson, H.G.: Spinal neurofibromatosis, AJR **126**:617-623, 1976.

29. Lefkowitz, D.M., and Quencer, R.M.: Vacuum facet phenomenon: a computed tomographic sign of degenerative spondylolisthesis, Radiology **144**:562, 1982.

30. Lott, I.T., and Richardson, E.P.: Neuropathological findings and the biology neurofibromatosis, Adv. Neurol. **29**:23-32, 1981.

31. McCrae, D.L., and Standen, J.: Roentgenologic findings in syringomyelia and hydromyelia, AJR **98**:695-703, 1966.

32. Meaney, T.F.: Magnetic resonance without nuclear, Radiology **150**:277, 1984.

33. Mitchell, G.E., Lourie, H., and Berne, A.A.: Various causes of scalloped vertebrae with notes on their pathogenesis, Radiology **89**:67-74, 1967.

34. Moe, J., et al.: Scoliosis and other spinal deformities, Philadelphia, 1978, W.B. Saunders Co., p. 215.

35. Naidich, T.P., McLane, D.G., and Harwood-Nash, D.C.: Spinal dysraphism. In Newton, T.H., and Potts, D.G., editors, Computed tomographyof the spine and spinal cord, San Anselmo, Calif., 1983, Clavadel Press, pp. 299-353.

36. Paushter, D.M., et al.: Clinical applications of nuclear magnetic resonance: central nervous system—brain stem and cord, RadioGraphics **4**(special edition):97-112, 1984.

37. Pettersson, H., et al.: Conventional metrizamide myelography (MM) and computed tomographic metrizamide myelography (CTMM) in scoliosis, Radiology **142**:111-114, 1982.

38. Resjo, I.M., et al.: Computed tomographic metrizamide myelography in syringohydromyelia, Radiology **131**:405-407, 1979.

39. Resjo, I.M., et al.: Normal cord in infants and children examined with computed tomographic metrizamide myelography, Radiology **130**:691-696, 1979.

40. Riccardi, V.M.: Von Recklinghausen neurofibromatosis, N. Engl. J. Med. **305**:1617-1627, 1981.

41. Rothman, S.L.G., and Glenn, W.V.: Spondylolysis and spondylolisthesis. In Newton, T.H., and Potts, D.G., editors: Computed tomography of the spine and spinal cord, San Anselmo, Calif., 1983, Clavadel Press, pp. 267-280.

42. Rubenstein, A.E., et al.: Neurological aspects of neurofibromatosis, Adv. Neurol. **29**:11-21, 1981.

43. Russel, D.S., and Rubenstein, L.J.: Pathologyof tumors of the nervous system, Baltimore, 1977, Williams and Wilkins.

44. Sackett, J.R., and Strother, C.M.: New techniques in myelography, Hagerstown, Md., 1979, Harper and Row.

45. Scotti, G., et al.: Diastematomyelia in children: metrizamide and CT metrizamide myelography, AJR **135**:1225-1232, 1980.

46. Shapiro, R.: Myelography, Chicago, 1975, Year Book Medical Publishers, pp. 293-309.

47. Sheldon, J.J., and Leborgne, J.M.: Computed tomography of the lumbar vertebral column. In Post, M.J.D., editor: Radiographic evaluation of the spine, New York, 1980, Masson Publishing Co., pp. 56-87.

48. Till, K.: Congenital malformations of the lower back in childhood, Proc. R. Soc. Med. **62**:727-729, 1969.

49. Williams, B.: Orthopaedic features in the presentation of syringomyelia, J. Bone Joint Surg. (Br.) **61**:314-323, 1979.

50. Winter, R.B., et al.: Diastematomyelia and congenital spine deformities, J. Bone Joint Surg. (Am.) **56**:27-39, 1974.

51. Yeates, A., et al.: Nuclear magnetic resonance imaging of syringomyelia, AJNR **4**:234-237, 1983.

Chapter Four

Spinal
Orthosis Treatment

*T*he treatment of scoliosis with orthotic devices such as braces can be traced back to Hippocrates, but the technique was rarely used until the nineteenth century.[39] Because they were cumbersome and difficult to wear, spinal orthoses were not commonly used for the treatment of scoliosis until the development of the Milwaukee brace by Drs. Blount and Schmidt during the 1950s.[7,8] The effectiveness and relative ease of use of the Milwaukee brace were quickly appreciated. Bracing is still the standard method for the treatment of children and adolescents with idiopathic scoliosis of a moderate degree.[25] The general principles of spinal orthosis will be discussed in this chapter with specific attention to idiopathic scoliosis. The other applications of bracing are discussed in later chapters on other forms of abnormal curvature.

Indications

Bracing is effective for the treatment of patients with infantile, juvenile, or adolescent-onset idiopathic scoliosis.[36] Patients with infantile idiopathic scoliosis are treated with braces for as long as possible, although this may require 10 to 15 years of treatment. If the curve cannot be maintained under 50 degrees, fusion is indicated regardless of the patient's age.[60] Although fusion in childhood will reduce the patient's adult trunk length, the shortening will still be less than that resulting from an untreated severe scoliosis.[60]

In general, bracing is ineffective in patients who are skeletally mature; therefore, children whose iliac apophyses have fused are not candidates for brace treatment.[60] The one uncommon exception may be the skeletally mature patient with an unstable curve that improves with application of a spinal orthosis. Bracing is also ineffective in large curves. Most authorities agree that infantile, juvenile, or adolescent curves over 60 degrees should be fused. The "gray zone" with regards to appropriate treatment is between 40 and 60 degrees. Many factors are used in deciding whether the patient should be braced or fused.

The success of spinal deformity orthosis treatment is best predicted by the extent of curve decrease achieved by orthosis application.[15] In addition, brace therapy is considered more likely to be successful if (1) the curve is flexible, (2) the rib hump is less than 3.0 cm, (3) the curve involves more than six to seven vertebrae, and (4) the patient has significant growth left.[60] The minimum curve size requiring brace therapy has been a subject of debate. As indicated in Chapter One, most curves less than 20 degrees will not progress, and only 46% to 80% of curves between 20 and 30 degrees will progress. Because of these data, a spinal orthosis is now recommended only for curves over 30 degrees or for curves between 20 and 30 degrees that show radiographic progression of more than 5 degrees.[44] There are only a few contraindications to bracing: (1) congenital scoliosis owing to a unilateral bar, (2) congenital kyphosis, (3) neurofibromatosis with dystrophic spinal changes, (4) rigid kyphosis owing to myelomeningocele, and (5) osteogenesis imperfecta not of the tarda type.[44,60]

Brace Construction

The most commonly used brace is the Milwaukee brace or one of its modifications (Fig. 4-1). Modern terminology refers to this as a CTLSO or a cervicothoracic lumbosacral orthosis based on the spinal segments crossed and the control desired.[2,4,44] The principles of construction have been described in detail.[10,58,60] The fundamental components are the pelvic girdle, the single anterior upright, the two posterior uprights, and the neck ring. A thoracic pad and lumbar pad are then attached at specific levels, depending on the underlying thoracic or lumbar curves. High thoracic curves associated with an elevated shoulder require a trapezius pad on the curve convexity which attaches to the anterior upright, passes over the trapezius muscle, and inserts onto the posterior upright on the concavity of the curve. Thoraco-lumbar curves are treated with an oval pad on the convexity of the curve and an axillary half-ring on the concavity.

Currently, the pelvic girdle is most commonly a high temperature thermoplastic that may be fabricated on a positive plaster of Paris mold of the patient or prefabricated on a plaster of Paris mold of a normal person of similar size.[21] The thermoplastic provides a comfortable, uniform fit with a lightweight material. The pelvic girdle is cut high anteriorly to allow thigh flexion for sitting but extends posteriorly to within approximately 2 cm of a chair seat when the patient is sitting. Shaping the pelvic girdle to provide flattening of the abdomen creates pelvic tilt to decrease lumbar lordosis. The posterior uprights are made of steel for structural strength. Since the anterior upright is in the midline, it is made of aluminum so that the spine can still be visualized on radiographs for measurement purposes. The uprights are closely fitting and allow room anteriorly for a deep inspiration only.

The neck ring theoretically provides a distraction force upon the occiput with only minimal, if any, force being transmitted anteriorly through the throat mold. The occipital pad should force the occiput upward and not forward. The neck ring must be centered over the pelvic ring. Reducing anterior neck forces prevents the mandibular growth deformities that occurred with the original brace design.[35]

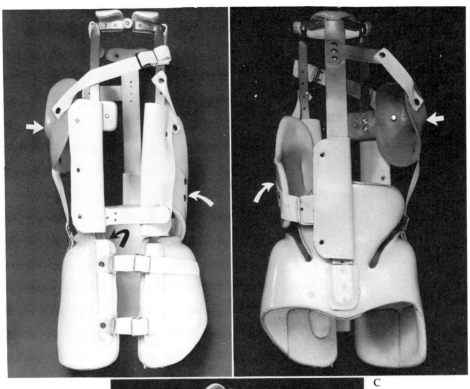

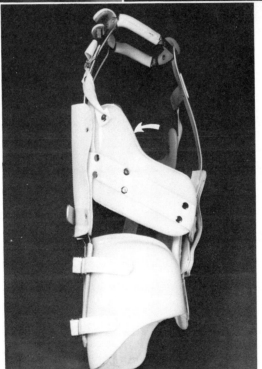

FIGURE 4-1
Milwaukee brace.
Posterior **(A)**, anterior **(B)**, and right side **(C)** views show the basic pelvic girdle,
neck ring, two posterior uprights, and one anterior upright. A right thoracic pad
(curved white arrow) and left axillary sling *(white arrow)* are attached. A left lumbar
pad would be placed inside the pelvic girdle at the level of the curved black arrow
(A).

The CTLSO devices are used for thoracic, thoracolumbar, double major thoracic, and double major thoracic and lumbar scoliosis. Single major lumbar, thoracolumbar, and lower thoracic curves can also be treated with a thoracolumbosacral orthosis (TLSO). These latter braces are cosmetically more acceptable to the patient since they are not visible when the patient is clothed (Fig. 4-2). There are a number of varieties of TLSO devices that end superiorly at the axilla and produce passive corrective forces.* The most popular type is the Boston brace (Fig. 4-2). For the single major lumbar curve, a lumbar pad is attached to the inside of the shell at the paralumbar region adjacent to the lumbar curve apex. The inferior counterforce to the lumbar pad comes from the inferior trochanter extension of the plastic shell on the side of the lumbar concavity. If the patient has a good "righting reflex," a superior counterforce is not needed. If a superior counterforce is necessary, a thoracic pad is attached on the side opposite to the lumbar curve convexity. A TLSO for a thoracolumbar curve is similarly constructed, but a second thoracic pad is added on the upper portion of the curve convexity.

---

*See references 14, 22, 48, 55, 58, 61.

A
B

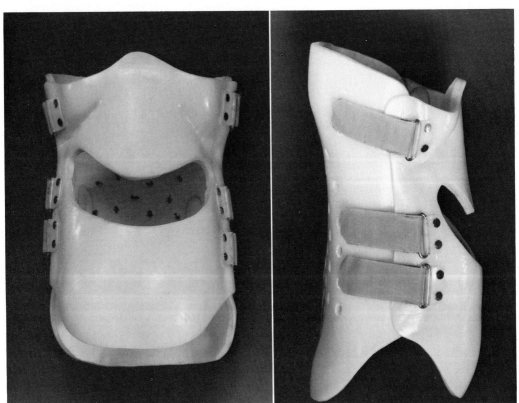

FIGURE 4-2
Boston brace.
Anterior **(A)** and right side **(B)** views demonstrate basic construction of the two large plastic half-shells.

Mechanical Principles

The neck ring of a CTLSO and the pelvic girdle are the upper and lower points that resist the lateral force from the thoracic pad (Fig. 4-3).[30] The neck ring and an axillary sling, if used, aid in inducing the righting reflex, which provides the superior counterforce to the thoracic pad. Without the resistance of these points, the patient would simply be pushed away from the thoracic pad without correction of the curve. This three-point principle is also used for correction of lumbar curves.[9] The lumbar pad force is balanced on the opposite side by the thoracic pad and pelvic girdle.

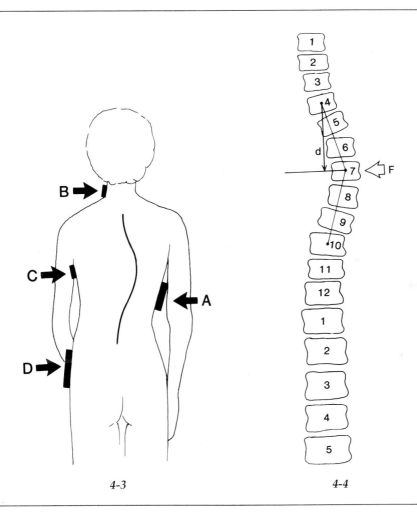

4-3   4-4

FIGURE 4-3
Milwaukee brace lateral forces.
The thoracic pad force (A) against the right thoracic curve is resisted by the neck ring (B), axillary sling (C), and pelvic girdle (D).

FIGURE 4-4
Corrective lateral force.
The lateral force (F) is proportional to the length of the lever arm (d). For curves less than 53 degrees, the lateral force is dominant over the distractive force of the Milwaukee brace.

The forces that result when wearing the Milwaukee brace are both distractive and lateral. The lateral forces come from the thoracic and lumbar pads. The distractive forces arise from the occipital pad and the upright supports. The mechanics of brace correction have been extensively analyzed.[3,20,30,40,56] With large curves of over 53 degrees, the lateral forces are less effective than the distractive forces. With the smaller curves that are usually treated with a brace, the lateral forces become dominant[30] (Fig. 4-4).

An important consideration in individual brace design is the presence of thoracic hyperkyphosis or hypokyphosis. The thoracic pad is most effective when it is positioned posteriorly and laterally. However, the typical posterior position results in a decrease in the thoracic kyphosis[29] (Fig. 4-8, C). Anteriorly directed forces are created by positioning the thoracic pad medial to the posterior upright and attaching it anteriorly to an outrigger (Fig. 4-5, B). In patients with thoracic hypokyphosis, the thoracic pad must be positioned more laterally than posteriorly. Forces are more laterally directed by attaching the thoracic pad lateral to the posterior upright and directly to the anterior upright (Fig. 4-5, A).

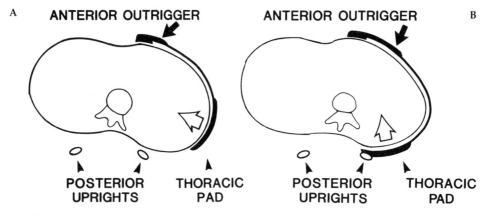

FIGURE 4-5
Milwaukee brace forces.
A, With thoracic hypokyphosis, the force *(open arrow)* is intentionally directed from the side by positioning the thoracic pad laterally and by attachment anteriorly to a short outrigger *(arrow)*.
B, Normally the force *(open arrow)* is directed more anteriorly with a posteriorly positioned thoracic pad attached to a long anterior outrigger *(curved arrow)*.
Modified from Winter, R.B., and Carlson, J.M.: Clin. Orthop. **126:**74-86, 1977.

Radiographic Evaluation

In addition to the routine posteroanterior (PA) film, a lateral spinal radiograph must be obtained prior to brace construction to evaluate the degree of thoracic kyphosis. This film is also used to exclude lumbar spondylolisthesis. In the presence of spondylolisthesis, the pelvic girdle must be carefully constructed to prevent an increase in lumbar lordosis.

After the brace has been constructed and the fit appears optimal externally, posteroanterior and lateral scoliosis radiographs are repeated with the patient standing in the brace. The degree of curve correction, the alteration of kyphosis and lordosis, and the position of the pads are evaluated. The thoracic pad contains rivets so that its position can be determined on the radiographs. The thoracic pad should be directed against the rib arising from the apex of the thoracic scoliosis[60] (Figs. 4-6 and 4-7). Since the delta-shaped lumbar pad is polystyrene and radiolucent, staples are embedded within it to localize its position. The lumbar pad should press against the paralumbar muscles at the level of the lumbar scoliosis apex but must be above the ilium and below the rib cage (Figs. 4-6 to 4-8). To allow easier adjustment, the lumbar pad is usually attached to the pelvic girdle with Velcro. The lateral radiograph should be evaluated to determine the changes, if any, in thoracic kyphosis and lumbar lordosis (Fig. 4-8, C).

After maximum correction is achieved, further radiographic evaluation with a PA radiograph is needed only every 6 months. The average patient wears the brace for 20 to 21 hours per day. Either exercise or swimming is recommended daily to increase trunk muscle strength.[60] Since the brace corrects both by passive brace forces and active muscle contraction, exercise while in the brace is thought to increase curve flexibility[16] and to increase curve correction, although this latter point has never been proven. Thoracic arching while in the orthosis does appear to reduce the thoracic rib depression.[53]

While the patient is skeletally mature, a period of weaning from the brace is begun.[18,60] Skeletal maturity is defined by fusion of the vertebral ring apophyses or fusion of the iliac crest apophyses.[17,60] A standing PA radiograph is obtained at skeletal maturity after the patient has been out of the brace for 4 to 6 hours. If the curve increases from its measurements in brace, full-time brace wearing must be resumed. If the curve is stable, the period of time out of brace can be increased periodically over a 6 to 12 month period with similar radiographic evaluation each time to verify curve stability. The patient then wears the brace only at nighttime for approximately 12 months. If the curve is still stable, the brace can be discontinued. The patient is then followed at 6 month intervals for 1 year and then yearly for 2 years. After this time, follow-up is optional but evaluation at 3 to 5 year intervals is suggested.

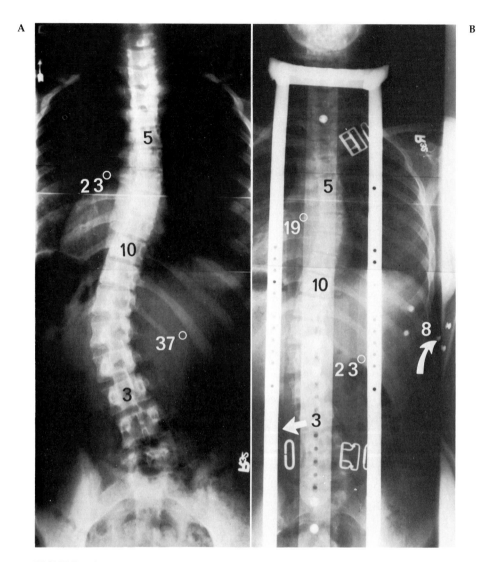

FIGURE 4-6

A, Thirty-seven-degree left thoracolumbar scoliosis with a compensatory right thoracic curve.

B, In Milwaukee brace the major curve reduces to 23 degrees. The middle rivet of the thoracic pad *(curved arrow)* is on the eighth rib below the optimal seventh rib at the curve apex. The faintly seen middle lumbar pad staple *(lower arrow)* is in good paraspinal location but at the third rather than the desired second lumbar level.

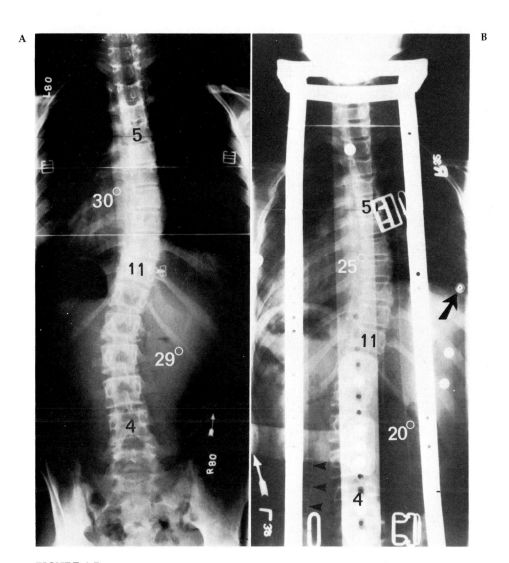

FIGURE 4-7
A, Double major right thoracic left lumbar scoliosis.
B, Milwaukee brace reduces both curves. The upper rivet level *(black arrow)* indicates correct thoracic pad placement on the eighth rib at the curve apex. The lumbar pad staples *(arrowheads)* indicate good close paraspinal placement but slightly low placement at the third lumbar level.

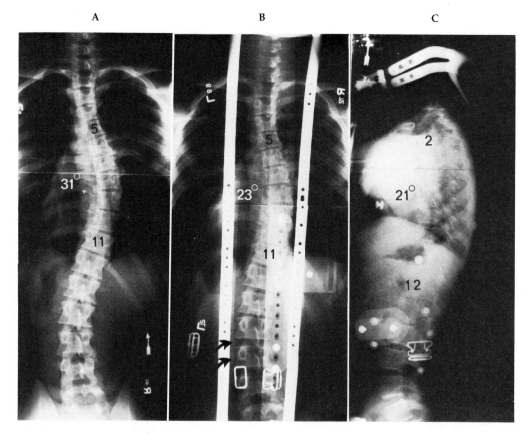

FIGURE 4-8
A, Right thoracic scoliosis.
B, Curve reduction with Milwaukee brace. The lumbar pad staples *(arrows)* show
good pad placement at the compensatory curve apex.
C, Lateral film in brace. Typical flattening of the thoracic kyphosis.

Effectiveness

The effectiveness of bracing can be measured by three parameters: the greatest curve reduction in brace, the percentage of curve reduction at the completion of brace therapy, and comparison of the prebrace curve size with the curve size after treatment when the patient has stopped growing. The full benefit of bracing cannot be quantitated because it cannot be determined how severe the scoliosis would have become without treatment. Initial curve reduction can be quantified by the decrease in curve size (pretreatment Cobb angle minus the posttreatment Cobb angle) or as the percent reduction in curve size (reduction in curve size divided by original curve size times 100). For example, a 40 degree curve reduced to 25 degrees with a brace has reduction in size of 15 degrees or 37.5% ($100 \times 15°/40°$). Curve reduction has been significant with both of the most commonly used braces, the Milwaukee and the Boston.

The best initial reduction in curve size with a Milwaukee brace is usually significant, with an average decrease in curve size of 30% to 50%.* In some patients, the curve is not decreased by the brace, but at least curve progression is halted. If curve progression continues in spite of brace treatment, surgical fusion of the spine is usually indicated.[15] Brace failure requiring surgical fusion may be due to development of thoracic lordosis[59] or low back pain in addition to curve progression.[15] Failure of brace therapy has occurred in 9% to 22% of compliant brace wearers.[15,38,45] In addition, surgical fusion may be necessary because 19% to 25% of adolescent girls are not compliant with the orthosis program, which lasts an average of 3 years.[15,38,45]

Although the initial reduction is large, there is usually some subsequent increase in curve size during the period of full-time brace wearing and weaning. The average curve reduction at the completion of brace therapy is 20% to 30%.[15,17,26,38]

Unfortunately, the large amount of curve reduction in brace is usually lost after treatment is discontinued. Although curve size may be stable during the 1 year weaning period from the brace, the curve frequently settles back to the prebrace measurement. Hassan and Bjerkreim found that the mean curve progression was 2 to 3 degrees per year for the first 4 years after treatment and 0.5 to 1 degree per year after that.[23] Most curves return to within a few degrees of their prebrace size within 5 years.[12,15,34,45] Although this loss of correction is discouraging, the important thing to remember is that a curve that had been progressive has been controlled during the period of rapid adolescent growth.[9] In contrast to this prevention of progression by bracing, many untreated scoliotic patients have marked curve worsening during their adolescent growth spurt. In addition, although the average gain for a group of patients is only a few degrees in permanent curve reduction, as many as one third of patients maintain a correction of 20% to 30%.[34]

Changes other than curve improvement with the Milwaukee brace have not been as thoroughly studied. Thulbourne and Gillespie found that the brace often elevated the depressed side of the thorax, thereby reducing the cosmetic deformity.[53] Recently, attention has been drawn to the issue of effects of bracing on balance, that is, decompensation of spinal alignment. While standing, patients with scoliosis may be balanced in the midline or out of balance to the left or right. Rudicel and Renshaw[50] studied the long-term effect of bracing in 22 patients who were treated for lumbar or thoracolumbar scoliosis. They found that the response to bracing did not correlate with restoration of spinal balance. Balance worsened or improved without correlation with length of brace wear, initial curve size, or curve correction. The long-term significance of this observation is unknown.

The results of multiple studies of Milwaukee braces have recently been summarized by Nash.[44] As a generalization, he found that curves smaller than 30 degrees, curves treated earlier, and longer curves do better. Curves can be expected to show an initial reduction of 30% to 40%, lose correction

---

*See references 15, 17, 26, 34, 38, 44.

during bracing to about 20%, and then progress by 1 to 2 degrees per year after the brace is discontinued. In addition to the absolute contraindications listed above, relative contraindications to bracing included loss of sensation, short angular curves, thoracic hypokyphosis, skeletal maturity, emotional problems, neuromuscular disease, and certain congenital anomalies.

Curve correction with the Boston brace or similar underarm braces has been as good as that achieved with a Milwaukee brace with an average best curve reduction in brace of 36% to 74%.[14,22,33,41,55] It was originally recommended that a Boston brace be used only for a curve whose apex was below the ninth thoracic vertebra.[13,48,55] Recently, the brace has been modified to reach under the axilla as far as possible to allow its use in midthoracic scoliosis.[54] Uden and coworkers[54] found an initial thoracic curve reduction of 41% with the Boston brace, which is comparable to the results of studies of the Milwaukee brace. This result is encouraging since patients prefer the Boston brace over the Milwaukee brace because the externally visible neck ring is not required. However, compliance is not better with the Boston brace than with the Milwaukee brace.[28] If the long-term results prove to be comparable for the Boston and Milwaukee braces, the Boston brace may become the standard treatment. Biomechanical studies suggest that both braces should be effective because most of the curve correction for curves less than 40 degrees comes from the lateral forces (Fig. 4-4) rather than from the distraction of the neck ring.[3,20,43] Because of the inability to produce sufficient lateral forces at a high enough level, both braces are usually ineffective in high thoracic curves.[37] Recently, the Boston brace was found to be as effective as the Milwaukee brace for thoracic curves whose apices were as high as the sixth thoracic vertebra.[27] Curves with higher apices did not correct as well, and a Milwaukee brace was recommended in these cases.

Complications

The only serious physical complication of bracing had been mandibular growth deformities caused by pressure on the mandible by the neck ring.[35,38] The lower molars were depressed, and there was extrusion of the lower incisors with loss of height of the anterior lower face and an increase in the mandibular angle.[1] It was assumed that these dental deformities were an unavoidable complication of prolonged brace wearing.[35] However, in 1965 it was observed that bracing was still effective in patients with a low set chin rest as long as the occiput pad was properly positioned.[35] This observation prompted revisions of the chin rest. By 1969, modifications were made in the original Milwaukee brace that relieved the pressure on the mandible.[35] The anterior throat mold was shaped and positioned to relieve the mandibular pressure. As a result of these brace design changes, abnormal dental and facial development have been almost completely eliminated.[46,49]

Since that time, the only medical complications have consisted of skin irritation and even ulceration if pressure is excessive on bony prominences.[13,26] Early in the brace fitting, the patient's skin is carefully examined for areas of redness, and padding is placed over these areas. Skin-softening agents should not be used, because the skin must thicken at the pressure points. Pressure on the anterior femoral cutaneous nerve may cause frontal thigh numbness, and padding is then required over the anterior superior iliac spine.

Although the medical complications are minimal, the psychological problems of bracing are significant.[42,57] Most of these patients are in their early adolescence with developing awareness of their bodies and self-image. They resist looking different from their peers and being limited by the restrictive brace. To lessen the emotional trauma, it is important for the medical team to respect the ordeal associated with treatment and to support the patient as well as the family. Most reports indicate that 19% to 25% of patients refuse to undergo or fail to complete a course of brace treatment.[15,38,45] In these noncompliant patients, curve progression can only be monitored and surgery undertaken if the curve becomes severe.

Electrical Stimulation

Nighttime electrical stimulation of the trunkal musculature is a recent development in the treatment of idiopathic scoliosis of a mild degree.[6,19,24,32] Preliminary animal investigation revealed that stimulation of the paraspinal muscles with implanted electrodes resulted in correction of surgically induced scoliosis.[11,47] Biomechanical analysis has shown that electrical stimulation to attain scoliosis correction is quite feasible on theoretical grounds considering the known mechanical properties of the axial muscles and the skeleton.[51] Subsequently, multiple small clinical studies using electrical stimulation for treatment of idiopathic scoliosis have been reported.[6,11,24,32] Electrical stimulation devices are recommended only in patients with single or double major curves of less than 40 degrees since it was found that 50% of patients with curves over 40 degrees had curve progression during electrical stimulation treatment.[11]

The first electrospinal instrumentation developed consists of an implanted receiver with three electrodes. The receiver is energized by a radiofrequency transmitter. The transmitter produces a muscle contraction lasting 1.5 seconds, with a 9 second interval between contractions.[11,19] Muscle stimulation is performed only at night during the sleeping hours. Recently, muscle stimulation has been performed using external electrodes attached by adhesive pads, thereby avoiding the need for surgical implantation of electrodes[6,31,32] (Fig. 4-9). Both external and internal stimulation have had a greater than 80% success in arresting or partially correcting idiopathic scoliosis.[6,19,24,31,32] Enthusiasm for this new technique must be tempered by the fact that relatively small numbers of patients have been studied and by the realization that many of the treated small magnitude curves may have been nonprogressive without any treatment. In addition, the long-term effects and stability of the spine after treatment have not been determined. As an example, a potential worrisome problem is the recent preliminary observation that patients with idiopathic scoliosis treated by electrical stimulation developed increased rib humps rather than the decrease in hump size seen with Milwaukee bracing.[52]

FIGURE 4-9
A 15-year-old girl with double major idiopathic adolescent scoliosis and transcutaneous stimulation electrodes in place. The upper right thoracic electrodes should be more lateral and about the apical eighth rib. The lower left lumbar electrodes are in a good lateral location but their separation should be increased.

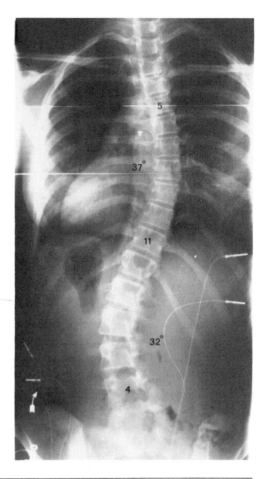

The principles and experimental background for placement of transcutaneous electrical muscle stimulation have been thoroughly presented by Axelgaard et al.[5] Maximal curve correction is achieved by placing the pair of electrodes over the lateral trunk musculature in the midaxillary line (Fig. 4-9). A positive and a negative electrode are placed on the convex side of the curve about its apex. Depending on the length of the curve, the electrodes are separated by 7 to 14 cm, with the most common separation in the range of 8 to 10 cm. If the electrodes are outside of the end vertebrae, muscle contraction spillover may worsen an adjacent curve. If double major scoliosis is present, a pair of electrodes should be placed on the convexity of each curve.

Summary

1. Indications
   a. Skeletally immature patient (occasionally in older patient with a flexible progressive curve)
   b. Curves less than 40 degrees (occasionally 40 to 60 degrees)
2. Milwaukee brace principles
   a. Components: neck ring, uprights, pelvic girdle, thoracic pad, lumbar pad
   b. Thoracic pad placement: usually posterior; lateral if hypokyphosis is present
3. Radiographic evaluation
   a. Serial PA films
   b. Initial lateral film in brace to look for sagittal plane changes
   c. Thoracic pad at ribs about curve apex
   d. Lumbar pad—paraspinal at curve apex
4. Milwaukee bracing effectiveness
   a. Average initial curve reduction, 30% to 50%
   b. Average curve reduction at completion, 20% to 30%
   c. Final curve usually equals pretreatment magnitude
5. Complications
   a. Mandibular deformities minimal with modern brace
   b. Local pressure effects
   c. Noncompliance
6. Transcutaneous electrical stimulation
   a. Lateral midaxillary line about curve apex
   b. Two sets of electrode pairs if thoracic and lumbar curves are present

REFERENCES

1. Alexander, R.G.: The effects on tooth position and maxillofacial vertical growth during treatment of scoliosis with the Milwaukee brace, Am. J. Orthod. **52:**161-189, 1966.
2. American Academy of Orthopaedic Surgeons: Atlas of orthotics. Biomechanical principles and application, St. Louis, 1975, The C.V. Mosby Co.
3. Andriacchi, T.P., et al.: Milwaukee brace correction of idiopathic scoliosis, J. Bone Joint Surg. (Am.) **58:**806-815, 1976.
4. Asher, M.A., and Whitney, W.H.: Orthotics for spinal deformity. In Redford, J.B., editor: Orthotics etcetera, Baltimore, 1979, The Williams & Wilkins Co.
5. Axelgaard, J., Nordwall, A., and Brown, J.C.: Correction of spinal curvatures by transcutaneous electrical muscle stimulation, Spine **8:**463-481, 1983.
6. Axelgaard, J., et al.: Transcutaneous electrical muscle stimulation for the treatment of idiopathic scoliosis—preliminary results, Orthop. Trans. **4:**29-30, 1980.
7. Blount, W.P.: Scoliosis and the Milwaukee brace, Bull. Hosp. Joint Dis. **19:**152-165, 1958.
8. Blount, W.P.: The Milwaukee brace in nonoperative scoliosis treatment, Acta Orthop. Scand. **33:**398-401, 1963.
9. Blount, W.P.: Use of the Milwaukee brace, Orthop. Clin. North Am. **3:**3-16, 1972.
10. Blount, W.P, and Moe, J.H.: The Milwaukee brace, Baltimore, 1973, The Williams & Wilkins Co.
11. Bobechko, W.P., Herbert, M.A., and Friedman, H.G.: Electrospinal instrumentation for scoliosis: current status, Orthop. Clin. North Am. **10:**927-941, 1979.
12. Bonnett, C.A., and Tosoonian, R.: Results of Milwaukee brace treatment in seventy patients, Orthop. Rev. **7:**79-83, 1978.
13. Bunnell, W.P.: Treatment of idiopathic scoliosis, Orthop. Clin. North Am. **10:**813-827, 1979.
14. Bunnell, W.P., MacEwen, G.D., and Jayakumar, S.: The use of plastic jackets in the non-operative treatment of idiopathic scoliosis, J. Bone Joint Surg. (Am.) **62:** 31-38, 1980.
15. Carr, W.A., et al.: Treatment of idiopathic scoliosis in the Milwaukee brace, J. Bone Joint Surg. (Am.) **62:**599-612, 1980.
16. Dickson, R.A., and Leatherman, K.D.: Cotrel traction, exercises, casting in the treatment of idiopathic scoliosis, Acta Orthop. Scand. **49:**46-48, 1978.
17. Edmonson, A.S., and Morris, J.T.: Follow-up study of Milwaukee brace treatment in patients with idiopathic scoliosis, Clin. Orthop. **126:**58-61, 1977.
18. Farady, J.A.: Current principles in the nonoperative management of structural adolescent idiopathic scoliosis, Phys. Ther. **63:**512-523, 1983.
19. Friedman, H.G., Herbert, M.A., and Bobechko, W.P.: Electrical stimulation for scoliosis, Am. Fam. Physician **25:**155-160, 1982.
20. Galante, J., et al.: Forces acting in the Milwaukee brace on patients undergoing treatment for idiopathic scoliosis, J. Bone Joint Surg. (Am.) **52:**498-506, 1970.
21. Hall, J.E., and Miller, W.: Prefabrication of Milwaukee braces, J. Bone Joint Surg. (Am.) **8:**1763, 1974.
22. Hall, J., et al.: A refined concept in the orthotic management of scoliosis, Orthot. Prosthet. **29:**7-13, 1975.
23. Hassan, I., and Bjerkreim, I.: Progression in idiopathic scoliosis after conservative treatment, Acta Orthop. Scand. **54:**88-90, 1983.
24. Herbert, M.A., and Bobechko, W.P.: Electrical stimulation of the spinal muscles to correct scoliosis, Orthop. Trans. **1:**76-77, 1977.
25. Hungerford, D.S.: Spinal deformity in adolescence, Med. Clin. North Am. **59:** 1517-1525, 1975.
26. Keiser, R.P., and Shufflebarger, H.L.: The Milwaukee brace in idiopathic scoliosis, Clin. Orthop. **118:**19-24, 1976.

27. Laurnen, E.L., Tupper, J.W., and Mullen, M.P.: The Boston brace in thoracic scoliosis, Spine **8:**388-395, 1983.
28. Lehner, J.T., and Lorber, C.: A community experience with the Boston thoraco-lumbar spinal orthosis: 130 consecutive cases, Orthop. Trans. **6:**361-362, 1982.
29. Lindh, M.: The effect of sagittal curve changes on brace correction of idiopathic scoliosis, Spine **5:**26-35, 1980.
30. Lonstein, J.E., and Winter, R.B.: Mechanics of the deformity and treatment in scoliosis, kyphosis, and spine fractures. In Ghista, D.N., editor: Osteoarthro-mechanics, New York, 1982, McGraw-Hill Book Co.
31. Macek, C.: Electrical stimulation of muscles replaces braces for scoliosis, JAMA **247:**1097-1098, 1982.
32. McCollough, N.C., III, Friedman, H., and Bracale, R.: Surface electrical stimulation of the paraspinal muscles in the treatment of idiopathic scoliosis, Orthop. Trans. **4:**29, 1980.
33. McCollough, N.C., III, et al.: Miami TLSO in the management of scoliosis: preliminary results in 100 cases, J. Pediatr. Orthop. **1:**141-152, 1981.
34. Mellencamp, D.D., Blount, W.P., and Anderson, A.J.: Milwaukee brace treatment of idiopathic scoliosis, Clin. Orthop. **126:**47-57, 1977.
35. Moe, J.H.: The Milwaukee brace in the treatment of scoliosis, Clin. Orthop. **77:**18-31, 1971.
36. Moe, J.H.: Indications for Milwaukee brace non-operative treatment in idiopathic scoliosis, Clin. Orthop. **93:**38-43, 1973.
37. Moe, J.H.: Modern concepts of treatment of spinal deformities in children and adults, Clin. Orthop. **150:**137-153, 1980.
38. Moe, J.H., and Kettleson, D.N.: Idiopathic scoliosis: analysis of curve patterns and the preliminary results of Milwaukee-brace treatment in one hundred sixty-nine patients, J. Bone Joint Surg. (Am.) **52:**1509-1533, 1970.
39. Moe, J., et al.: Scoliosis and other spinal deformities, Philadelphia, 1978, W.B. Saunders Co.
40. Mulcahy, T., et al.: A follow-up study of forces acting on the Milwaukee brace on patients undergoing treatment of idiopathic scoliosis, Clin. Orthop. **93:**53-68, 1973.
41. Murphy, J.: The Lexan jacket in the conservative treatment of scoliosis: a comparison of results obtained with the Milwaukee brace, J. Bone Joint Surg. (Am.) **57:**136, 1975.
42. Myers, B.A., Friedman, S.B., and Weiner, I.B.: Coping with a chronic disability: psychosocial observations of girls with scoliosis treated with the Milwaukee brace, Am. J. Dis. Child. **120:**175-181, 1970.
43. Nachemson, A., and Elfstrom, G.: Intravital wireless telemetry of axial forces in Harrington distraction rods in patients with idiopathic scoliosis, J. Bone Joint Surg. (Am.) **53:**445-465, 1971.
44. Nash, Jr., C.L.: Scoliosis bracing, J. Bone Joint Surg. (Am.) **62:**848-852, 1980.
45. Nordwall, A.: Early results in 159 patients treated with the Milwaukee brace, Acta Orthop. Scand. (Suppl.) **150:**99-124, 1973.
46. Northway, R.O., Jr., Alexander, R.G., and Riolo, M.L.: A cephalometric evaluation of the old Milwaukee brace and the modified Milwaukee brace in relation to the normal growing child, Am. J. Orthod. **65:**341-363, 1974.
47. Olsen, G.A., et al.: Electrical muscle stimulation as a means of correcting induced canine scoliotic curves, Clin. Orthop. **125:**227-235, 1977.
48. Park, J., et al.: A modified brace (Prenyl) for scoliosis, Clin. Orthop. **126:**67-73, 1977.
49. Persky, S.L., and Johnston, L.E.: An evaluation of dentofacial changes accompanying scoliosis therapy with a modified Milwaukee brace, Am. J. Orthod. **65:**364-371, 1974.

50. Rudicel, S., and Renshaw, T.S.: The effect of the Milwaukee brace on spinal decompensation in idiopathic scoliosis, Spine **8:**385-387, 1983.

51. Schultz, A., Haderspeck, K., and Takashima, S.: Correction of scoliosis by muscle stimulation, Spine **6:**468-476, 1981.

52. Steinway, M., Gillespie, R., and Koreska, J.: Vertebral rotation and rib hump deformity in idiopathic thoracic scoliosis, Orthop. Trans. **7:**11, 1983.

53. Thulbourne, T., and Gillespie, R.: The rib hump in idiopathic scoliosis, J. Bone Joint Surg. (Br.) **58:**64-71, 1976.

54. Uden, A., Willner, S., and Pettersson, H.: Initial correction with the Boston thoracic brace, Acta Orthop. Scand. **53:**907-911, 1982.

55. Watts, H.G., Hall, J.E., and Stanish, W.: The Boston brace system for the treatment of low thoracic and lumbar scoliosis by the use of a girdle without superstructure, Clin. Orthop. **126:**87-92, 1977.

56. White, A.A., Panjabi, M.M.: The clinical biomechanics of scoliosis, Clin. Orthop. **118:**100-112, 1976.

57. Wickers, F.C., Bunch, W.H., and Barnett, P.M.: Psychological factors in failure to wear the Milwaukee brace for treatment of idiopathic scoliosis, Clin. Orthop. **126:**62-66, 1977.

58. Winter, R.B., and Carlson, J.M.: Modern orthotics for spinal deformities, Clin. Orthop. **126:**74-86, 1977.

59. Winter, R.B., Lovell, W.W., and Moe, J.H.: Excessive thoracic lordosis and loss of pulmonary function in patients with idiopathic scoliosis, J. Bone Joint Surg. (Am.) **57:**972-977, 1975.

60. Winter, R.B., and Moe, J.H.: Orthotics for spinal deformity, Clin. Orthop. **102:**72-91, 1974.

61. Zamosky, I.: New concepts in the corrective bracing of soliosis, kyphosis, and lordosis, Orthot. Prosthet. **32:**3-10, 1978.

Chapter Five

Surgical Correction of Spinal Deformity

Marc A. Asher and Arthur A. De Smet

*S*urgical correction of a spinal deformity is usually performed to eliminate pain, to correct a cosmetically unacceptable appearance, or to prevent further progression of the deformity. Spinal fusion alone may be adequate, but internal fixation is now frequently used to increase the degree of correction and to maintain this correction until the bony fusion is solid.[16,23]

The selected method of internal fixation and fusion varies with the severity of the underlying deformity and its etiology. Familiarity with these methods allows one to determine radiographically if the postoperative appearance is satisfactory and to detect if a complication has occurred. All of the internal fixation devices are readily seen on radiographs, and their position can be easily ascertained. Spinal fusion is usually performed posteriorly because of the easier access to the posterior elements than to the anterior vertebral bodies. Posterior internal fixation is achieved using either Harrington rods or, less commonly, segmental spinal instrumentation (SSI) such as Luque rods. Anterior fusion may be indicated when the patient has deficiency of the posterior spinal elements, neuromuscular disease, or severe deformity requiring staged correction. Anterior interbody fusion is usually employed, although anterior strut grafts are desirable in the management of fixed kyphosis. Although used less commonly than posterior fixation, anterior fixation devices such as Dwyer or Zielke instrumentation may be indicated.

The methods of anterior and posterior fusion will be reviewed briefly with emphasis on the principles of technique and the use of radiographs to select the fusion area. The correct radiographic appearance of the internal fixation devices will also be stressed.

Posterior Fusion and Instrumentation
PREOPERATIVE RADIOGRAPHIC EVALUATION

Prior to the operation, a basic radiographic evaluation consists of upright posteroanterior (PA), or anteroposterior (AP), and lateral films. If there is any question about the curve pattern, nonstressed supine AP left and right bending films are obtained as well.[18] If an indication of the expected correction is desired, bending films with a physician stressing the bend can be obtained. The percentage correction achieved on the stress bending films is the most that can be expected from the surgery.[30]

The upright film is used to determine the extent of fusion.[17] As a general rule, the fusion should extend from one vertebral body above the superior end vertebra down to two vertebrae below the inferior end vertebra for thoracic and thoracolumbar curves (Fig. 5-1).[24] For lumbar curves, the fusion should extend from one vertebra above the superior vertebra down to the inferior end vertebra.[24] The end vertebrae are those that are most tilted relative to the horizontal as previously described for measuring the Cobb angle.

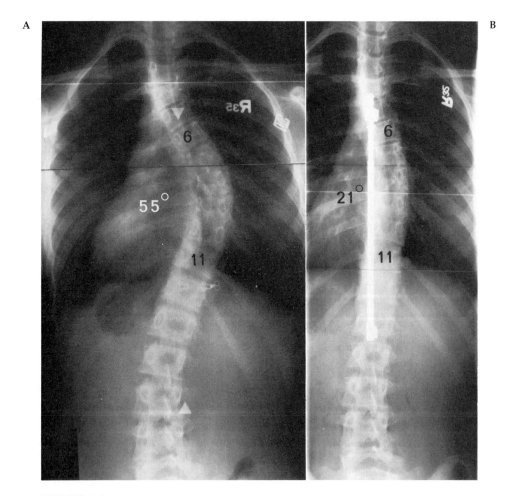

FIGURE 5-1

A, A 12-year-old girl with a 55 degree right sixth thoracic to eleventh thoracic (T6-11) idiopathic scoliosis.

B, Postoperative radiographic showing curve reduction to 21 degrees with the hooks of a Harrington distraction rod at T5 and the first lumbar level (L1).

Selection of the lower level of the fusion is also influenced by additional considerations.[58] All of the rotated vertebrae must be included in the fusion (Fig. 5-2).[10,16,38,40] If Harrington instrumentation is planned, the lower hook site on the concave side lamina must be within the stable zone. The stable zone is defined by parasagittal lines extending vertically from the sacral superior facets (Fig. 5-3).[24]

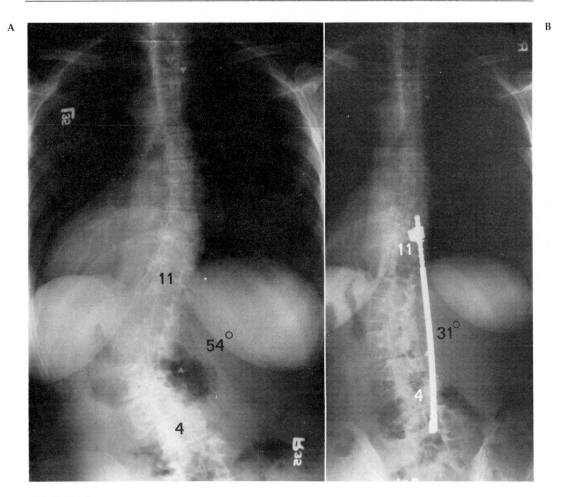

FIGURE 5-2

A, A 52-year-old woman with a 54 degree left T11-L4 lumbar scoliosis, secondary degenerative joint disease, and frontal plane translational shift of L3 on L4.

B, Postoperative radiograph showing curve reduction to 31 degrees with the Harrington distraction rod hooks at T10 and L5. L4 and L5 were included in the fusion because of their rotation and the L4-5 disk disease.

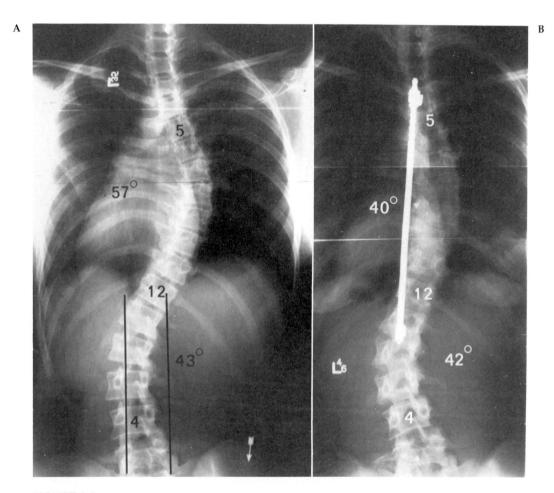

FIGURE 5-3

A, A 57 degree right thoracic T5-12 scoliosis with flexible 43 degree left lumbar T12-L4 scoliosis. Harrington stable zone is indicated by vertical lines through the sacral facets.

B, Postoperative Harrington distraction rod with distal hook in the center of the stable zone.

The lateral film is used to determine if there is abnormal kyphosis or lordosis. The distraction rod should be contoured to minimize the secondary spinal straightening that occurs with a straight Harrington distraction rod. Since the Harrington compression rod considerably reduces thoracic kyphosis, it should not be used in patients with thoracic hypokyphosis or thoracic lordosis.[3]

Supine, nonstress bending films are used to help determine whether a single curve or double curve needs to be fused.[24,28,29] As an alternative, Kleinman et al.[30] suggested that a prone film with physician stressing at the apex of each curve could be used to determine curve flexibility. The advantages of supine bending versus prone push films has not been determined. The importance of these films arises in determining whether a lumbar minor curve should be fused. If a lumbar curve is highly structural, that is, corrects poorly with side bending, it should be included in the fusion.[39] If a highly structural lumbar curve is not included in the fusion, the patient may develop one or more of the following complications: (1) worsening of the lumbar curve, (2) pain at the lower end of the fusion, or (3) permanent tilt of the torso to one side. On the other hand, unnecessary fusion of a lumbar curve increases the complexity of the surgery and leaves the patient with limited spinal flexibility. There is also an increased incidence of subsequent low back pain if the fusion is extended down to the fourth or fifth lumbar levels,[8] so unnecessary lumbar fusion should be avoided.

Recently, King et al.[28,29] presented the results of their important study of the appropriate fusion levels in thoracic scoliosis. They found that the correction achieved on supine, nonstress bending films was a good estimate of the subsequent amount of operative correction. More importantly, they showed that all patients with both thoracic and lumbar curves did not need to have fusion of both spinal segments. A flexibility index was used to determine when lumbar fusion was necessary. The flexibility index was defined as lumbar curve flexibility minus the thoracic curve flexibility. For example, 10% lumbar flexibility minus 50% thoracic flexibility = −40% index. Combined thoracic and lumbar scoliosis where the lumbar curve was larger and less flexible than the thoracic curve (negative flexibility index) required fusion of both curves. Combined scoliosis in which the thoracic curve was larger and less flexible than the lumbar curve (positive flexibility index) was successfully treated by fusion of the thoracic curve alone. The upper level of the fusion was the first nonrotated vertebra above the curve. The lower fusion level was determined by a vertical line through the midline of the sacrum, the center sacral line. The "stable vertebra" or lower fusion level was the vertebra that was most closely bisected by the midsacral line.

SURGICAL TECHNIQUE

For the interested reader, the surgical technique for posterior spinal fusion has been extensively reviewed.[16,18,24,39,58] The patient is positioned prone on a special frame or padded blocks with the abdomen hanging free. If the abdomen is not dependent, the raised intraabdominal pressure increases the paravertebral venous pressure and increases the intraoperative bleeding. A posterior, midline, longitudinal incision is made and carried down to the tips of the spinous processes, care being taken to avoid the paraspinal muscles. The posterior elements are exposed by subperiosteal dissection out to the tips of the transverse processes. All of the ligaments and capsular attachments posteriorly except for the ligamenta flava are removed.

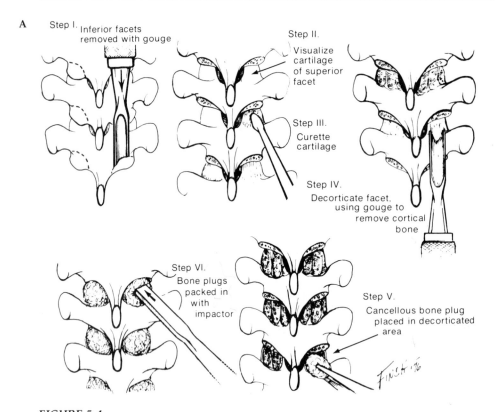

FIGURE 5-4

A, Posterior facet fusion technique. In the first step, the inferior facet joint is sharply cut with a semicircular gouge in the manner outlined. The bone fragment with underlying articular cartilage is removed in one piece. The superior facet cartilage is then easily visualized and is removed with a sharp curette. A trough is created by removing the outer cortex of the superior facet. Cancellous bone is then taken from the outer table of the ilium and snugly impacted into the decorticated area previously created.

An important element of any posterior spinal fusion is the need to destroy the cartilage of the facet joints and place cancellous bone within the joints. After the facet joints are packed with bone graft, all the spinous processes are removed, and the posterior surfaces of the lamina are decorticated (Fig. 5-4). Bits of this graft as well as small linear fragments of iliac bone graft are placed longitudinally across the lamina of the fused segments (Fig. 5-4). These general principles of surgical technique are used with various modifications in all methods of posterior fusion.

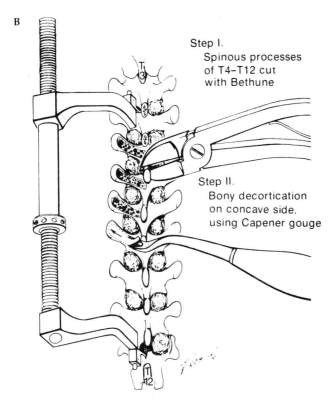

FIGURE 5-4, cont'd
B, Posterior bony decortication is carried out after the facet joints have been prepared and packed with bone. Spinous processes are first cut with a Bethune bone cutter, and bony decortication on the concave side is carried out to the tips of the transverse processes.

From Moe, J.H., et al.: Scoliosis and other spinal deformities, Philadelphia, 1978, W.B. Saunders.

HARRINGTON INSTRUMENTATION

Harrington instrumentation consists of both distraction and compression devices.[21] The distraction device consists of a 6.35 mm (¼ inch) diameter rod and two hooks (Fig. 5-5). One end of the rod has a series of notches to function as a ratchet and allow distraction of the spine.[22] Following the completion of distraction, a small safety washer is placed on the rod to prevent slippage.[23] The compression device consists of a flexible 4.76 mm (³/₁₆ inch) diameter threaded rod and multiple hooks (Fig. 5-5). Each compression hook is secured on its closed end by a nut to prevent retraction of the hook.

If a Harrington distraction rod is to be used, posterior spinal fusion is begun as described before, but the instrumentation is inserted prior to the facet joint fusion (Fig. 5-6). The distraction hooks are placed on the concavity of a scoliosis. The upper hook is inserted under the lamina and superior facet

FIGURE 5-5
Harrington instrumentation
Compression rod with hooks *(right)*
and distraction rod with hooks *(left)*.

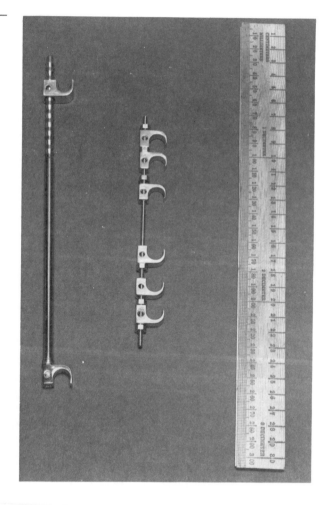

joint that has been selected as the upper level of the fusion. A small portion of the lamina and inferior articulating facet is cut away to seat the hook properly. The lower hook is then placed under the lamina of the lower-most vertebral body to be included within the fusion. The laminar border is frequently notched to secure the hook. Removal of a portion of the inferior lamina and facet process of the vertebra above is often necessary to allow placement of the hook. Once the hooks are inserted, a large outrigger is inserted into both hooks, providing distraction of the spine and thus reducing the degree of scoliosis. A special bracket is available that allows the outrigger to remain in place during the subsequent rod insertion.

In single major curves, usually only one distraction rod is used, passing from the superior to the most inferior segment across the concavity of the curve (Figs. 5-1 and 5-3). In the absence of thoracic hypokyphosis, convex

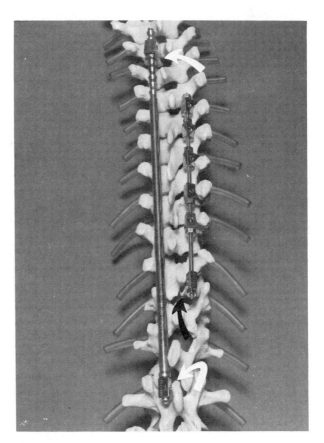

FIGURE 5-6
Distraction rod and compression rods in place on specimen spine.
The two distraction hooks *(white arrows)* and lowest compression hook *(black arrow)* are sublaminar in position. The other compression hooks are over the transverse processes.

side compression instrumentation may be added. However, improvement in coronal plane curve correction can only be expected in flexible, small (<70 degree) curves.[3] Transverse traction (Cotrel-DTT) between the compression and distraction rods improves stability but at the expense of increased vertebral body rotation toward the convexity.[44] In the presence of severe structural thoracic lordosis associated with decreased pulmonary function, staged anterior and posterior correction should be considered. The principle is to create a kyphosis by producing a flail posterior chest wall and realigning the spine using a combined Harrington-segmental spinal instrumentation technique.[5]

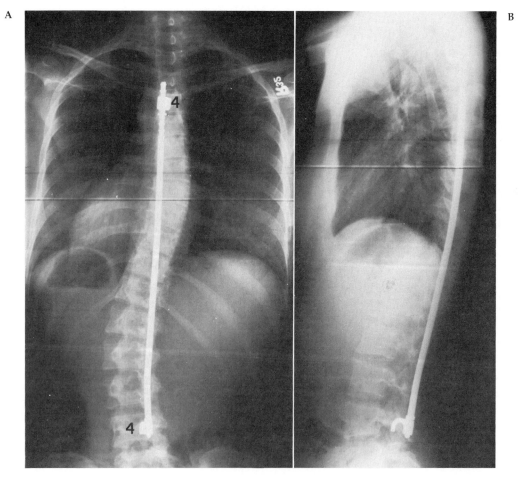

FIGURE 5-7

A, Patient with double major T5-11 thoracic and T11-L4 lumbar scoliosis treated with a single Harrington distraction rod across the concavity of each curve with its hooks at T4 and L4.

B, Lateral film showing the straightening of the spine that occurs with a noncontoured rod.

In curves that are double major or single major with highly structural minor curves, the so-called dollar sign or cross-over rod is placed with the upper hook at one vertebra above the superior level of the thoracic curve and the lower hook at the inferior level of the lumbar curve (Fig. 5-7).[24] This single rod is superior to overlapping rods on the concavity of each curve, because two separate rods may cause a kyphosis at the junction between the two rods. If the curve is very severe, with a rigid apex, two rods can be placed across the concavity of the curve with the innermost rod across the inflexible portion and a longer rod to allow greater correction of the more flexible portion of the curve (Fig. 5-8). Sublaminar wires attached between a distraction rod and the

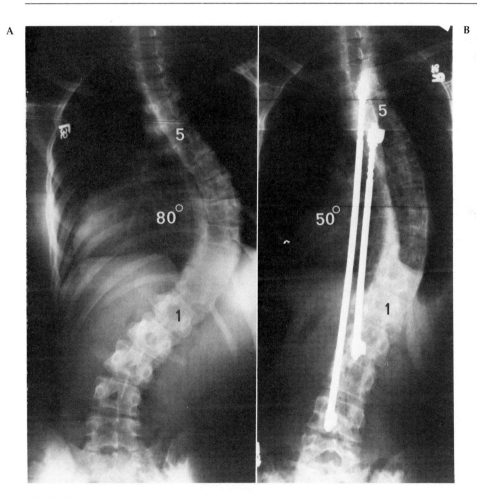

FIGURE 5-8
A, Highly structural 80 degree T5-L1 right thoracic scoliosis.
B, Correction with an inner distraction rod across the rigid apical portion and a longer rod across the outer, more flexible portion of the curve.

Harrington instrumentation can be extended to the sacrum by use of a transilial bar or, as became available later, a large hook to place over the sacral ala. If severe lumbar lordosis is present, the sacral bar can be used (Fig. 5-9). However, loss of normal lumbar lordosis is a more common problem, and this, plus the high incidence of pseudarthrosis with sacral insertion of Harrington rods, has resulted in a recent trend toward Luque instrumentation when fusion to the sacrum is required.[31] In most cases, fusion to the sacrum, or even to L5, in idiopathic scoliosis is not indicated or beneficial and therefore is not recommended.[13] This is especially true in the adolescent and young adult.

The rod is now frequently contoured to decrease the amount of straightening that occurs in the sagittal plane (Fig. 5-10). If the rod is not contoured,

FIGURE 5-10
Lateral radiograph of contoured T1-L4 distraction rod and T9-L4 compression rod. Contrast to Figure 5-7, *B*.

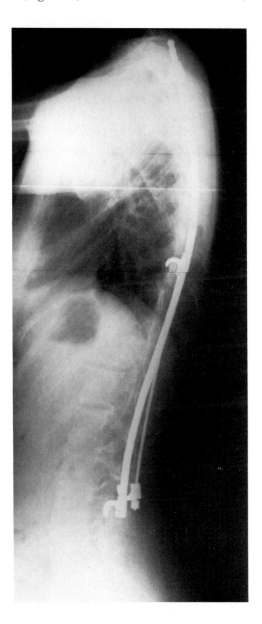

there is flattening of both the thoracic kyphosis and the lumbar lordosis (Fig. 5-7, *B*) with particularly marked decrease in the lumbar lordosis.[1,8] Rod contouring should only be done in the smooth portion as the ratcheted portion may fatigue fracture in vivo if it is bent. A contoured rod must be square on the nonratcheted end if a lordosis preserving effect is desired. The one exception to this is the double curve where the kyphosis contour of the thoracic portion of the rod tends to stabilize the lordosis contour of the lumbar portion of the rod. Currently, square shouldered rods can be identified radiographically by the absence of a protrusion of a small portion of the rod through the hook, whereas there is a small protrusion of the round-ended rod (Fig. 5-11).

A potential use for Harrington rods is for control of a scoliotic curve in the young child without the addition of posterior fusion so that spinal growth is not stopped in the fused segment. The subcutaneously placed rod is then lengthened at periodic intervals (about 6 months), changed as necessary because of growth or rod breakage, and fusion eventually performed when spine growth is more nearly complete. Moe et al.[42] reported an experience in 20 such patients with an average age at treatment onset of 9 years. A Milwaukee brace was worn full-time. Rod breakage or hook dislocation occurred in 50% of the patients. Although these results are preliminary, the technique appears to offer an alternative to extensive spinal fusion at an early age in children with long or double curves.

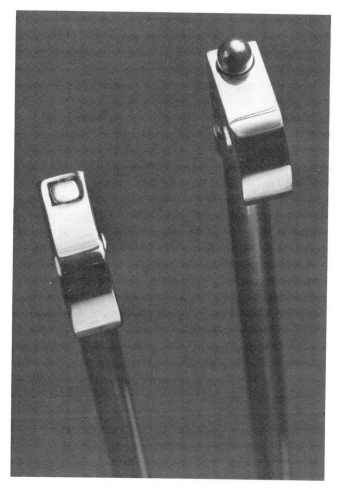

FIGURE 5-11
Close-up of square-ended and round-ended Harrington rods. Note the round rod
tip protrudes slightly beyond the hook.

RADIOGRAPHIC EVALUATION

The initial evaluation of the surgical use of Harrington instrumentation begins with the intraoperative films. After initial dissection down to the spine, the previously selected upper and lower vertebral bodies of the fusion are determined by placing a metallic marker on the spinous process of the lower vertebra. A PA radiograph is obtained to verify that the desired lower level of the fusion has been correctly located (Fig. 5-12). The upper level can then be identified by counting spinous processes on the exposed spine. Because these films are obtained with mobile x-ray units through a thick body part, adequate radiographs may be hard to obtain. Use of a grid for these films is difficult because of the problems of centering the x-ray tube with the grid unless a special tunnel such as used for operative cholangiography has been constructed.[50] Without a grid, there is increased scatter radiation and the vertebral bodies are poorly defined. In this situation, the use of a high contrast film such as Ortho M (Eastman Kodak, Rochester, NY) is helpful. A high contrast film improves edge definition and aids in identifying the vertebral levels. The use of a single, high-speed Kodak Lanex regular screen with the Ortho M film provides a 200 speed system that is sufficiently fast for most patients. In larger patients, a 400 speed system such as Kodak Ortho G film and double screen Kodak Lanex Regular cassette may be necessary, although bony detail is compromised without the use of a grid. In very obese patients, an 800 speed system (Ortho H and double Lanex Regular) can be used.

An immediate postoperative AP film is obtained to verify that the rod has been seated properly at the desired levels and to determine the initial degree of correction. When the patient is later mobilized, upright PA and lateral films are obtained to document that there has been no loss of correction or hook dislodgement during the postoperative period.

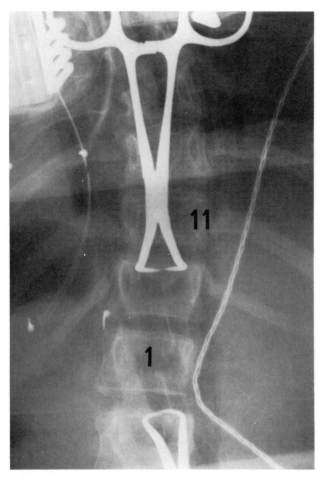

FIGURE 5-12
PA intraoperative radiograph showing towel clips attached to the spinous processes
of T11 and L1. Note that the spinous processes project below the labeled vertebral
bodies.

In addition to determining the percentage of correction achieved, proper placement of the internal fixation devices should be verified (Fig. 5-1). All rotated lumbar vertebrae should be included in the fusion (Fig. 5-2). The one possible exception may be the double thoracic and lumbar curve with a positive flexibility index being treated with selective fusion of the thoracic spine. In this instance, when the lower hook is in the stable zone, the neutral vertebra may not be included.[29] The lower hook should be in the stable zone, that is, medial to a parasagittal line through each sacral facet (Fig. 5-3) and ideally be in the vertebra most nearly bisected by the center sacral line. Each compression rod hook should be under the convex side transverse process down to T11 and over the convex side lamina below T11 (Figs. 5-6 and 5-13).

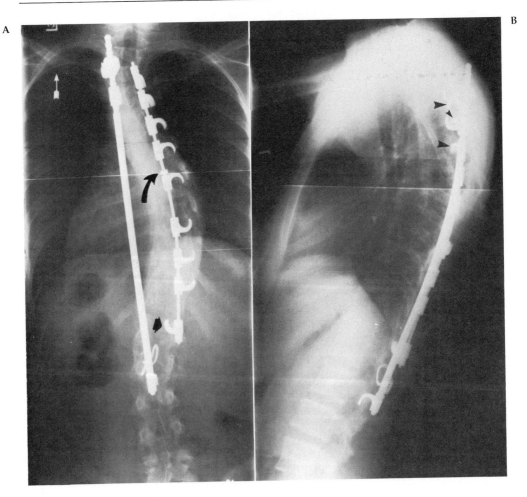

A   B

FIGURE 5-13
PA **(A)** and lateral **(B)** radiographs of Harrington distraction rod on the curve concavity and compression rod on the curve convexity. The lower compression hook *(arrow)* is on the lamina of T12 rather than under the transverse processes as at other levels. Each compression hook is secured by a retaining nut. One nut (**A,** *curved arrow*) has unscrewed slightly. Note on **B** how the upper compression hooks appear pointed anteriorly *(arrowheads)* while the others appear directed laterally owing to vertebral rotation.

LUQUE INSTRUMENTATION

Although Harrington instrumentation is the most widely used method for posterior fixation of the spine, it has theoretical disadvantages. The Harrington system is limited in its ability to correct a curve because the principal force is distraction only and because the bone-metal interface has a limited strength, especially in patients with neuromuscular paralysis.[53] This limitation has been shown theoretically,[49] clinically,[54] and in laboratory experiments.[56] Biomechanical studies have shown that almost complete curve correction is best achieved by transverse forces rather than the vertical forces of the Harrington rod.[55]

The advantages of transverse forces were stressed by Luque who developed an L-shaped rod for posterior internal fixation.[34,35] The short right angle bend of the end of the rod prevents its migration, a significant complication of the straight rod technique described by Resina and Alves.[45] A Luque rod is positioned posteriorly along the left and the right sides of the spine. Transverse forces are created by passing a wire under each lamina and then twisting the wire around its respective rod. By securing the spine at multiple points, the force is distributed across multiple levels with resultant greater curve stability.[55,56] Greater curve stability results in less postoperative motion of the arthrodesed spinal segment that is beneficial for solid fusion of the bone graft. The rods can also be contoured to maintain a normal thoracic kyphosis and lumbar lordosis. Although the Harrington distraction rod can also be contoured, the degree of contouring is limited. As the bending is increased with the Harrington rod, the distractive force is reduced, and the risk of rod breakage as well as hook pull-out or cut-out increases. The multisegmental transverse nature of the Luque rod forces is unaffected by bending the rods.

In spite of these considerations, the percent correction is similar for Harrington and Luque instrumentations. Average correction with Luque rods was reported in a small series of patients to be 40.1% with an average loss of correction of 7 degrees,[25] comparable to an average correction of 30% to 55% with Harrington instrumentation.

The disadvantages of Luque rod instrumentation are the increased operative time, increased blood loss, and increased neurologic complications owing to the passage of sublaminar wires.[43] Long-term studies of the stability of the fusion and pseudarthrosis rate are also not available. A potential but unproven use for Luque instrumentation is in the treatment of progressive scoliosis in childhood. If posterior fusion and Harrington instrumentation are used, curve progression is halted but so is spinal growth over the fused segment resulting in less adult height than is theoretically possible. In an experiment using laboratory dogs, McAfee et al.[37] found that by using Luque instrumentation without arthrodesis much of the spine's growth potential was preserved.

The surgical technique for Luque rod insertion has been presented in detail.[2,32,36] The general technique of posterior spinal fusion is used as described above with two exceptions. The ligamentum flavum is removed to allow passage of the sublaminar wires, and the laminae are not decorticated. Removing both the ligamentum flavum and decorticating the laminae could result in spinal stenosis owing to bone graft narrowing the spinal canal.[36] Also, laminar decortication prior to rod placement would result in even greater blood loss. If the fusion is to extend down to the sacrum, each rod is driven into a drill hole placed in the ipsilateral posterior iliac crest (Fig. 5-14). For all other levels of fusion, the L end of one rod passes across the spinous process of the superiorly fused vertebra, and the L end of the other rod passes across the spinous process of the inferior vertebra (Fig. 5-15). The rods are contoured prior to insertion to provide a lumbar lordosis and thoracic kyphosis. Each

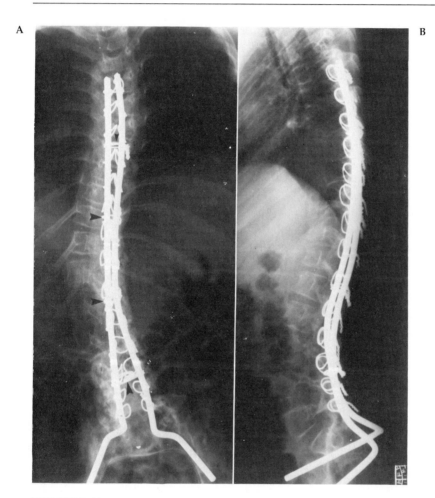

A　　　　　　　　　　　　　　　　　　　　　　　　　B

FIGURE 5-14

PA **(A)** and lateral **(B)** radiographs of an 8-year-old boy with cerebral palsy and long thoracolumbar scoliosis after Luque rod instrumentation and fusion. The distal rod ends are placed into the ilia. Contouring the rods produces normal thoracic kyphosis and lumbar lordosis. Four wires *(arrowheads)* join the two rods posteriorly. The other wires are sublaminar and attach each rod to ipsilateral laminae.

rod is then wired onto the lamina at each level. The two rods are then wired together (Fig. 5-16).

The same intraoperative and postoperative film sequences are used for both Luque and Harrington instrumentation. The only major difference in film interpretation from Harrington instrumentation is that the L-shaped rods are evaluated for slippage, and the retaining wires are checked for proper placement and fracture. The percentage of correction is determined by comparing the preoperative and postoperative upright PA films.

FIGURE 5-15
Cerebral palsy patient in a cast after Luque rod correction of right thoracic scoliosis. The overlapping short L ends *(arrowheads)* and sublaminar wires are clearly seen as are the wires uniting the rods *(arrows)*.

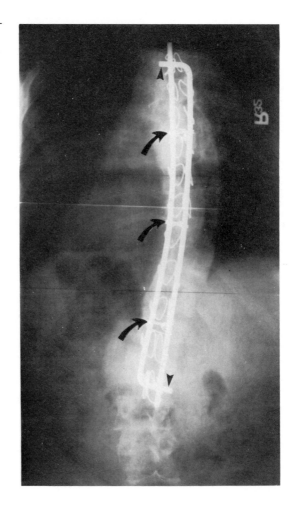

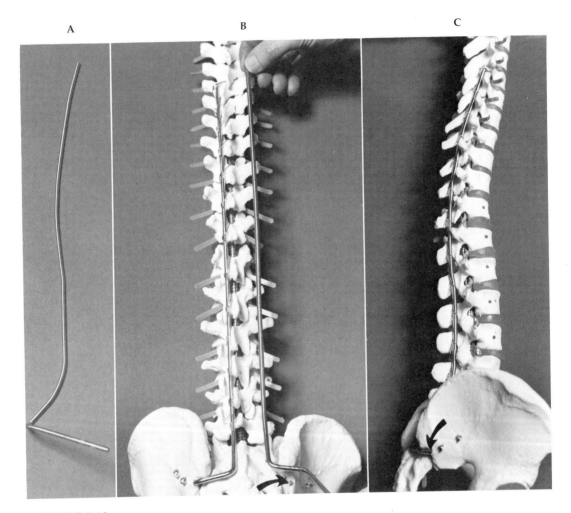

FIGURE 5-16
Positioning of Luque rods on assembled skeleton spine and pelvis.

A, Lateral view of contoured rod showing upper left convexity for the thoracic region, lower right convexity for the lumbar region, and contoured end for ilial insertion.

B, Posterior view. Compare left rod wired into position with right rod held above desired position. Drill hole for L end of right rod is seen *(arrow)*.

C, Lateral view illustrates the posterior iliac entry of the L end *(arrow)* and the rod contouring for the thoracic and lumbar regions.

Anterior Fusion and Instrumentation

Although posterior instrumentation and fusion is the safest and most commonly used method for correction of spinal deformities, anterior fusion is necessary in certain circumstances. Anterior fusion is generally recommended in the following conditions: (1) paralytic lumbar and thoracolumbar scoliosis over 75 degrees with pelvic obliquity, (2) scoliosis with deficient posterior elements owing to myelomeningocele or extensive laminectomy, (3) scoliosis with spastic cerebral palsy, (4) idiopathic lumbar or thoracolumbar scoliosis over 80 degrees, (5) congenital scoliosis owing to hemivertebra or unsegmented bar, and (6) severe congenital or acquired kyphosis.[4,19,33,46] In these conditions, posterior fusion even with internal fixation results in a high frequency of pseudarthrosis. Anterior fusion is usually performed first followed by posterior instrumentation and fusion with resultant greater curve correction and stability.

SURGICAL TECHNIQUE

Depending on the levels to be fused, either a transthoracic[4,6,7,9] or thoracoabdominal approach is used.[4,6,19,46] If the deformity is limited to the thoracic spine, a transthoracic approach is used, and the rib one level above the uppermost level of the fusion is removed. The parietal pleura is incised, and the lung and pleura are retracted away from the spine. If both thoracic and lumbar spine are to be fused, the thoracolumbar approach is used with transthoracic exposure of the thoracic spine and retroperitoneal exposure of the lumbar spine so the abdominal cavity need not be entered. The diaphragm must also be divided peripherally and reattached at the completion of the procedure. A retroperitoneal iliolumbar approach may be used for the lumbar spine and an anterior transabdominal exposure for the lumbosacral junction.

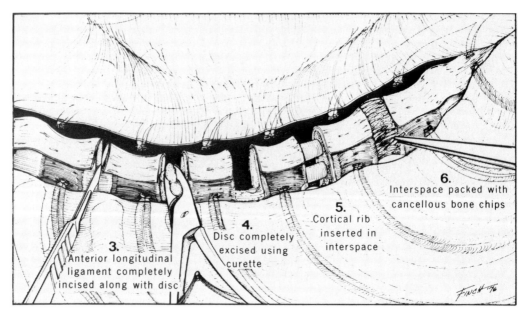

FIGURE 5-17
Anterior interbody fusion is accomplished by complete excision of the anterior longitudinal ligament along with removal of the disk. The disk is removed to the posterior annulus, and the intervening cartilage is removed to the bony endplates. If correction of the kyphosis is necessary, one should remove the posterior annulus along with the endplates up to the posterior longitudinal ligament. Generally, however, this will not be essential, since removal of the disk material up to the posterior annulus will make it possible to hinge open the kyphosis and significantly correct the angular deformity. The rib bone that has been removed during the thoracotomy is cut into small pieces and wedged into each intervertebral space, hinging the vertebral bodies open and correcting the kyphosis. Remaining rib strips are then placed into the interspace, or, if desirable, cancellous bone from the iliac crest may be used to supplement the fusion mass.
From Moe, J.H., et al.: Scoliosis and other spinal deformities, Philadelphia, 1978, W.B. Saunders.

The intervertebral disk and cartilaginous endplates at each selected level are removed with curettes. Into each of these disks, bits of bone from either the resected rib or the iliac crest are embedded (Fig. 5-17). If there is absence or marked deficiency of the vertebral bodies, as in cases of congenital kyphosis, an anterior "inlay" strut can be used for reinforcement.[6] A large trough is cut in the anterior aspect of the vertebral bodies. Undercut notches are created in the superior and inferior end vertebral bodies. The spine is distracted after insertion of the strut at one end to key it into the other notch.

Anterior strut fusion without the inlay technique can also be used for severe kyphosis.[6] Struts are created from the resected rib. The resected rib is usually cut into several pieces of varying lengths to span the kyphotic segment at several levels and increase the mechanical rigidity (Fig. 5-18). The

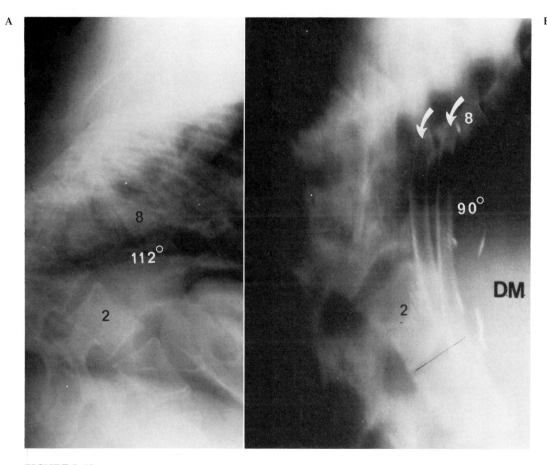

A   **B**

FIGURE 5-18

A, Severe 112 degree posttuberculosis T8-L2 kyphosis and apical vertebral destruction.

B, Reduction of the kyphosis to 90 degrees with two anterior rib strut grafts *(arrows).*

Courtesy Robert B. Winter, MD, Minneapolis, Minnesota.

advantage of such anterior graft material is that it is under compression from the kyphosis, which aids in graft union while a posterior graft would be under tension from distractive forces.[27]

DWYER INSTRUMENTATION

Dwyer instrumentation was the first commonly used method for internal fixation of an anterior spinal fusion. The technique produces excellent correction and fixation of thoracolumbar and lumbar scoliosis.[11,12] Because the technique draws the vertebral bodies together and increases kyphosis, it should not be used when there is hyperkyphosis.[47,51,52] Since it requires an anterior exposure, its use is not recommended in high thoracic curves where anterior exposure is technically difficult.[26,47] Although Dwyer instrumentation allows dramatic correction of idiopathic thoracolumbar and lumbar scolioses,[26,52] one authority[4] prefers the use of Harrington instrumentation, which has fewer complications and is easier to insert. Despite these difficulties, others[20,26,47] prefer the Dwyer instrumentation because it more completely corrects both the lateral deviation and rotation of the spine. In patients with combined thoracic and lumbar scoliosis where the lumbar curve is painful, progressive, and larger than the thoracic curve, a two-stage procedure with both Dwyer and Harrington instrumentations has been suggested.[57]

The instrumentation consists of screws, vertebral staples or plates, and a braided cable (Fig. 5-19). The staples fit around each vertebral body to be fused, and a screw passes through a hole in the staple into the center of the vertebral body. Each screw has a vertical opening in its head to allow passage of the cable.

The transthoracic or, more commonly, thoracolumbar approach is used for this type of instrumentation. Diskectomies are performed at all the levels. The staples are placed about the vertebral bodies. After placing the staples, screws are selected that are just long enough to penetrate through both sides of the vertebral body, thereby achieving the most rigid cortical fixation possible. The cable is then slid through the opening in the top screw, and the disk space is closed tightly upon the inserted bone graft (Fig. 5-20). The screw head is then crimped with a special crimper to prevent sliding of the cable.[48] The same procedure is followed at each level from the superior to the most inferior vertebral body to be included in the fusion. A reinforcing collar is placed on the cable just below the lower-most screw and then crimped in place. A second reinforcing collar can be crimped over the cut end of the cable to cover the free wire strands which could cut into retroperitoneal structures.

A 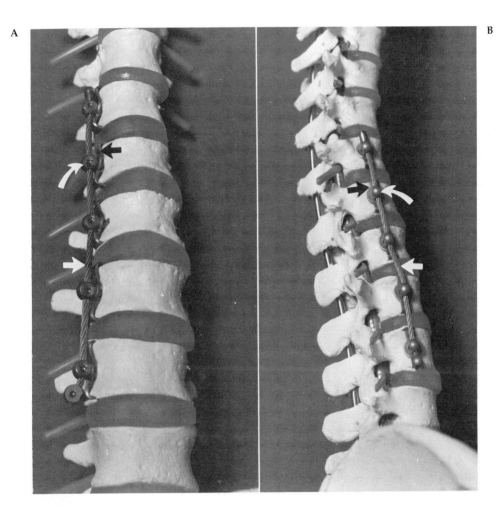 B

FIGURE 5-19
Anterior **(A)** and right lateral **(B)** views of Dwyer instrumentation inserted onto an
assembled spine. The cable *(white arrow)*, one staple *(black arrow)*, and one screw
(curved white arrow) are marked.

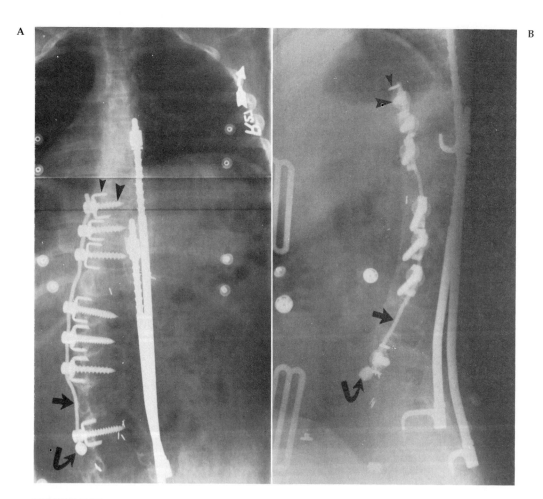

FIGURE 5-20
PA **(A)** and lateral **(B)** radiographs of an 8-year-old girl with a repaired myelomeningocele and surgical correction of a thoracolumbar scoliosis with Harrington rods and Dwyer instrumentation. The Dwyer system consists of screws *(large arrowhead)*, staples *(small arrowhead)*, cable *(arrow)*, and crimped-on reinforcing collar *(curved arrow)* at the cut end of the cable.

ZIELKE INSTRUMENTATION

In 1976, a new form of anterior spinal instrumentation was introduced by Zielke.[41] Operative series are now just being reported, but early results show results comparable to those achieved with Dwyer instrumentation.[41] Because of its greater ability to correct vertebral rotation, Zielke instrumentation is now generally preferred over Dwyer instrumentation whenever anterior internal fixation is desired.

The operative technique has been described in detail by Moe et al.[41] The instrumentation consists of single screws inserted in each vertebral body to be fused (Figs. 5-21 and 5-22). Each screw is then linked by a flexible 4.76 mm (³/₁₆ inch) stainless-steel threaded rod. Two locking nuts are placed around

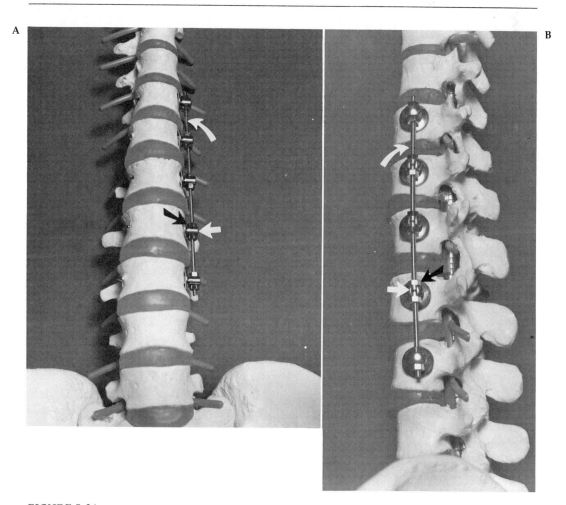

A   B

FIGURE 5-21
Anterior **(A)** and lateral **(B)** views of Zielke instrumentation placed on assembled spine specimen. The flexible, threaded rod *(curved white arrow)*, one screw *(white arrow)*, and one retaining nut *(black arrow)* are marked.

A

B

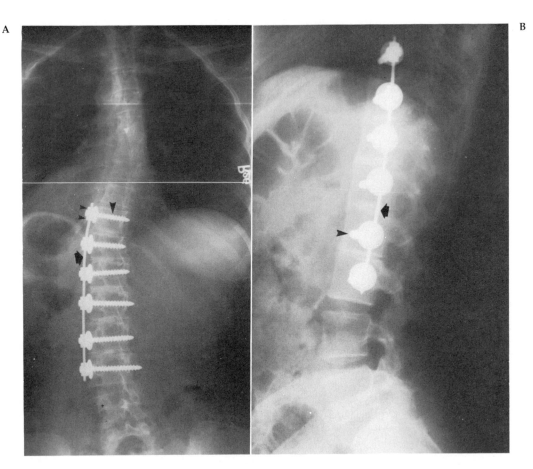

FIGURE 5-22
PA **(A)** and lateral **(B)** radiograph of a solid anterior fusion with intact Zielke instrumentation. Note the transvertebral screws *(large arrowhead)*, flexible rod *(arrow)*, and two retaining nuts *(small arrowheads)* about each screw.

each screw (Figs. 5-21 and 5-22). After curve correction is complete, the threads of the rod around the locking nuts are destroyed to prevent the nuts from unwinding.

All vertebrae that are wedged open to the convexity of the curve or that are translated laterally more than 0.5 cm are instrumented. The screws are placed as far posteriorly in the vertebral body as possible and pass in a slight posteroanterior direction. This positioning causes vertebral body derotation when the screws are drawn onto the rod. Screw length is selected so that the distalmost thread of the screw just engages the concave vertebral cortex. Exposure and fusion techniques are similar to those used for Dwyer instrumentation, although wedge-shaped disk space bone graft is recommended to reduce the resultant kyphosis if an increase in kyphosis is not desired.

In a series of 45 patients with idiopathic scoliosis, an average curve correction of 75% was achieved with a subsequent average loss of curve correction of 4 degrees.[41] Rotation and lateral translation were usually completely corrected in these same patients. Mechanical failures have been frequent with a 5% incidence of pseudarthrosis, 12.5% incidence of rod fracture, and a 47.5% incidence of partial pull-out of one or more screws.[41] Despite these complications, loss of curve correction has been low, and patient satisfaction with the procedure has been good.[41]

RADIOGRAPHIC EVALUATION

As for the posterior instrumentation and fusion, intraoperative radiographs are obtained for level localization. Postoperative films are then obtained to verify the degree of correction and to ensure proper placement of either the strut grafts or the instrumentation devices. Lateral tomograms are useful to delineate the location of strut grafts (Fig. 5-18, *B*). Each Dwyer staple should be within the excised superior and inferior disk space. The Dwyer and Zielke screws should penetrate through both cortices, without an excessive amount of screw protruding through into the retroperitoneum. On the upright postoperative films, continued proper seating of the various staples and screws is verified.

Summary

I. Posterior fusion and instrumentation
   A. Preoperative radiographic evaluation
      1. Upright PA film to determine length of fusion and Harrington hook placement
      2. Supine left and right bending films
         a. To determine if both thoracic and lumbar curves need fusion
         b. To estimate achievable operative correction
      3. Lateral film—use compression rod if thoracic hyperkyphosis
   B. Surgical technique
      1. Remove facet joint cartilage and pack with bone chips
      2. Decorticate laminae and lay longitudinal "matchstick" graft from the ilium
   C. Posterior instrumentation
      1. Harrington
         a. Distraction and compression rods available
         b. Contour distraction rod for normal sagittal plane contour
      2. Luque
         a. Offers greater curve stability but increased difficulty of insertion
         b. Both L ends in ilia if lumbosacral fusion
II. Anterior fusion and instrumentation
   A. Indications
      1. Deficient posterior elements

  2. Many forms of neuromuscular scoliosis
  3. Severe deformity requiring staged fusion
 B. Surgical technique
  1. Completely remove disks and endplates
  2. Place bone graft
 C. Dwyer and Zielke instrumentations
  1. Both use transvertebral screw that should just penetrate the oppo-
    site cortex
  2. Both increase kyphosis

REFERENCES

1. Aaro, S., and Ohlen, G.: The effect of Harrington instrumentation on the sagittal configuration and mobility of the spine in scoliosis, Spine 8:570-575, 1983.
2. Allen, B.L., Jr., and Ferguson, R.L.: The Galveston technique for L rod instrumentation of the scoliotic spine, Spine 7:276-284, 1982.
3. Asher, M.A., Gilbert, J., and Orrick J.: Harrington distraction (D) versus distraction plus compression (D + C) for the correction of right thoracic idiopathic scoliosis, Orthop. Trans. 2:272, 1978.
4. Bradford, D.S.: Anterior spinal surgery in the management of scoliosis, Orthop. Clin. North Am. 10:801-812, 1979.
5. Bradford, D.S., Blatt, J.M., and Rasp, F.L.: Surgical management of severe thoracic lordosis. A new technique to restore normal kyphosis, Spine 8:420-428, 1983.
6. Bradford, D.S., et al.: Techniques of anterior spinal surgery for the management of kyphosis, Clin. Orthop. 128:129-139, 1977.
7. Burrington, J.D., et al.: Anterior approach to the thoracolumbar spine: technical considerations, Arch. Surg. 111:456-463, 1976.
8. Cochran, T., Irstam, L., and Nachemson A.: Long-term anatomic and functional changes in patients with adolescent idiopathic scoliosis treated by Harrington rod fusion, Spine 8:576-584, 1983.
9. Cook, W.A.: Transthoracic vertebral surgery, Ann. Thorac. Surg. 12:54-68, 1971.
10. Crawford, A.H., MacEwen, G.D., and Lokietek, W.: Surgical management of idiopathic scoliosis at the Alfred I. Dupont Institute, Ohio State Med. J. 75:513-517, 1979.
11. Dwyer, A.F.: Experience of anterior correction of scoliosis, Clin. Orthop. 93:191-206, 1973.
12. Dwyer, A.F., and Schafer, M.F.: Anterior approach to scoliosis: results of treatment in fifty-one cases, J. Bone Joint Surg. (Br.) 56:218-224, 1974.
13. Fisk, J.R., Winter, R.B., and Moe, J.H.: The lumbosacaral curve in idiopathic scoliosis, J. Bone Joint Surg. (Am.) 62:39-45, 1980.
14. Gaines, R.W., and Leatherman, K.D.: Benefits of the Harrington compression system in lumbar and thoracolumbar idiopathic scoliosis in adolescents and adults, Spine 6:483-488, 1981.
15. Gaines, R.W., McKinley, L.M., and Leatherman, K.D.: Intraoperative comparison of relative corrections of rib hump comparing the use of Harrington distraction rod with Harrington combined distraction and compression systems, Orthop. Trans. 2:272, 1978.
16. Goldstein, L.A.: Surgical management of scoliosis, J. Bone Joint Surg. (Am.) 48:167-196, 1966.
17. Goldstein, L.A.: The surgical management of scoliosis, Clin. Orthop. 77:32-56, 1971.
18. Goldstein, L.A.: The surgical treatment of idiopathic scoliosis, Clin. Orthop. 93:131-157, 1973.

19. Hall, J.E.: The anterior approach to spinal deformities, Orthop. Clin. North Am. **3:**81-98, 1972.

20. Hall, J.E.: Current concepts review: Dwyer instrumentation in anterior fusion of the spine, J. Bone Joint Surg. (Am.) **63:**1188-1190, 1981.

21. Harrington, P.R.: Surgical instrumentation for management of scoliosis, J. Bone Joint Surg. (Am.) **42:**1448, 1960.

22. Harrington, P.R.: Treatment of scoliosis: correction and internal fixation by spine instrumentation, J. Bone Joint Surg. (Am.) **44:**591-610, 1962.

23. Harrington, P.R.: The management of scoliosis by spine instrumentation: an evaluation of more than 200 cases, South. Med. J. **56:**1367-1377, 1963.

24. Harrington, P.R.: Technical details in relation to the successful use of instrumentation in scoliosis, Orthop. Clin. North Am. **3:**49-67, 1972.

25. Herring, J.A., and Wenger, D.R.: Segmental spinal instrumentation, Spine **7:**285-298, 1982.

26. Hsu, L.C.S., et al.: Dwyer instrumentation in the treatment of adolescent idiopathic scoliosis, J. Bone Joint Surg. (Br.) **64:**536-541, 1982.

27. Johnson, J.T.H., and Robinson, R.A.: Anterior strut grafts for severe kyphosis, Clin. Orthop. **56:**25-36, 1968.

28. King, H.A., et al.: Selection of fusion levels in thoracic idiopathic scoliosis, Orthop. Trans. **5:**25, 1981.

29. King, H.A., et al.: The selection of fusion levels in thoracic idiopathic scoliosis, J. Bone Joint Surg. (Am.) **65:**1302-1313, 1983.

30. Kleinman, R.G., et al.: The radiographic assessment of spinal flexibility in scoliosis: a study of the efficacy of the prone push film, Clin. Orthop. **162:**47-53, 1982.

31. Kostuik, J.P., and Hall, B.B.: Spinal fusions to the sacrum in adults with scoliosis, Spine **8:**489-500, 1983.

32. Lahde, R.E.: Luque rod instrumentation, AORN J. **38:**35-43, 1983.

33. Leatherman, K.D.: Current status of anterior spine surgery for scoliosis, Clin. Orthop. **126:**93-99, 1977.

34. Luque, E.R.: Segmental correction of scoliosis with rigid internal fixation: preliminary report, Orthop. Trans. **1:**136, 1977.

35. Luque, E.R.: Treatment of scoliosis without external support, Orthop. Trans. **1:**37, 1977.

36. Luque, E.R.: Segmental spinal instrumentation for correction of scoliosis, Clin. Orthop. **163:**192-198, 1982.

37. McAfee, P.C., et al.: The use of segmental spinal instrumentation to preserve longitudinal spinal growth, J. Bone Joint Surg. (Am.) **65:**935-942, 1983.

38. Moe, J.H.: A critical analysis of methods of fusion for scoliosis: an evaluation in two hundred and sixty-six patients, J. Bone Joint Surg. (Am.) **40:**529-554, 1958.

39. Moe, J.H.: Methods of correction and surgical techniques in scoliosis, Orthop Clin. North Am. **3:**17-48, 1972.

40. Moe, J.H.: The classic: a critical analysis of methods of fusion for scoliosis: an evaluation in two hundred and sixty-six patients, Clin. Orthop. **126:**4-16, 1977.

41. Moe, J.H., Purcell, G.A., and Bradford, D.S.: Zielke instrumentation (VDS) for the correction of spinal curvature, Clin. Orthop. **180:**133-153, 1983.

42. Moe, J.H., et al.: Subcutaneous Harrington instrumentation without fusion plus external orthotic support for the treatment of difficult curvature problems in young children, Clin. Orthop. **185:**35-45, 1984.

43. Neuwirth, M.G.: Segmental spinal instrumentation. A historic review and current concepts, Bull. Hosp. Joint Dis. Orthop. Inst. **63:**49-55, 1983.

44. Ogilvie, J.W., and Millar, E.A.: Comparison of segmental spinal instrumentation devices in the correction of scoliosis, Spine **8:**416-419, 1983.

45. Resina, J., and Alves, A.F.: A technique of correction and internal fixation for scoliosis, J. Bone Joint Surg. (Br.) **59:**159-165, 1977.

46. Riseborough, E.J.: The anterior approach to the spine for the correction of deformities of the axial skeleton, Clin. Orthop. **93**:207-214, 1973.
47. Schafer, M.F.: Dwyer instrumentation of the spine, Orthop. Clin. North Am. **9**:115-122, 1978.
48. Schafer, M.F., Page, D., and Shen, G.: Mechanical evaluation of the Dwyer screw-cable attachment, Spine **4**:398-400, 1979.
49. Schultz, A.B., and Hirsch, C.: Mechanical analysis of techniques for improved correction of idiopathic scoliosis, Clin. Orthop. **100**:66-73, 1973.
50. Shipps, F., and McKirdie, M.: Operative cholangiography using a 6:1 crisscrossed grid, AJR **119**:46-51, 1973.
51. Simmons, E.H., et al.: An analysis of Dwyer instrumentation of the spine with assessment of its place in spinal surgery, J. Bone Joint Surg. (Br.) **59**:117, 1977.
52. Stephen, J.P., Wilding, K., and Cass, C.A.: The place of Dwyer anterior instrumentation in scoliosis, Med. J. Aust. **1**:206-208, 1977.
53. Ulin, R.I., and McGinniss, G.H.: Segmental spinal instrumentation at the Mount Sinai Hospital, Mt Sinai J. Med. **50**:348-350, 1983.
54. Waugh, T.R.: Intravital measurements during instrumental correction of idiopathic scoliosis, Acta Orthop. Scand. (Suppl.) **93**:1-87, 1966.
55. Wenger, D.R., Carollo, J.J., and Wilkerson, J.A., Jr.: Biomechanics of scoliosis correction by segmental spinal instrumentation, Spine **7**:260-264, 1982.
56. Wenger, D.R., et al.: Laboratory testing of segmental spinal instrumentation versus traditional Harrington instrumentation for scoliosis treatment, Spine **7**:265-269, 1982.
57. Winter, R.B.: Combined Dwyer and Harrington instrumentation and fusion in the treatment of selected patients with painful adult idiopathic scoliosis, Spine **3**:135-141, 1978.
58. Winter, R.B.: Posterior spinal fusion in scoliosis: indications, technique, and results, Orthop. Clin. North Am. **10**:787-800, 1979.

Chapter Six

Radiologic Evaluation of Surgical Complications

*T*he radiologically detectable skeletal complications of spinal arthrodesis are internal fixation device failure, pseudarthrosis, and loss of curve correction.[15,50] These complications are interrelated in that fixation device failure frequently occurs if a pseudarthrosis develops, and there is often resultant loss of curve correction. However, each of these complications may occur independently and, hence, will be discussed separately. The frequency, clinical implications, and radiologic evaluation of the skeletal complications of spinal arthrodesis will be stressed.

The other complications of spinal fusion include infection, hemorrhage, spinal cord injury, thrombophlebitis, nerve entrapment, and rod pressure effects and have been thoroughly reviewed.[6,17,43] They will not be discussed, as they are evaluated primarily clinically and not radiographically.

In evaluating the frequency of spinal arthrodesis complications, it should be remembered that both skeletal and nonskeletal complications are increased when surgery is performed for adult scoliosis.[28,44,48] In a recent review, Swank reported a complication rate of 50% for surgical correction of adult scoliosis.[47] The most frequent reported complications were instrument failure (11% to 25%), pseudarthrosis (10% to 17.6%), and infection (4.5% to 8.7%). Complications are considerably less frequent with surgical correction of adolescent idiopathic scoliosis during the second decade of life.

Internal Fixation Device Fracture
HARRINGTON INSTRUMENTATION

Constant bending or loading of a metallic fixation device results in metal fatigue and subsequent fracture. All metal will eventually fracture if subjected to continued stress. For this reason, spinal instrumentation is intended only to obtain initial reduction of the spinal deformity and to maintain reduction until the bony fusion becomes solid. If the metal fractures, there are three major causes: (1) inadequate immobilization while the fusion is solidifying, (2) failure of the fusion, that is, a pseudarthrosis, or (3) location of a fixation device hook outside of the extent of the fusion.

Each cause of failure has different clinical implications so that metal failure is not necessarily indicative of an unsuccessful surgical procedure. If the spine was inadequately immobilized with a cast or brace during fusion maturation and the fixation device fractures, there will usually be a loss of curve correction. Only if curve worsening is significant will removal of the fractured metal and insertion of a new rod to regain the lost correction be necessary. Further cast or brace treatment until the fusion is solid may be all that is needed. The length of the period of postoperative spinal immobilization with a brace or cast is controversial, with a recommended range of 6 to 12 months.[29,35,47,52] Spinal fusions are usually solid by 7 to 10 months postoperatively, although a few require 15 to 18 months.[53] For this reason, metal fracture occurring more than 1 year postoperatively suggests that the bone fusion is not solid and that a pseudarthrosis is present.[51] In this situation, reoperation and repair of any pseudarthrosis is indicated. However, an alternative cause for metal failure may be that the fusion did not extend over the entire length of the fixation device.[25] This most commonly occurs about the upper hook of a Harrington distraction rod. Because the rod extends beyond the length of the fusion, it is subjected to bending forces from the still mobile segment of the spine. The repetitive flexion results in metal fatigue. In this situation, the rod may fracture, but it is clinically insignificant unless the curve progresses to include the nonfused spinal segment or the fractured rod causes local pain.

Compression rod fracture is uncommon, occurring in only one of 888 patients when current fusion techniques were used.[14] There may be loss of curve correction of 3 to 5 degrees, but operative intervention is not recom-

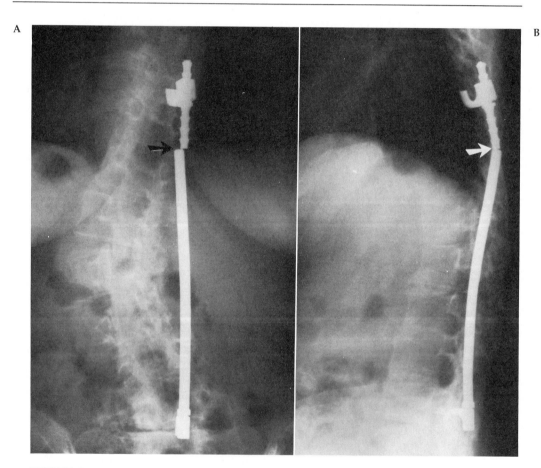

FIGURE 6-1

Anteroposterior (AP) (A) and lateral (B) radiographs of a 51-year-old woman with a tenth thoracic (T10) to first sacral (S1) fusion for left lumbar scoliosis and severe lumbar degenerative disk disease. The Harrington distraction rod has fractured at the junction of the smooth and ratcheted portions (arrows).

mended.[24] If the broken ends irritate overlying tissues, the fractured rods should be removed or the protruding portions cut off.

The distraction rods fracture more commonly than the compression rods. The usual fracture site is at the junction of the smooth and notched portions of the rod[24] (Fig. 6-1). The reported incidence of rod fracture is highly variable, ranging from 0% to 12%,[18,49,51] but most series report an incidence of 2.1% to 7.0%.* The reduction in rod fracture over the past two decades reflects extensive clinical studies defining the optimal techniques for spinal fusion. As a generalization, a spinal fusion is more likely to be successful if the facet joints are decorticated and packed with bone chips, if autogenous graft is used for posterolateral fusion, and if the spine is immobilized postoperatively with a cast or brace.[25] Prolonged postoperative bedrest is of no benefit,[35] and most authorities now maintain enforced bedrest for only 3 to 14 days postoperatively with an average of 7 days.[5,47,52,53] The arthrodesis appears to heal more strongly with the vertical loading that occurs when the patient is upright in a cast or brace.[24,52]

As discussed in the beginning of this section, the clinical significance of a rod fracture depends on its cause and the effect on the curve.[14] If the rod fractures early without a significant loss of correction and healing of the bone is progressing, further observation is all that is necessary. If the rod fractures after 1 year, pseudarthrosis must be suspected but may not be present. Harrington has recommended that these patients be monitored by follow-up radiographs at 3 to 6 month intervals.[23,25] If the rod ends do not overlap or if the curve does not worsen, presumably at least one end of the rod is outside of the bone graft, but the extent of the fusion is sufficient to prevent curve progression.[24] In this situation, further surgery is not needed. However, with current surgical techniques, insufficient length of fusion is infrequent, so most fractured rods now reflect an underlying pseudarthrosis.

LUQUE INSTRUMENTATION

Because of the segmental nature of the force distribution with the Luque rod, rod fracture is uncommon (Fig. 6-2). More commonly, one of the sublaminar retaining wires fractures.[30] Because of the multiple fixation points, a single fractured wire is often insignificant unless there is local irritation or wire migration. Wire fracture occurred in two of Luque's original 65 patients.[30] Wire migration into the spinal canal with subsequent neurologic symptoms has been reported in one patient.[2]

DWYER AND ZIELKE INSTRUMENTATIONS

Although the Dwyer instrumentation also has multiple fixation points, instrumentation fractures are more common than with Luque instrumentation.[46] The increased incidence of fracture probably reflects the preselection of more complex and intractable spine deformities for this type of instrumenta-

---

*See references 7, 14, 17, 22, 25, 48.

A

B

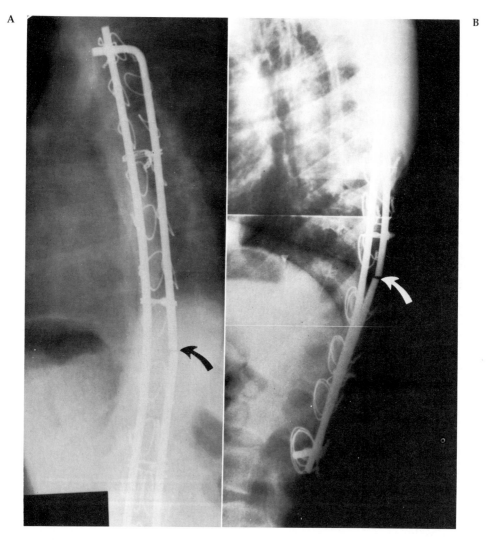

FIGURE 6-2
AP **(A)** and lateral **(B)** radiographs of a fractured Luque rod near the curve apex in
a 16-year-old boy with cerebral palsy.

tion. The generated forces are larger and the incidence of pseudarthrosis is
higher than with Luque instrumentation, ranging from 6.5%[46] to 12%[20] to
19.4%.[13] It has been suggested that the incidence of pseudarthrosis will be
decreased by more thorough removal of the disk-space material and subperiosteal exposure of the spine.[19] Fractures usually develop through the cable at
the apex of the curve (Fig. 6-3).

Because of its recent development, few reports are available on the complications associated with Zielke instrumentation. Moe et al.[38] reported that
the rods fractured in 12.5% (5/40) of their patients who had Zielke instrumentation.

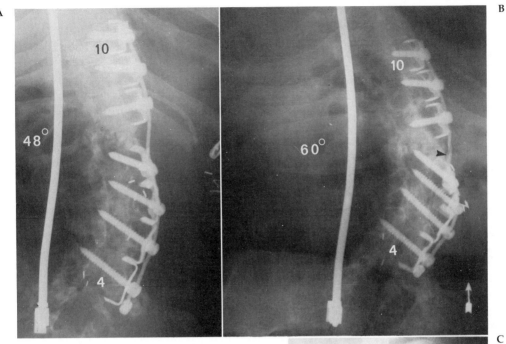

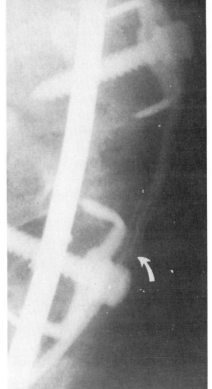

FIGURE 6-3
Spinal dysraphism and scoliosis in a
27-year-old man.
A, Initial radiograph after two-stage anterior
  fusion with Dwyer instrumentation and
  posterior fusion with Harrington rod.
B, One year later, the curve has increased
  and the cable is frayed *(arrowhead).*
C, Coned-down lateral radiograph better
  showing fractured cable *(arrow).*

Internal Fixation Device Displacement
HARRINGTON INSTRUMENTATION

In the early series of patients treated with Harrington distraction rods, several of the upper hooks slipped on the ratched portion of the rod resulting in loss of curve correction.[3,23,26,42] Because the effective distraction length of the rod decreases with retraction of the hook, the curve usually worsens. To solve this problem, a washer or retaining wire is now placed beneath the upper hook. Because the upper edge of the hook catches on the ratchets and the length of the hook is not proportional to the length of a ratchet, a full or half notch gap may normally be seen between the hook and the washer (Fig. 6-4).

Hook dislodgement is still a problem occurring in 1.4% to 8.8% of patients.* The hook may slip from the facet joint onto the transverse process, which results in 5 to 7 degrees of curve worsening. Reoperation may not be necessary. More commonly, the hook rotates off the spine into the overlying soft tissues (Fig. 6-4). Usually, the hooks dislodge during the immediate postoperative period with movement of the patient. The hook should be reinserted surgically in this situation. The postoperative radiographs should be carefully scrutinized for this complication. Anteroposterior (AP) and lateral postoperative radiographs are recommended because the dislodged hook may be detectable on only one of these projections.

LUQUE INSTRUMENTATION

Luque rod displacement is uncommon and generally occurs only with crossing double L rods. The short, bent end of the L-shaped rod is not fixed into bone so the rod can shift in the soft tissues if the spine is not immobilized in the postoperative period or if the spinal fusion is not solid.[2] In the absence of a pseudarthrosis, repositioning of the rod is usually not necessary. If the rods have been driven into the ilia as part of a lumbosacral fusion, displacement is rare.

DWYER AND ZIELKE INSTRUMENTATIONS

The most common cause of displacement of either Dwyer or Zielke instrumentation is pulling free of a transvertebral screw. Each screw should pass through the right and left sides of the vertebral body cortex. If only one cortex is penetrated because the screw is too short, screw pull-out can occur. The screws at the ends of the device are the most common site for pull-out with both Dwyer[11] and Zielke[38] instrumentations.

---

*See references 3, 7, 10, 18, 22, 23, 29, 35, 42, 44, 49, 51.

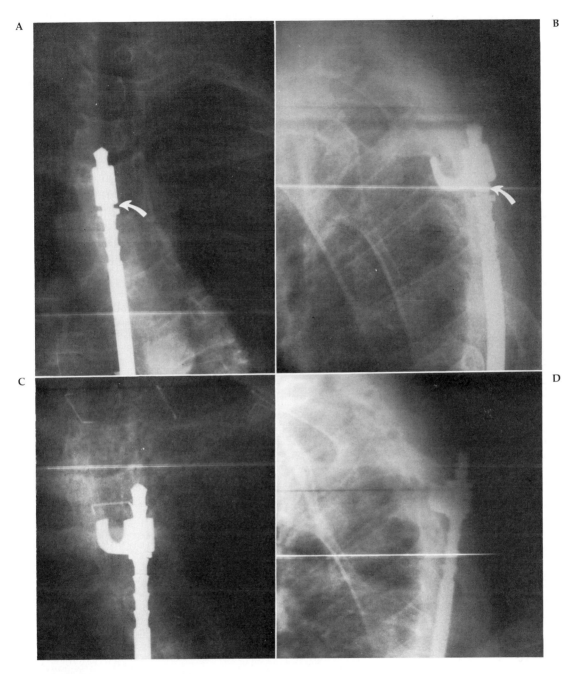

FIGURE 6-4
Coned-down AP **(A)** and lateral **(B)** postoperative radiographs of the upper end of a Harrington distraction rod. Note the normal gap *(arrows)* between the hook and the washer. After cast placement, AP **(C)** and lateral **(D)** radiographs show the hook settled onto the washer and rotated off the lamina.

Pseudarthrosis

Pseudarthrosis or failure of graft union is the most common skeletal complication of spinal fusion. Early attempts at spinal fusion resulted in a high incidence (10% to 39%) of pseudarthrosis even in patients with idiopathic scoliosis.* As a consequence, some authorities routinely explored all spine fusions 6 months later and placed bone graft at any poorly healing sites.[33] As experience was gained, the incidence of pseudarthrosis after fusion for idiopathic scoliosis has been reduced to less than 10%.† A 6 month exploration is no longer recommended.[32] The improved results reflect the development of better methods of facet joint fusion and the use of supplementary autogenous bone graft for the posterolateral fusion.[24,36]

Even with the best technique, pseudarthrosis may still occur. It is usually manifested clinically by localized pain over the pseudarthrosis site or radiographically by loss of curve correction. If a curve progresses in the postoperative period when the curve should be stable, the site of the pseudarthrosis can be determined by radiologic examination prior to surgical repair.

*See references 4, 6, 8, 16, 23, 28, 36, 37, 43, 44.
†See references 7, 18, 29, 34, 39, 42, 49.

FIGURE 6-5
Oblique lumbar radiograph after internal fixation and posterior fusion for spondylolisthesis. The posterior graft is evident *(arrowheads)* and solid from the fourth lumbar (L4) to the sacrum.

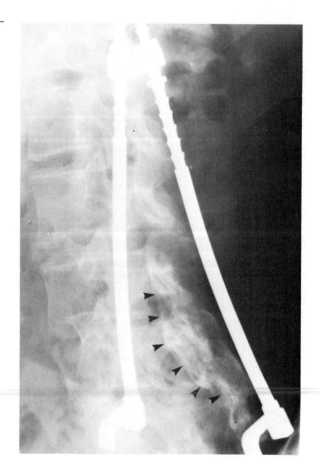

As a first step for pseudarthrosis detection, coned-down AP, lateral, and oblique films of the fusion should be obtained. The bone graft is best visualized on the oblique films (Fig. 6-5). A pseudarthrosis presents as a radiolucent defect with well defined borders all the way across the bone mass. However, because of the thickness of the graft, a pseudarthrosis may be obscured on routine radiographs, or an apparent defect may actually be incomplete in a functionally solid graft. In these circumstances, tomograms may be useful.

CONVENTIONAL TOMOGRAPHY

In general, multidirectional tomograms provide better delineation of bone graft material than linear tomograms. The linear ghost artifacts of linear tomography across a pseudarthrosis may mimic bridging spicules. However, if a metal device is present, linear tomograms are preferable (Fig. 6-6). Because of the extreme radioopacity of the metal, it is incompletely blurred out by any pattern of tomographic motion. Multidirectional tube motion generates metal shadows that overlie most of the image (Fig. 6-7). If linear tube motion is along the axis of the metal rod, there is less metal artifact, and the

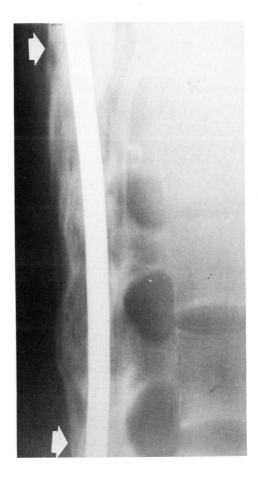

FIGURE 6-6
Linear lateral tomogram clearly reveals solid bony fusion *(between arrows)* posterior to the distraction rod with no blurring of the rod.

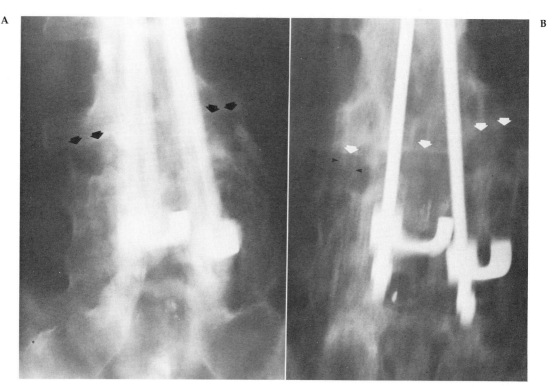

FIGURE 6-7
L4-5 pseudarthrosis.
A, Hypocycloidal tomogram sharply defines lateral margins *(arrows)* of the
  pseudarthrosis but central portion is obscured by tomographic blurring of
  distraction rods.
B, Linear tomogram creates several linear "ghosts" *(arrowheads)*, but complete
  pseudarthrosis defect is visualized *(arrows)*.

graft can at least be visualized (Fig. 6-7). On tomography, a pseudarthrosis
appears as a linear well defined radiolucent defect throughout the full-thick-
ness of the graft (Fig. 6-7). Dawson et al.[9] found that plain film evaluation for
pseudarthrosis correlated with the operative findings in only 54% of cases,
but tomographic findings correlated with operative findings in 95% of cases.
They recommended using tomography as a diagnostic predictor with the
following guidelines. If a single unilateral bone graft defect is found, only
close observation is suggested. In those patients with multiple unilateral defects, activity should be restricted. A second operation to augment the fusion
is recommended whenever complete bilateral defects are detected.

A

B

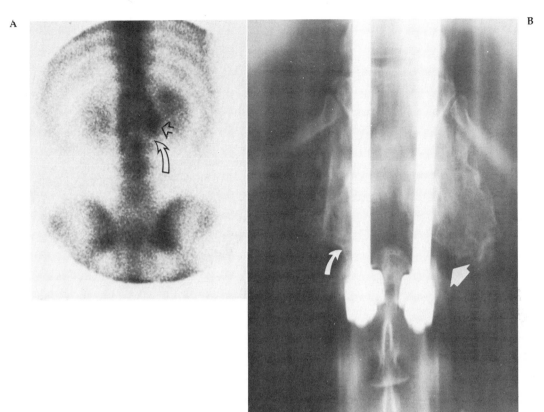

FIGURE 6-8
Right L1-2 pseudarthrosis.
A, 99mTc methylene diphosphonate bone scan shows photopenic area *(curved arrow)*
   at site of pseudarthrosis just below increased uptake *(arrow)* at superior
   hypertrophic bone.
B, AP linear tomogram (reversed for comparison purposes) confirms pseudarthrosis
   (arrow) just below hypertrophic bone. The graft is solid on the left *(curved arrow)*.

BONE SCANS

Radionuclide bone scans have also been used to detect pseudarthrosis in
spinal fusion.[21,34] McMaster and Merrick thoroughly evaluated the usefulness
of bone scanning in an extensive prospective study of 110 scoliotic patients.[34]
They routinely performed bone scans and surgical exploration on all patients
6 months after the spinal arthrodesis. One of their nine patients with a
pseudarthrosis had a normal bone scan. The other eight patients had abnormal bone scans but so did one third of the patients with solid fusions. Diffuse
patchy radionuclide uptake was entirely nonspecific and was believed to be
caused by continued healing of immature fusions. A focal area of increased
uptake (Fig. 6-8) was more specific, but half of the patients with this pattern
still had a solid fusion at exploration. In two patients, a repeat bone scan at 1
year was helpful in that a focal area of uptake developed when there had been

previously diffuse patchy uptake. They speculated that bone scanning at 1 year may be more clinically useful. Bone scanning is not recommended in the diagnosis of well established pseudarthroses as the bone scans were normal in 11 patients with operatively confirmed pseudarthroses which were diagnosed and treated at an average of 45 months after the original spinal fusion.[21]

In summary, radionuclide scanning has limited usefulness for the detection of pseudarthrosis. Prior to 1 year postoperatively, areas of irregular graft maturation prevent detection of a pseudarthrosis, and after 2 to 3 years, the pseudarthroses become mature so increased bone activity is no longer detected. In the period between 1 and 2 years postoperatively, scanning may be useful if one remembers that there will still be frequent false positives. We prefer to use tomography if signs of a pseudarthrosis, such as localized pain, curve progression, or instrument failure, develop.

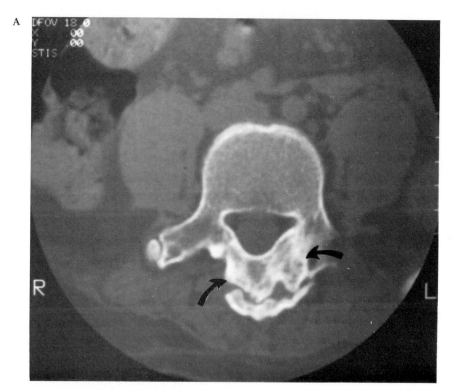

FIGURE 6-9
CT of L4-5 pseudarthrosis.
A, Scan at L5 shows solid posterior bone fusion mass *(arrows)* although a curvilinear posterior fragment is ununited.
B, Scan at L4-5 disk level demonstrates right hemilaminectomy. The left facet joint did not fuse and has an ununited fragment medially *(arrow)*.
C, Oblique longitudinal reconstruction confirms failure of facet fusion and pseudarthrosis *(arrowheads)*.

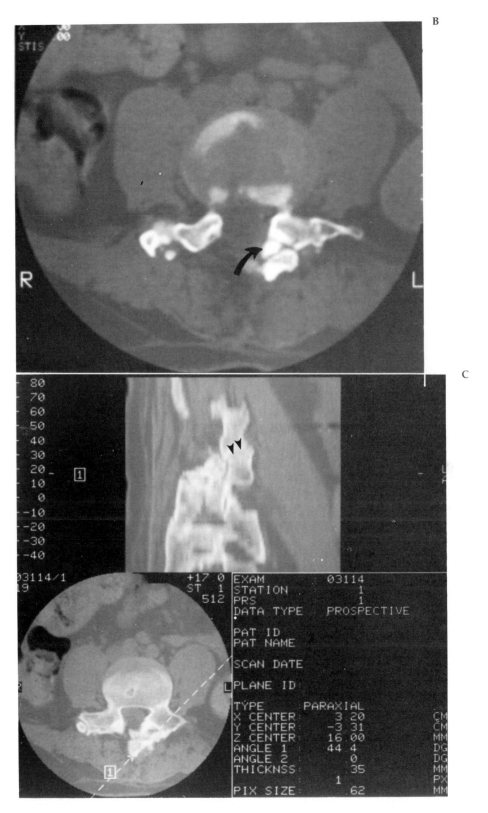

FIGURE 6-9, cont'd
For legend see opposite page.

COMPUTED TOMOGRAPHY (CT)

CT has recently been used to detect bone graft maturation. CT provides cross-sectional imaging, so it is useful for determining the quality of the bone fusion mass (Fig. 6-9). However, two factors significantly limit the use of CT scanning for the detection of spinal pseudarthrosis. First, metallic internal fixation devices cause significant streak artifacts although a space-enhancing algorithm minimizes these artifacts.[31] Second, pseudarthroses usually occur transversely in the plane of the CT sections so that the pseudarthrosis may not be detected owing to volume averaging across a narrow defect. Thin-section scans can be used to image a narrow pseudarthrosis (Fig. 6-9), but thin-section scans over a long fusion to locate an occult pseudarthrosis are not practical.

Loss of Curve Correction
HARRINGTON INSTRUMENTATION

The initial postoperative correction of an abnormal spinal curvature is usually quite dramatic. Curve correction is usually expressed as a percentage where the curve Cobb angle on the first postoperative standing radiograph is subtracted from the preoperative standing Cobb angle, and the result is divided by the preoperative angle multiplied by 100. For instance, a 70 degree preoperative curve corrected to a 28 degree curve represents a 60% curve correction ($100 \times [70° - 28°]/70°$).

Correction of idiopathic adolescent scoliosis with Harrington instrumentation has a reported range of correction of 38.5% to 65%.* With modern techniques, an average correction of 50% to 60% should be expected in idiopathic adolescent scoliosis.[52] The amount of curve correction that can be achieved surgically decreases with increasing patient age and increasing curve size.[7]

If a spinal arthrodesis were perfectly successful, the residual curvature in the immediate postoperative period would remain static for the remainder of the patient's life. Long-term follow-up of spinal fusions using modern techniques of internal fixation and bone grafting are available only in patients with Harrington instrumentation. In these patients, the long-term results have been excellent at an average 26 years' follow-up with loss of curve correction of less than 5 degrees in 84% of patients.[40]

Including those patients with fractured rods and pseudoarthrosis, the average loss of correction has been less than 10 degrees in multiple reported series.†

Loss of correction has three possible causes, including (1) "settling in" of the hooks, (2) progression of the curve above or below the fused spinal segment, and (3) combined pseudarthrosis and instrument failure. Loss of correction is best quantified by the increase in curvature degrees from the

---

*See references 1, 3, 6, 7, 10, 17, 18, 23, 24, 26, 28, 35, 39, 41, 42, 44.
†See references 3, 6, 7, 17, 18, 26, 29, 39, 42, 44, 48.

immediate postoperative film such as an increase of 5 from 40 degrees postoperative to 45 degrees on follow-up examination.

The most common cause of loss of correction with Harrington distraction rods is "settling in" of the hooks. Under the forces of weight-bearing, the hooks may impact into or erode the underlying bone (Fig. 6-10). Small losses of correction of 3 to 5 degrees are due to inherent settling of the instruments.[29]

If the fusion has not incorporated sufficient vertebrae, the curve may progress by increasing lateral curvature of the nonfused vertebrae at the ends of the curve (Fig. 6-11). Depending on the clinical significance of the progression, reoperation may be necessary to extend the fusion.[45]

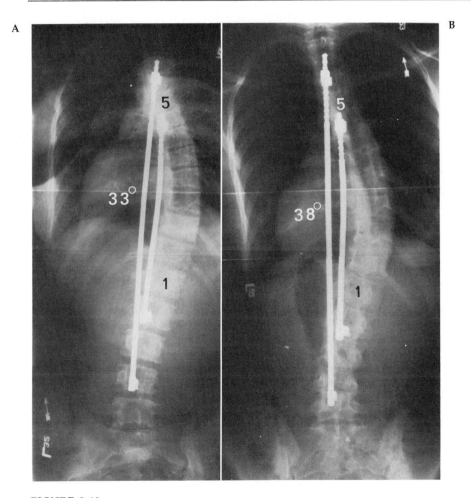

FIGURE 6-10
Immediate postoperative upright film in cast after double Harrington rod insertion for idiopathic scoliosis shows a 33 degree curve **(A)** which increases to 38 degrees 1 year later **(B)** owing to hook settling.

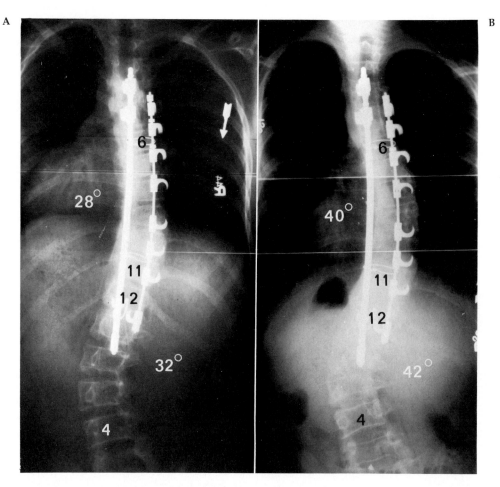

FIGURE 6-11
A 14-year-old boy with 60 degree right thoracic and 42 degree left lumbar scoliosis treated with fusion of the thoracic curve only. Initial postoperative film **(A)** shows good curve correction, but follow-up film 1 year later **(B)** shows curve progression. Although the lumbar curve was smaller than the thoracic preoperatively, it had limited flexibility, so, in retrospect, combined thoracic and lumbar fusion should have been performed.

All other cases of curve progression are caused by the combined development of pseudarthrosis and instrument failure. Instrument failure can consist of either fracture or displacement as discussed above. A scoliotic curve cannot progress if either the fusion or internal fixation is intact. Failed instrumentation in the presence of solid fusion should not result in significant curve progression. Even in the presence of a pseudarthrosis, the curve will not significantly worsen if the internal fixation is stable. However, a persistent pseudarthrosis eventually results in instrument failure. For this reason, bilateral pseudarthroses require repair even before loss of correction or instrument fracture.

LUQUE INSTRUMENTATION

In contrast to the well-documented effectiveness of Harrington instrumentation, large or long-term follow-up series of Luque instrumentation have not been published. Preliminary results have been encouraging. In Luque's original series of 65 patients, an average correction of 72% was achieved with an average loss of correction of 1.5 degrees.[30]

DWYER AND ZIELKE INSTRUMENTATIONS

Although not as extensively studied as Harrington instrumentation, a moderate number of short-term studies has been reported on the use of Dwyer instrumentation for anterior fixation of the spine. The range of reported correction has been from 36% to 70%.[12,27,46] In a series of patients followed by Dwyer, 79.7% of treated patients had curve progressions of 5 degrees or less, while 12.2% had progressions of more than 10 degrees.

Even less information is available on the loss of correction with Zielke instrumentation. Moe et al. reported an average loss of correction of 4 degrees at an average follow-up of 2 years.[38] One curve increased 12 degrees owing to a pseudarthrosis.

Summary

A. Fixation device failure
  1. Causes
     a. Inadequate immobilization
     b. Pseudarthrosis
     c. Device extending beyond the fusion
  2. Harrington distraction rod fracture (2.1% to 7.0% incidence), significant only with rod overlap, curve progression, or pseudarthrosis
  3. Harrington compression rod fracture usually causes only minor loss of correction
  4. Luque instrumentation failure
     a. Rod fracture—infrequent
     b. Sublaminar wire fracture more common
  5. Dwyer instrumentation failure—cable fracture commonly at curve apex
B. Fixation device displacement
  1. Harrington device displacement (1.4% to 8.8% incidence), usually in immediate postoperative period
  2. Luque rod—slipped or rotated rod
  3. Dwyer and Zielke instrumentations—usually screw pull-out at curve ends
C. Pseudarthrosis
  1. Detection (should be less than 10% incidence)
     a. Routine radiographs with oblique projections
     b. Radionuclide bone scans—only between 1 and 2 years postoperatively
     c. Linear tomograms—best with fixation devices

      d. Computed tomography—not good for detection of occult pseudar-
         throsis

   2. Significance—repair if bilateral, painful, or significant loss of correction

D. Loss of curve correction (average less than 10 degrees, 84% less than 5
   degrees)

   1. Causes

      a. Hook settling

      b. Inadequate length of fusion

      c. Instrument failure *plus* pseudarthrosis

   2. Indications for reoperation

      a. Pseudarthrosis

      b. Inadequate length of fusion causing curve progression

REFERENCES

1. Asher, M.A., Gilbert, J., and Orrick J.: Harrington distraction (D) versus distraction plus compression (D + C) for the correction of right thoracic idiopathic scoliosis, Orthop. Trans. **2:**272, 1978.

2. Bernard, T.N., et al.: Late complications due to wire breakage in segmental spinal
   instrumentation, J. Bone Joint Surg. (Am.) **65:**1339-1345, 1983.

3. Bjerkreim, I.: Operative treatment of scoliosis with the Harrington instrumentation technique, Acta Orthop. Scand. **47:**397-402, 1976.

4. Blount, W.P., et al.: The Milwaukee brace in the operative treatment of scoliosis, J.
   Bone Joint Surg. (Am.) **40:**511-525, 1958.

5. Bonnett, C.A., Brown, J.C., and Dietrich, T.: Postoperative immobilization with
   the Milwaukee brace after spinal fusion and Harrington instrumentation, Orthop.
   Rev. **5:**39-42, 1976.

6. Crawford, A.H., MacEwen, G.D., and Lokietek, W.: Surgical management of
   idiopathic scoliosis at the Alfred I. Dupont Institute, Ohio State Med. J. **75:**513-
   517, 1979.

7. Curtis, R.S., et al.: Results of Harrington instrumentation in the treatment of
   severe scoliosis, Clin. Orthop. **144:**128-134, 1979.

8. Dawson, E.G., Caron, A., and Moe, J.H.: Surgical management of scoliosis in the
   adult, J. Bone Joint Surg. (Am.) **55:**437, 1973.

9. Dawson, E.G., Clader, T.J., and Bassett, L.W.: The role of tomography in posterior
   spinal fusions, Orthop. Trans. **7:**24, 1983.

10. Dickson, J.H., and Harrington, P.R.: The evolution of the Harrington instrumenta-
    tion technique in scoliosis, J. Bone Joint Surg. (Am.) **55:**993-1002, 1973.

11. Dwyer, A.F.: Experience of anterior correction of scoliosis, Clin. Orthop. **93:**191-
    206, 1973.

12. Dwyer, A.F., and Schafer, M.F.: Anterior approach to scoliosis: results of treat-
    ment in fifty-one cases, J. Bone Joint Surg. (Br.) **56:**218-224, 1974.

13. Dwyer, A.F., et al.: The late complications after the Dwyer anterior spinal instru-
    mentation for scoliosis, J. Bone Joint Surg. (Br.) **59:**117, 1977.

14. Erwin, W.D., Dickson, J.H., and Harrington, P.R.: Clinical review of patients with
    broken Harrington rods, J. Bone Joint Surg. (Am.) **62:**1302-1307, 1980.

15. Foley, M.J., et al.: Thoracic and lumbar spine fusion: postoperative radiologic
    evaluation, AJR **141:**373-380, 1983.

16. Goldstein, L.A.: Results in the treatment of scoliosis with turnbuckle plaster cast
    correction and fusion, J. Bone Joint Surg. (Am.) **41:**321-335, 1959.

17. Goldstein, L.A.: Surgical management of scoliosis, J. Bone Joint Surg. (Am.) **48:**
    167-196, 1966.

18. Goldstein, L.A.: The surgical treatment of idiopathic scoliosis, Clin. Orthop. **93:** 131-157, 1973.
19. Hall, J.E.: Current concepts review: Dwyer instrumentation in anterior fusion of the spine, J. Bone Joint Surg. (Am.) **63:**1188-1190, 1981.
20. Hall, J.E., Gray, J., and Allen, M.: Dwyer instrumentation and spinal fusion. A follow-up study, J. Bone Joint Surg. (Br.) **59:**117, 1977.
21. Hannon, K.M., and Wetta, W.J.: Failure of technetium bone scanning to detect pseudarthroses in spinal fusion for scoliosis, Clin. Orthop. **123:**42-44, 1977.
22. Harrington, P.R.: Treatment of scoliosis: Correction and internal fixation by spine instrumentation, J. Bone Joint Surg. (Am.) **44:**591-610, 1962.
23. Harrington, P.R.: The management of scoliosis by spine instrumentation: An evaluation of more than 200 cases, South. Med. J. **56:**1367-1377, 1963.
24. Harrington, P.R.: Technical details in relation to the successful use of instrumentation in scoliosis, Orthop. Clin. North Am. **3:**49-67, 1972.
25. Harrington, P.R., and Dickson, J.H.: An eleven-year clinical investigation of Harrington instrumentation, Clin. Orthop. **93:**113-130, 1973.
26. Horlyck, E., and Thomasen, E.: Operative treatment of scoliosis with Harrington instrumentation technique, Acta Orthop. Scand. **49:**350-353, 1978.
27. Hsu, L.C.S., et al.: Dwyer instrumentation in the treatment of adolescent idiopathic scoliosis, J. Bone Joint Surg. (Br.) **64:**536-541, 1982.
28. Kostuik, J.P., Israel, J., and Hall, J.E.: Scoliosis surgery in adults, Clin. Orthop. **93:**225-234, 1973.
29. Leider, L., Jr., Moe, J.H., and Winter, R.B.: Early ambulation after the surgical treatment of idiopathic scoliosis, J. Bone Joint Surg. (Am.) **55:**1003-1015, 1973.
30. Luque, E.R.: Segmental spinal instrumentation for correction of scoliosis, Clin. Orthop. **163:**192-198, 1982.
31. Mack, L.A., et al.: CT of acetabular fractures: postoperative appearances, AJR **141:**891-894, 1983.
32. McMaster, M.J.: Stability of the scoliotic spine after fusion, J. Bone Joint Surg. (Br.) **62:**59-64, 1980.
33. McMaster, M.J., and James, J.I.P.: Pseudarthrosis after spinal fusion for scoliosis, J. Bone Joint Surg. (Br.) **58:**305-312, 1976.
34. McMaster, M.J., and Merrick, M.V.: The scintigraphic assessment of the scoliotic spine after fusion, J. Bone Joint Surg. (Br.) **62:**65-72, 1980.
35. Mir, S.R., et al.: Early ambulation following spinal fusion and Harrington instrumentation in idiopathic scoliosis, Clin. Orthop. **110:**54-62, 1975.
36. Moe, J.H.: A critical analysis of methods of fusion for scoliosis: An evaluation in two hundred and sixty-six patients, J. Bone Joint Surg. (Am.) **40:**529-554, 1958.
37. Moe, J.H., and Gustilo, R.B.: Treatment of scoliosis: results in 196 patients treated by cast correction and fusion, J. Bone Joint Surg. (Am.) **46:**293-312, 1964.
38. Moe, J.H., Purcell, G.A., and Bradford, D.S.: Zielke instrumentation (VDS) for the correction of spinal curvature, Clin. Orthop. **180:**133-153, 1983.
39. Moe, J.H., and Valuska, J.W.: Evaluation of treatment of scoliosis by Harrington instrumentation, J. Bone Joint Surg. (Am.) **48:**1656-1657, 1966.
40. Moskowitz, A., et al.: Long-term follow-up of scoliosis fusion, J. Bone Joint Surg. (Am.) **62:**364-375, 1980.
41. Nachemson, A., and Nordwall, A.: Effectiveness of preoperative Cotrel traction for correction of idiopathic scoliosis, J. Bone Joint Surg. (Am.) **59:**504-508, 1977.
42. Piggott, H.: Treatment of scoliosis by posterior fusion, Harrington instrumentation and early walking, J. Bone Joint Surg. (Br.) **58:**58-63, 1976.
43. Pinto, W.D.C.: Complications of the surgical treatment of scoliosis, Israel J. Med. Sci. **9:**837-846, 1973.
44. Ponder, R.C., et al.: Results of Harrington instrumentation and fusion in the adult idiopathic scoliosis patient, J. Bone Joint Surg. (Am.) **57:**797-801, 1975.

45. Risser, J.C., and Norquist, D.M.: A follow-up study of the treatment of scoliosis, J. Bone Joint Surg. (Am.) **40:**555-569, 1958.
46. Stephen, J.P., Wilding, K., and Cass, C.A.: The place of Dwyer anterior instrumentation in scoliosis, Med. J. Aust. **1:**206-208, 1977.
47. Swank, S.M.: The management of scoliosis in the adult, Orthop. Clin. North Am. **10:**891-904, 1979.
48. Swank, S., et al.: Surgical treatment of adult scoliosis, J. Bone Joint Surg. (Am.) **63:**268-287, 1981.
49. Vesely, D.G., Blaylock, H.I., and Harrison, J.: Scoliosis treatment by spinal fusion, Harrington instrumentation, and Milwaukee brace, Ala. J. Med. Sci. **16:**370-373, 1979.
50. Wilkinson, R.H., et al.: Radiographic evaluation of the spine after surgical correction of scoliosis, AJR **133:**703-709, 1979.
51. Wilson, R.L., Levine, D.B., and Doherty, J.H.: Surgical treatment of idiopathic scoliosis, Clin. Orthop. **81:**34-47, 1971.
52. Winter, R.B.: Scoliosis and other spinal deformities, Acta Orthop. Scand. **46:**400-424, 1975.
53. Winter, R.B.: Posterior spinal fusion in scoliosis: indications, technique, and results, Orthop. Clin. North Am. **10:**787-800, 1979.

Chapter Seven

Secondary Scoliosis

*A*lthough idiopathic scoliosis accounts for 80% to 90% of the patients with scoliosis, the secondary forms remain an important problem because they are often the most severe and intractable cases. Appropriate treatment requires accurate diagnosis of the underlying etiology. Current classification lists of the forms of secondary scoliosis are quite lengthy.[85] The largest general categories are congenital, neuropathic, myopathic, mesodermal, skeletal dysplasias, and acquired asymmetric trunkal growth. Each of these major categories will be discussed with a brief review of the entity, the frequency and significance of the associated scoliosis, and its radiographic presentation.

Congenital Scoliosis

Congenital scoliosis is lateral spinal curvature resulting from anomalous asymmetric development of one or more vertebrae. Patients with myelomeningocele alone are not included in this classification because their posterior spinal element deficiency does not cause asymmetric spinal growth. An extensive review of congenital scoliosis and other congenital spinal anomalies can be found in the recent text by Winter.[127]

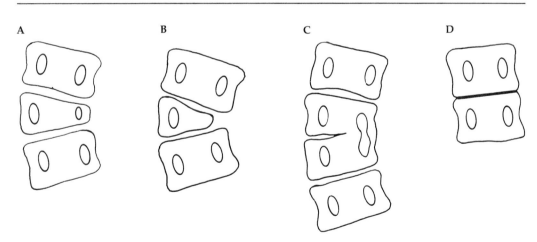

FIGURE 7-1
Causes of congenital scoliosis.
A, Wedged vertebra.
B, Hemivertebra.
C, Unsegmented bar.
D, Block vertebra.
Modified from Winter, R.B., et al.: J. Bone Joint Surg. (Am.) **50:**1-15, 1968.

189

RADIOGRAPHIC APPEARANCE

Simplifying the previously proposed classifications of congenital scoliosis,[82,86,130,131] there are four fundamental types: (1) wedge vertebra due to partial unilateral failure of formation, (2) hemivertebra due to complete unilateral failure of formation, (3) unilateral unsegmented bar due to failure of segmentation, and (4) block vertebra due to bilateral failure of segmentation (Fig. 7-1). Isolated block vertebrae seldom cause significant scoliosis, but the fused vertebrae may be larger on one side than the other, creating a mild congenital scoliosis. These basic anomalies can occur singly or in combination with each other. A hemivertebra may be fused along its superior or inferior surface to an adjacent vertebra (Fig. 7-2). Tomography is often necessary to define fully the vertebral anomalies in congenital scoliosis (Fig. 7-3). A unilateral, unsegmented bar appears as a curvilinear bridge of bone at the apex of the scoliosis with merging of the pedicles and loss of the disk space at the site of the bar[76] (Fig. 7-4).

FIGURE 7-2
Left lumbar 15 degree congenital scoliosis with an accessory hemivertebra *(arrow)* fused to the inferior surface of the second lumbar (L2) vertebra.

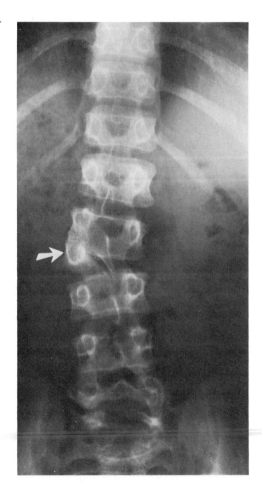

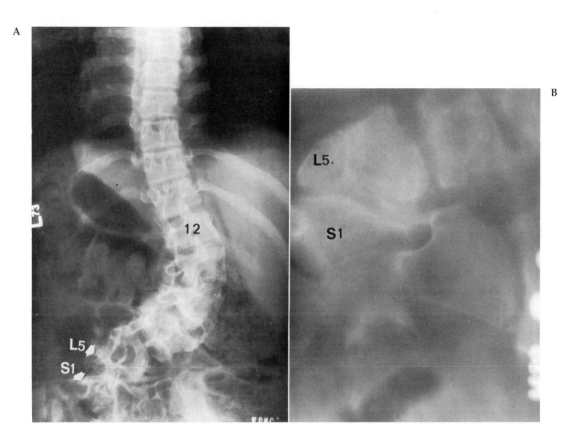

FIGURE 7-3
Twelve-year-old girl with a 60 degree twelfth thoracic (T12) to fourth lumbar (L4) right lumbar scoliosis. The left hemivertebrae at L5 and S1 are poorly seen on the PA film **(A)** but clearly seen on the AP tomogram **(B),** which has been reversed for comparison purposes.

A 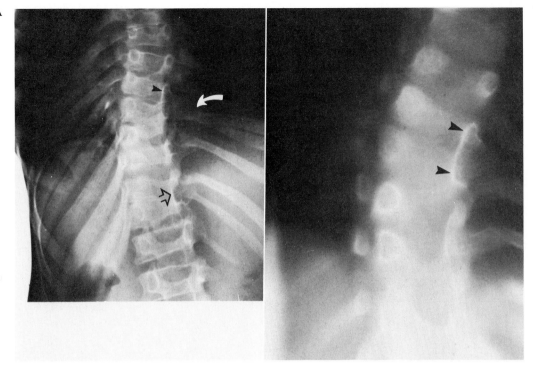 B

FIGURE 7-4

A, An 8-year-old boy with 42 degree left thoracic scoliosis due to a right congenital bar from T6 to T8 *(arrowhead)* and another from T10 to T11 *(open arrow)*. A frequently associated anomaly, rib fusion, is also present on the right *(curved arrow)*.

B, AP tomogram clearly shows upper unsegmented bar *(arrowheads)*.

ASSOCIATED CONGENITAL ANOMALIES

Because of the embryologic origin of these anomalies, it is not surprising to find a high frequency of associated congenital anomalies. The most common associated conditions have been congenital heart disease and genitourinary anomalies, although head and neck, gastrointestinal, and peripheral skeletal anomalies have also been associated with congenital scoliosis.[46,54,86,130,131] Genitourinary abnormalities are among the anomalies most frequently associated with congenital scoliosis, having been found in 13% to 34%[27,77,125] of patients when excretory urograms were performed routinely. The most common renal anomalies in order of frequency are unilateral renal agenesis (36%), collecting system duplication (22%), hydronephrosis (14%), and renal ectopia (14%).[77] Because some of these anomalies can result in an increased incidence of subsequent renal disease, several authors recommend that excretory urograms be performed on all patients with congenital scoliosis to detect those anomalies requiring correction.[46,54,77] Although one study found an association between cardiac defects and thoracic anomalies and between genitourinary anomalies and lumbar anomalies,[130,131] a larger prospective study with routine excretory urograms on all patients found no correlation between the level of the spinal anomaly and the types of associated extraspinal defect.[77]

An important anomaly associated with congenital scoliosis is diastematomyelia, or sagittal division of a segment of the spinal cord.[57,132] Diastematomyelia is one of a spectrum of abnormalities including diplomyelia, dermoid sinus, dermoid cyst, arachnoid cyst, tethered cord, cord angioma, and lipoma that are grouped under the term *spinal dysraphism*.[124] Winter et al.[132] found a 4.9% incidence of diastematomyelia in congenital scoliosis. The split spinal cord may be divided by a fibrous, cartilaginous, or osseous septum.

If a congenital scoliosis is detected, diastematomyelia must be excluded radiographically and clinically. The radiographic findings of diastematomyelia are presented in detail in Chapter Three. The radiographs must be carefully scrutinized for localized widening of the interpedicular space or spina bifida in the area of the scoliosis. One or both of these findings are present in most patients with diastematomyelia. A sagittal intraspinal bony spur is, of course, diagnostic of diastematomyelia. Clinically, about three fourths of patients with diastematomyelia have an overlying cutaneous abnormality such as a hairy patch, sinus or skin dimple, myelomeningocele, lipoma, hemangioma, or nevus.[57] In a thorough literature review, Keim and Green[57] found that lower extremity neurologic defects were reported in 89 (87.3%) of 102 patients. If diastematomyelia is suspected because of radiologic findings, a cutaneous abnormality, or a neurologic deficit, then conventional or computed tomography are recommended to search for a bony septum. Although about one half of the midline septa are found between the first and third lumbar vertebrae, they have been reported to occur at any level in the thoracic or lumbar spine.[57] Diastematomyelia must be recognized and the septum removed prior to scoliosis correction or else corrective distraction may result in permanent neurologic damage.[46,130-132]

PATTERNS AND PROGRESSION

For an unknown reason, congenital scoliosis is two to three times more common in girls than in boys.[77,82,130,131] The lateral curves usually become evident either in infancy or during the postpubertal growth spurt.[82] The curves are thoracic or thoracolumbar in location 65% to 84% of the time.[77,82,130,131] The curves are usually distinct from idiopathic curves in that they are often short in length and demonstrate little correction with bending.

The likelihood of progression of untreated congenital scoliosis is high, with as many as 84% of these children developing curves of over 40 degrees.[130,131] Curve progression depends on the type of vertebral anomaly, curve location, and the age of curve presentation. Curve progression is more likely with thoracic and thoracolumbar curves,[82,130,131] unilateral unsegmented bars,[82,130,131] and when presenting in infancy.[82] The worst prognosis for developing a severe curve in a congenital scoliosis is seen with a unilateral, unsegmented bar with contralateral hemivertebrae.[82,86]

TREATMENT

Early treatment with a spinal orthosis to hold the curve until growth is complete is advised for progressive congenital scoliosis.[53,130,131] The purpose of the brace is to correct and hold the flexible portions of the curve above and below the rigid segment containing the congenital anomaly. If the curve continues to progress or is cosmetically unacceptable, posterior arthrodesis is recommended.[53,130,131] Because these curves tend to be short, angular, and inflexible,[31,86] the correction achieved by surgery is usually not as large as that achieved in idiopathic scoliosis. The average percent correction by surgery has ranged from 26.7% to 36.6%.[46,54,129-131] The reported average loss of correction has been small, averaging 6 to 13 degrees.[54,129-131] Although fusion does prevent growth over the fused segment,[130,131] fusion is recommended even in early childhood if curve progression cannot be controlled by bracing.[129]

Neuropathic Scoliosis

Patients with neuropathic scoliosis are affected by either spastic or flaccid muscle paralysis. Because of the lack of corrective muscle forces in response to positional imbalance, the curves are often rapidly progressive. As a consequence of the severe, fixed deformities that develop, care of the handicapped patient, including feeding and bathing, becomes difficult. The deformed torso causes bony prominences to be subjected to uneven pressures when sitting or lying, so decubitus ulcers are frequent and often intractable. Many patients with neuropathic scoliosis ultimately require spinal fusion to be able to sit upright, to preserve respiratory function, and to facilitate nursing care.

These patients differ considerably from those with idiopathic scoliosis. Progression is much more likely in neuropathic scoliosis. Neuropathic scoliosis usually develops first during early childhood with rapid progression during the adolescent growth spurt. Many of the curves have the paralytic or "C-shaped" pattern, that is, are long and sweeping with their apex at the thoracolumbar junction. Pelvic obliquity (tilting) is often associated with the scoliosis. Management often consists of a spinal deformity orthosis during childhood followed by spinal fusion after adolescence or if the curve progresses during orthosis treatment. Unlike the situation in idiopathic scoliosis, fusion is often extended down to the sacrum because of the associated pelvic obliquity[101] (Fig. 7-5).

Radiography of the patient with neuropathic or myopathic scoliosis is particularly challenging. Obtaining good radiographs is difficult because of demineralization and because many patients are overweight and are unable to stand or sit unassisted. Yet upright films are needed to assess the spinal deformity that may hinder the patient's function and care in a wheelchair. Most of the films are obtained with the patient sitting on a stool while being supported by a family member. One should be aware that, if the patient is not consistently positioned, marked changes in curvature may reflect positioning difference only (Fig. 7-6). In patients with their own wheelchair insert, a sitting radiograph can be obtained in the wheelchair (Fig. 7-6). This technique

FIGURE 7-5
An 8-year-old boy with cerebral palsy and a typical long, paralytic pattern thoracolumbar scoliosis. The iliac crests *(arrows)* are at different heights due to associated pelvic obliquity (18 degrees). The angle created by a horizontal line and a tangential line to the crests quantifies the pelvic obliquity.

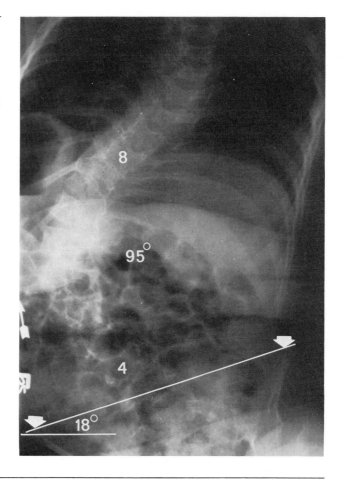

provides a more secure support for the patient and allows reproducible evaluation of the abnormal curvature.

One classification divides neuropathic scoliosis into upper motor neuron, lower motor neuron, and dysautonomia forms, as given below.[85] The severity and pattern of spinal deformity, however, vary within each class and overlap between classes.

1. Upper motor neuron
   a. Cerebral palsy
   b. Spinocerebellar degeneration
   c. Syringomyelia
   d. Spinal cord tumor
   e. Spinal cord trauma
2. Lower motor neuron
   a. Poliomyelitis and other viral myelitides
   b. Spinal muscular atrophy
      (1) Werdnig-Hoffman
      (2) Kugelberg-Welander
   c. Myelomeningocele
3. Dysautonomia (Riley-Day syndrome)

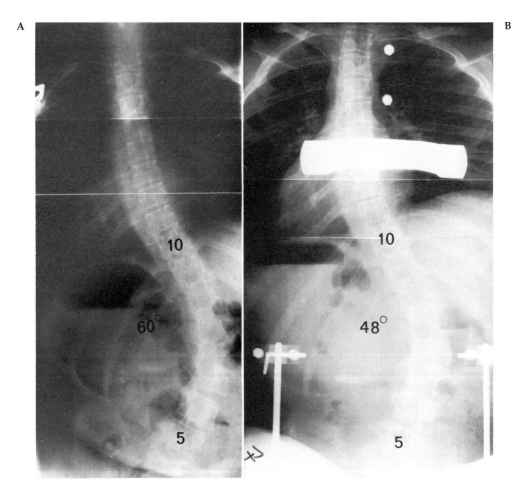

FIGURE 7-6
A 12-year-old boy with Duchenne's muscular dystrophy and right thoracolumbar
scoliosis. Curve is larger while supported on stool *(A)* than when seated in
wheelchair *(B)* due to leaning to the left **(A)** when held by his parent.

CEREBRAL PALSY

Cerebral palsy is a generic term used to describe patients with nonprogressive impaired brain and motor function manifesting itself at birth or during the first year of life. Both the mental retardation and motor deficit can vary from mild to severe. The voluntary motor deficit may be classified as spastic (with increased muscle tone), athetoid (with involuntary movements), or the uncommon ataxic form (with cerebellar incoordination). The most common form is spastic paralysis, which may be quadriplegic, hemiplegic, diplegic, paraplegic, monoplegic, or triplegic. The athetoid form is slightly less common than the spastic and is usually associated with spastic tetraplegia.

Among cerebral palsy patients, the prevalence of scoliosis has been found to range from 16.4% to 38%.[7,85,106,108,110] The prevalence of scoliosis does not vary with the type of cerebral palsy[106,108,110] or the patient's sex.[106,110] The curves are most commonly the long thoracolumbar pattern (45%), followed by the lumbar (25%), thoracic (16%), and double major (14%) patterns.[110] The largest and most clinically significant curves are the unilateral thoracic and thoracolumbar (Fig. 7-7) because of the resultant respiratory compromise and severe trunkal deformity.[74,110]

Management of these patients is begun with a brace but is often difficult. Many cerebral palsy patients with scoliosis require spinal fusion.[101] The fusion should be extended to the sacrum in patients who have pelvic obliquity (Fig. 7-5) or who are unbalanced when sitting.[22,74] The degree of pelvic obliquity in these patients is quantified by measuring the angle between a horizontal line and a second line drawn tangentially across the tops of the iliac crests[92] (Fig. 7-5). The goal of surgery is to create a vertical torso centered over a level pelvis.[85] Posterior instrumentation and fusion may be satisfactory in younger patients with smaller degrees of scoliosis (Fig. 7-7). This is especially true since the advent of segmental spinal instrumentation (Luque rods). For the older patient and patients with larger curves, some studies have found that a two-stage procedure usually results in the best correction and lowest incidence of pseudarthrosis.[17,18,22,74] Anterior fusion with Dwyer or, now, Zielke instrumentation is performed first, followed by posterior fusion and Harrington instrumentation 2 to 3 weeks later. We agree that two-stage fusion is indicated in older children with large curves but believe that posterior fusion with Luque instrumentation is preferable for younger children with smaller curves. Even with these modern techniques, pseudarthroses occur in 17% to 18% of patients.[22,74]

A

B

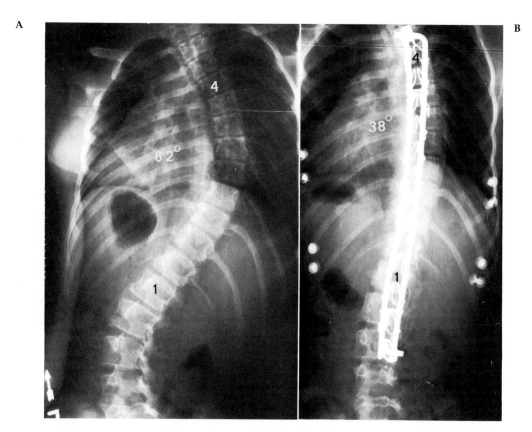

FIGURE 7-7
A 14-year-old girl with cerebral palsy with right thoracic curve before **(A)** and after
(B) correction with posterior fusion and Luque instrumentation.

SPINOCEREBELLAR DEGENERATION

Spinocerebellar degeneration refers to several diseases characterized by a variable rate of progressive loss of balance and neural degeneration. The most common forms of degeneration associated with scoliosis are Friedreich's ataxia and Charcot-Marie-Tooth disease.[49] Unlike most neuropathic curves, the scoliosis in patients with spinocerebellar degeneration is usually thoracic in level.[49] Treatment is especially difficult in these patients because the progressive neurologic deficit often continues to worsen the scoliosis.

Scoliosis is a particularly difficult management problem in patients with Friedreich's ataxia (Fig. 7-8). They have a 56% to 88% incidence of scoliosis,[47] and the curves are often large. Bracing can disturb their balance and interfere with their gait.[49] Surgery is effective, but the benefits of surgery must be balanced against the expected lifespan in a given patient. The mean age at death of these patients is 36 years due to heart failure from the associated cardiomyopathy.[47] Scoliosis is less frequently associated with Charcot-Marie-Tooth disease (10.1% prevalence).[49] It is often mild, requiring no treatment, or responds well to bracing during childhood.[49] In the infrequent cases where it is necessary, posterior spinal fusion is usually successful without special problems or complications.[49]

FIGURE 7-8
A 17-year-old with Friedreich's ataxia and right thoracic, left thoracolumbar scoliosis.

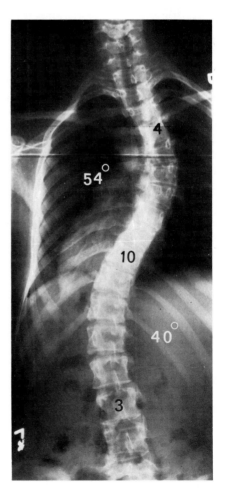

SYRINGOMYELIA

Syringomyelia is a progressive cavitary degeneration of the spinal cord with predominant involvement of the cervical spine. Eccentric expansion of the syrinx into the spinal cord regions controlling the trunk muscles has been postulated as the cause for scoliosis in these patients.[51] In a series of 43 children with syringomyelia, scoliosis was found in 63%, with almost one half of the curves over 25 degrees.[51] The incidence of scoliosis was lower when neurologic symptoms were first noted in late adolescence. Because the upper trunkal muscles are primarily involved, the majority of the curves are thoracic (78%), with the rest being thoracolumbar (11%) or lumbar (11%).[51]

An underlying syrinx in a patient presenting with scoliosis is usually first suspected by the detection of abnormal neurologic findings. In a series of 75 patients with syringomyelia, the plain films were abnormal only in 32% of the cases.[73] However, one patient with syringomyelia has been described who presented with scoliosis at age 5 years at a time when she was neurologically normal.[6] The diagnosis was first made by noting characteristic widening of the cervical spinal canal (Fig. 7-9) on cervical spine radiographs. The special radiographic studies used to diagnose this condition are described in detail in Chapter Three.

SPINAL CORD TUMORS

A slow-growing spinal cord tumor is a rare cause of scoliosis, being reported only in several small series. Curtiss and Collins[29] described three children with low-grade spinal astrocytomas and progressive scoliosis. Boldrey et al.[16] found three patients with thoracic angiomas and progressive scoliosis. None of these patients had abnormal plain films. The diagnosis of spinal cord tumor was suspected clinically because of the associated progressive neurologic deficits. Since idiopathic scoliosis is associated with neurologic dysfunction rarely, and then only with severe curves, any patient with scoliosis and an abnormal neurologic examination should be evaluated for underlying spinal pathology as described in Chapter Three.

FIGURE 7-9
Syringomyelia.
The interpedicular distances are
widened and the pedicles are
flattened in the cervical and upper
thoracic spine.

Courtesy Dr. Solomon Batnitzky,
Kansas City, Kansas.

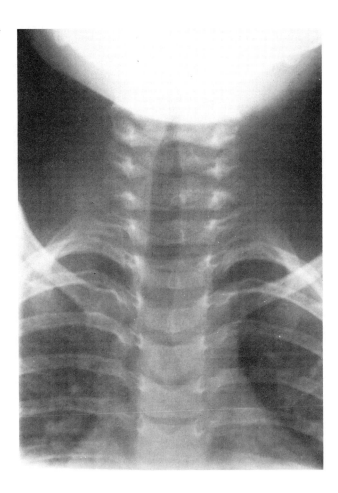

SPINAL CORD TRAUMA

The radiographic findings and treatment for children with scoliosis due to posttraumatic paralysis (Fig. 7-10) are similar to those for children who have poliomyelitis.[21] The scoliosis develops below the level of paralysis and is seldom severe when the trauma occurs in adulthood. The etiology of the scoliosis is easily determined from the clinical history and the radiographs if vertebral fractures are present.

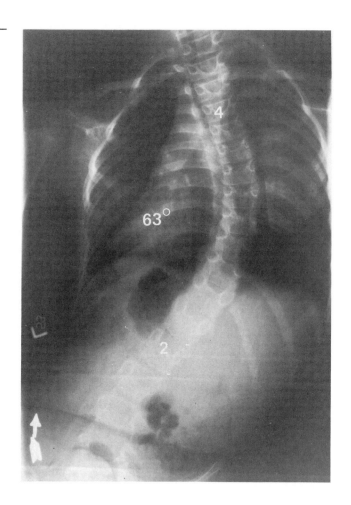

FIGURE 7-10
Posttraumatic quadriplegia and right thoracic scoliosis similar to that commonly seen in poliomyelitis.

VIRAL MYELITIS

Poliomyelitis is the prototype for these dreaded viral infections. Although immunization has eliminated the epidemic infections in some countries, poliomyelitis is still a major health problem in many parts of the world. The large number of these children with paralytic scoliosis was a major stimulus for the development of modern orthoses and surgical treatment for scoliosis.

Paralytic scoliosis differs dramatically from idiopathic scoliosis in its clinical course and treatment implications. These curves can develop as late as 12 years after the onset of paralysis,[26] but most curves develop within 2 years.[52] A major problem in the management of these patients is the associated pelvic obliquity. Fixed tilt of the pelvis to one side (pelvic obliquity) can develop due to imbalance of thigh abductor and adductor muscles or imbalance of trunk muscles.[90] There are multiple complications of this obliquity, including (1) difficulty walking even with braces and crutches, (2) painful impingement of the iliac crest on the rib cage, (3) hip dislocation, (4) progressive lumbar scoliosis, and (5) ischial decubiti.[90]

The radiographic pattern of curves is similar to that seen in idiopathic scoliosis, with thoracic curves being the most common (Fig. 7-11). Combining the extensive data from two large series, the approximate distribution of curve types was thoracic, 51%; thoracolumbar, 28%; lumbar, 17%; and double major, 4%.[26,52] Although the relative importance of specific muscle groups is debated, the curve location reflects the asymmetric muscle paralysis in the region of the curve.[26,52,103] Right-sided curves are more common than left-sided ones. Unlike idiopathic curves, however, both thoracic and thoracolumbar curves in these patients are often very long, encompassing much of the spine. These long, C-shaped curves are not found in patients with idiopathic scoliosis. Another distinctive curve feature is the severe collapse or "telescoping" of the spine occurring in some patients. This phenomenon reflects marked curve flexibility so that a moderate curve in the supine position becomes severe when the patient is upright. Patients with this marked curve flexibility have severe but symmetric muscle paralysis.[52,103]

Current practice for management of paralytic scoliosis consists of a spinal deformity orthosis during childhood followed by surgery after spinal growth is complete or if the curve progresses with brace treatment. The brace is not significantly modified for the paralyzed patient, but the pelvic girdle and thoracic pad are made larger to compensate for the patient's lack of muscle control.[23]

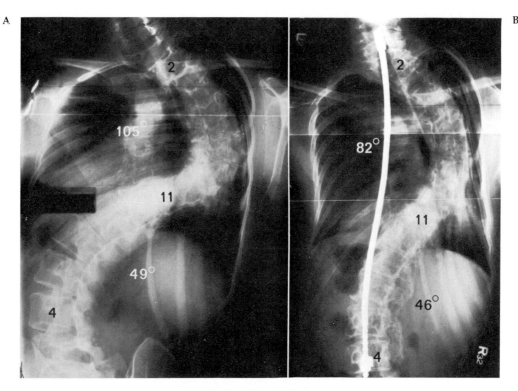

FIGURE 7-11

A, A 41-year-old woman with severe paralytic right thoracic scoliosis due to old poliomyelitis.

B, After posterior fusion and Harrington instrumentation. Pseudarthrosis later developed, so two-stage initial fusion may have been preferable.

Surgical correction is dramatically different here than it is for idiopathic scoliosis in that a two-stage spinal fusion is often recommended rather than posterior fusion. Although smaller thoracic curves can do well with posterior fusion, posterior fusion alone (Fig. 7-11) results in a high incidence (28%) of pseudarthrosis with large curves and thoracolumbar curves.[19] An anterior fusion with internal fixation followed in 2 weeks by posterior fusion and Harrington instrumentation is now the recommended procedure for these curves.[30,70,90,91,126] If fixed pelvic obliquity is present, the fusion must be extended to include the sacrum, thereby reducing the obliquity and preventing its progression.[42,126] If surgical fusion is required prior to skeletal maturity, spinal growth is stopped thereby reducing the potential height of the patient. To compensate for this problem, Luque[75] has suggested the use of internal fixation without arthrodesis. He found that using two Harrington distraction rods with segmental sublaminar wiring resulted in significant curve correction and stability while allowing for continued spinal growth. A definite disadvantage, though, is that the rods usually fractured or dislodged as the patient grew, so multiple operations were required.

SPINAL MUSCULAR ATROPHY

Spinal muscular atrophy is an autosomal recessive, hereditary neuro-muscular disorder caused by anterior horn degeneration and characterized by severe trunkal and proximal muscle weakness.[2,49,111] The disease runs a spectrum from the infantile Werdnig-Hoffman with early onset and death to the juvenile Kugelberg-Welander with later onset and potential long-term survival. Respiratory insufficiency is the major medical problem of these patients, and long-term survival relates primarily to sparing of the respiratory muscles by the disease.

The major orthopedic complication of this disease is scoliosis, which occurs in 58% to 70% of patients.[49,111] The curves are larger than 60 degrees in half of the patients.[111] The most common curve patterns are single major thoracolumbar and lumbar, usually convex to the right.[2,49,111] Treatment of the scoliosis is desirable because severe curvature worsens pulmonary function and hinders wheelchair sitting.

These benefits must be balanced against the current motor function and anticipated length of survival before beginning treatment of the scoliosis. Although bracing is suggested for those patients with scoliosis progressing before skeletal maturity, it has only occasionally been successful.[2,49,111] The most effective treatment appears to be posterior instrumentation and a long posterior fusion.[2] Luque instrumentation is currently preferred over Harrington instrumentation.[128] As is the case for patients with poliomyelitis, the fusion must be extended down to the sacrum if there is pelvic obliquity, which is almost always present.

MYELOMENINGOCELE

Prior to the 1950s, spinal deformity in myelomeningocele patients was seldom a clinical problem because of these patients' short life expectancy. In 1959, Norton and Foley[89] correctly predicted the current situation in which many patients born with a myelomeningocele can now expect to live into adulthood and develop satisfactory ambulation using crutches and braces. A recent study found that almost all such patients who had lower extremity innervation to the fourth lumbar level or below had functional ambulation.[3]

The scoliosis that develops in these patients can be congenital or neuropathic in origin.[45] Congenital scoliosis due to vertebral bars or hemivertebrae accounts for 25% to 38% of myelomeningocele scoliosis[59,95] and has been discussed previously. The neuropathic scoliosis results from the severe, symmetric paralysis that these patients have. In three large case studies of myelomeningocele patients, the incidence of scoliosis was found to range from 50% to 57%.[8,59,95] Scoliosis can begin at any age but most often becomes greater than 30 degrees in late childhood and adolescence.[114] Scoliosis is unlikely to develop if the bony or neurologic defect is not above the fifth lumbar level but is almost certain to develop if both defects reach the fourth lumbar level.[95]

The typical radiographic appearance of a neuropathic scoliosis secondary to a myelomeningocele is a long, sweeping thoracolumbar curve extending down to the sacrum with associated pelvic obliquity[37,84,92] (Fig. 7-12).

Spinal orthotic treatment is useful in treating small curves and in delaying, but not eliminating, the need for surgery. Because of the deficient osteoporotic vertebral bone mass in these patients, surgical fusion is always difficult. The most widely recommended procedure is a two-stage fusion beginning with anterior discectomy fusion and sometimes Zielke or Dwyer instrumentation. Because this instrumentation increases kyphosis, it is especially useful when there is a lordotic component to the curve and when the curve can be largely corrected at this first stage. The anterior procedure is followed in 2 to 3 weeks by posterior fusion with Harrington distraction rods[20,92] or, more recently, segmental spinal instrumentation[75] with fixation to the pelvis using the Galveston technique.[128] The anterior fusion should be centered at the curve apex and extended as far as possible, preferably to include the lumbosacral junction. The posterior fusion must include the sacrum to correct pelvic obliquity and restore a balanced sitting posture.[20,37,92,119] Using the two-stage technique, an average correction of 61.7% was found, with a subsequent loss of correction of only 5 degrees.[92] However, the incidence of pseudarthrosis is still high (23%).[92]

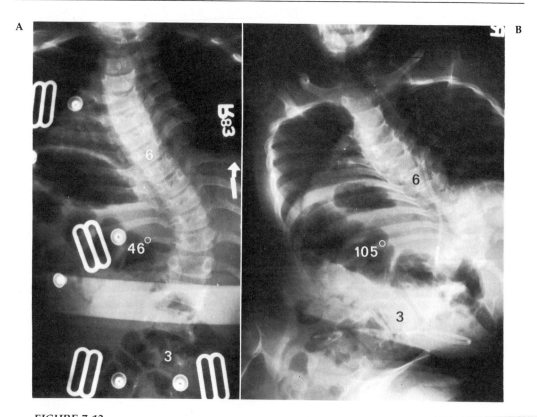

FIGURE 7-12
A 6-year-old girl with a myelomeningocele and a right thoracolumbar paralytic scoliosis. Despite the use of a brace **(A)** the curve and associated pelvic obliquity dramatically progressed in 18 months **(B)** requiring surgery.

FAMILIAL DYSAUTONOMIA

Familial dysautonomia (Riley-Day syndrome) is an idiopathic disease with focal demyelination in the brain, spinal cord, and nerves resulting in muscular incoordination, a stumbling gait, and a high incidence of scoliosis.[135] The disease is most common in Jewish children of Eastern European extraction, and often there is associated vasomotor instability. Most patients die in childhood of pulmonary disease.

In a large survey of 65 patients, Yoslow et al.[135] found a 60% incidence of scoliosis with 83% of the curves greater than 20 degrees and 5% greater than 50 degrees. Girls are affected twice as often as boys. Most of the curves are thoracic (Fig. 7-13) with an equal number of right and left convexity curves. Because of the systemic autonomic dysfunction, these patients do not respond well to bracing or surgery. In view of this factor, as well as the short lifespan and low frequency of large curves, treatment is not commonly indicated.

FIGURE 7-13
An 8-year-old boy with familial dysautonomia and minimal left thoracic scoliosis.

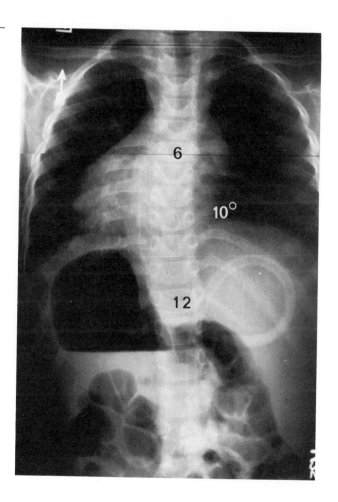

Myopathic Scoliosis
MUSCULAR DYSTROPHY

The muscular dystrophies are inherited disorders characterized by progressive skeletal muscle degeneration and subsequent weakness.[117] The major types are pseudohypertrophic (Duchenne), facioscapulohumeral, limb-girdle, and myotonic.[117] Patients with myotonic and limb-girdle dystrophy rarely develop significant scoliosis.[116] Patients with facioscapulohumeral dystrophy occasionally develop scoliosis. Because of the better prognosis of their underlying disease, these patients can be treated with orthotics or spinal fusion (Fig. 7-14) in a fashion similar to that used for idiopathic scoliosis.[116]

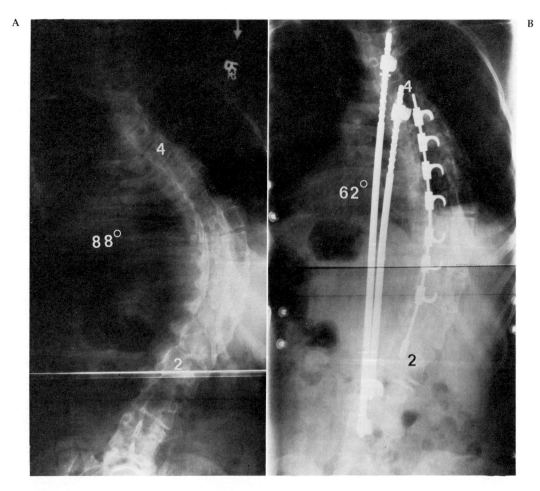

FIGURE 7-14

A 30-year-old woman with facioscapulohumeral muscular dystrophy and right thoracic scoliosis **(A)**. Operative correction with posterior fusion and Harrington compression and distraction rods **(B)**.

Patients with Duchenne-type muscular dystrophy pose a major therapeutic dilemma regarding the treatment of their scoliosis. They seldom develop significant scoliosis while ambulatory, presumably due to the symmetric paraspinal muscle flexing that occurs when walking with braces and crutches.[116] Once the patient is wheelchair-bound, the scoliosis progresses rapidly in 80% to 85% of patients.[40,106] The curves can increase 20 to 30 degrees per year, with almost half of the nonambulatory scoliotic patients having curves over 90 degrees.[104]

The most common curve pattern is the long thoracolumbar with associated pelvic obliquity.[104] Treatment with standard braces and wheelchair pads and supports has been ineffective.[40,104,117] Recently, Gibson et al.[40] described and recommended an effective spinal support device for mounting on a standard wheelchair base.

If the curve is already larger than 35 degrees or progresses despite spinal orthosis, posterior surgical fusion has been recommended,[40] but it is controversial due to the shortened lifespan of these patients.[113]

ARTHROGRYPOSIS MULTIPLEX CONGENITA

Arthrogryposis is a nonfamilial disorder characterized by muscle weakness and fibrous replacement of muscle. Its most common manifestations are club feet, joint contractures, and congenital hip dislocations.[39,72,97] Because these children have normal to above-normal intelligence, their overall prognosis is reasonable if surgical management is directed at soft tissue releases for early ambulation. The underlying skeletal structures are normal except for osteoporosis and overtubulation due to prolonged immobility.[72]

Scoliosis is commonly seen in association with arthrogryposis with a frequency ranging from 7% to 40%.[32,39,72,97,115] The most commonly reported curve pattern has been the long C-shaped neuromuscular curve. Drummond and Mackenzie[32] stressed that congenital scoliosis due to vertebral anomalies and scoliosis due to pelvic obliquity from unilateral hip contracture or dislocation can also occur. The Milwaukee brace is usually used in mild scoliosis with Harrington instrumentation, and posterior fusion is indicated in larger and progressive curves.

Mesodermal Scoliosis

Because the embryonic mesoderm forms the osseous and ligamentous structures that are key mechanical elements of spinal stability, inherited mesodermal disorders such as neurofibromatosis and Marfan's syndrome are associated with an increased incidence of scoliosis. The patterns and significance of the associated scoliosis vary greatly and will be discussed in detail.

NEUROFIBROMATOSIS

Neurofibromatosis is an autosomal dominant inherited disease of the neuroectodermal and mesodermal tissues with a population frequency of about 1 in 3000 births.[25] The skeletal anomalies have been grouped into four categories: (1) bone erosion by tumor, (2) osteomalacia from a renal tubular defect, (3) congenital abnormalities such as macrocranium, and (4) mesodermal dysplasias such as pseudarthrosis and scoliosis.[24,80] Scoliosis is the most common skeletal abnormality, occurring in 10% to 41% of patients with neurofibromatosis.[25,50] It represents 1% to 3% of all cases of scoliosis.[100,133]

Although the curves have typically been described as short and angular in configuration[63,69] (Fig. 7-15), two large series found that 57% to 70% of the curves involved more than five vertebrae. However, Holt[50] believes that the presence of a short, angular scoliosis with five or fewer vertebrae primarily involved is virtually diagnostic of neurofibromatosis. Most of the curves (63% to 75%) occur in the thoracic spine with one series reporting almost exclusively right convexity curves[100] and another reporting an equal frequency of right

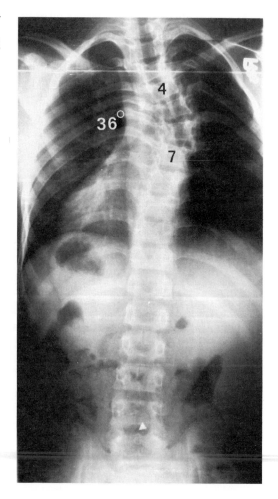

FIGURE 7-15
A 13-year-old boy with neurofibromatosis and short-segment right thoracic scoliosis.

and left curves.[25] Notably, both series reported an absence of lumbar curves, with the nonthoracic curves being cervical or thoracolumbar. The frequency of scoliosis and kyphoscoliosis has been equal with no cases of pure lumbar hyperlordosis.[100,133]

The prognosis of the spinal deformity varies widely depending on the size of the curve, age at presentation, and the presence of associated bony defects. Mild curves (less than 15 degrees) presenting in childhood are usually not progressive and require no treatment.[25,100] However, once a curve starts to progress it tends to worsen rapidly with an average increase of 5 to 7 degrees per year.[25,133] Braces have been uniformly ineffective in progressive curves. Posterior fusion with Harrington instrumentation (Fig. 7-16) is now the recommended treatment for these patients with progressive scoliosis[25,100,133] unless, as described below, there is significant hyperkyphosis.

Recently Winter et al.[133] emphasized that scoliosis in neurofibromatosis patients should be considered in three basic categories. Curves without axial dystrophic changes such as rib penciling, transverse process spindling (Fig.

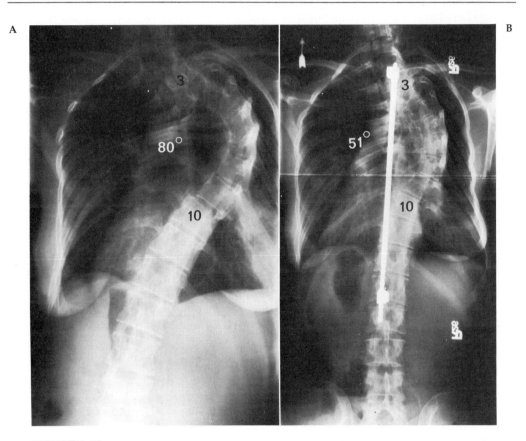

FIGURE 7-16
A 22-year-old girl with neurofibromatosis and short right thoracic scoliosis (A). Posterior fusion and Harrington distraction rod were chosen for treatment (B) because of the absence of dystrophic skeletal changes and hyperkyphosis.

7-17, *A*), vertebral body scalloping (Fig. 7-17, *B*), foraminal enlargement, and paraspinal masses could be treated as idiopathic scoliosis. Patients with scoliosis and axial dystrophic changes did best with Harrington instrumentation and posterior fusion. In contrast, dystrophic kyphoscoliosis required combined anterior and posterior fusion to prevent the high frequency of pseudarthrosis (64%) seen with posterior fusion alone (Fig. 7-18). Cord compression due to spinal angulation occurred only with kyphoscoliosis. Patients with cord compression due to their kyphoscoliosis could not be treated by decompression laminectomy alone since their deformity rapidly worsened.

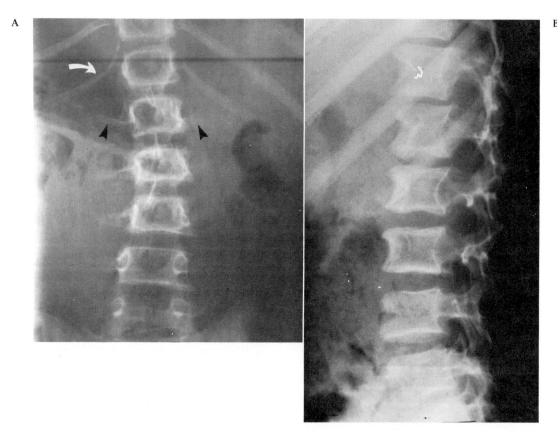

A

B

FIGURE 7-17
Neurofibromatosis in an 8-year-old boy.
A, Anteroposterior film shows spindled lumbar transverse processes *(arrowheads)* and a penciled right twelfth rib *(arrow).*
B, Lateral film shows marked anterior and posterior scalloping of lumbar and lower thoracic vertebrae.

MARFAN'S SYNDROME

Marfan's syndrome is a hereditary connective tissue disorder frequently associated with dislocated lenses, aortic aneurysms, and skeletal anomalies. Common skeletal anomalies include arachnodactyly, pes planus, high arched palate, pectus excavatum, pectus carinatum, and scoliosis.[105] The features of the associated scoliosis were thoroughly summarized by Robins et al.[105] Scoliosis occurred in 55% of their 64 patients. The most common curve patterns were double major right thoracic–left lumbar (48%) and single right thoracic (33%) (Fig. 7-19). The curves are very rigid, resisting Milwaukee brace treatment, and are routinely progressive. In contrast to idiopathic scoliosis, almost one half of the cases began in the infantile and juvenile periods.

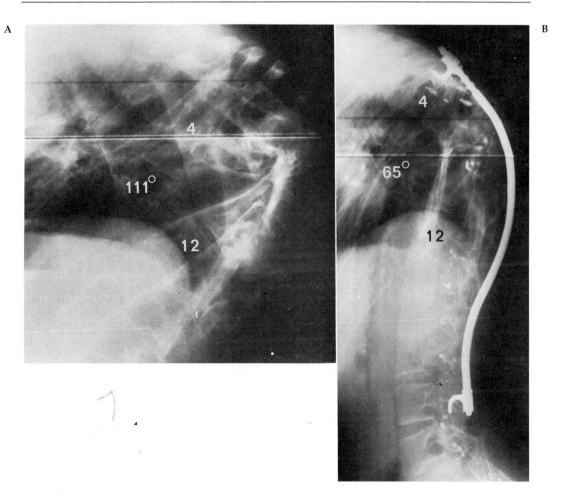

FIGURE 7-18
A 10-year-old girl with neurofibromatosis and dystrophic kyphoscoliosis **(A)** requiring anterior fusion and posterior fusion with Harrington instrumentation **(B)**.

FIGURE 7-19
A 13-year-old boy with Marfan's disease and
mild right thoracic scoliosis.

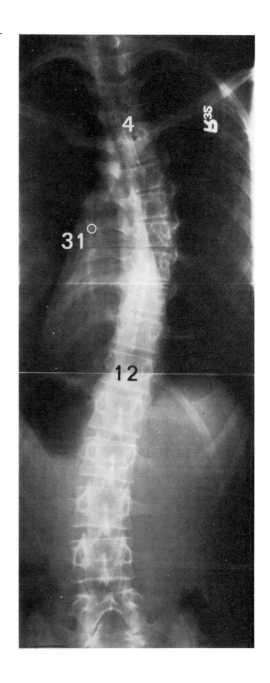

Scoliosis in the Skeletal Dysplasias

Many of the patients with congenital abnormalities of bone formation develop scoliosis. The clinical significance of the scoliosis varies with the prognosis of the underlying disorder and the progressive or nonprogressive nature of the scoliosis. The term *skeletal dysplasia* has been selected as a unifying phrase to emphasize the common feature of abnormal bone formation in such diverse conditions are osteogenesis imperfecta, dwarfism, and mucopolysaccharidosis.

OSTEOGENESIS IMPERFECTA

Osteogenesis imperfecta is a connective tissue disorder characterized by deficient collagen formation both in soft tissues and in osteoid. The faulty osteoid formation results in weak, easily fractured bones. The major clinical problems in these patients have been extensively summarized.[10,36,60] The disease is characterized by blue sclerae, abnormal tooth dentin formation, osteoporotic bones, deafness, ligamentous laxity, excessive sweating, and easy bruisability with two basic subtypes. The first subtype, osteogenesis imperfecta congenita, is not hereditary, often lethal, and manifests itself at birth by deformities due to prenatal fractures. The other form, osteogenesis imperfecta tarda, is inherited with an autosomal dominant pattern and manifested by varying susceptibility to fractures. Many schemes for subdividing this second group have been proposed, but the basic distinction is whether the patients have multiple, early childhood fractures or infrequent, later onset fractures.[10,60]

Common skeletal anomalies include long bone bowing, radial head dislocation, protrusio acetabuli, coxa vara, genu valgum, pes planovalgus, vertebral compression fracture, and scoliosis.[60] The bones are usually severely demineralized with thin cortices, but cortical thickening and hyperplastic callus can also be seen.[10]

Spinal radiography reveals osteoporotic vertebrae with frequent compression fractures. The depressed endplates can create the biconcave or "codfish" vertebra appearance (Fig. 7-20). Scoliosis occurs in 30% to 70% of patients with 36% of the curves over 50 degrees.[12] As the children reach adolescence, the incidence of scoliosis approaches 80%.[12] The most common pattern of curve is uncertain, with three studies reporting that the single thoracic curves (Fig. 7-21) were the most common.[10,60,88] Two other studies reported that the double major pattern was the most common.[28,134] In osteogenesis imperfecta congenita, the curves begin about age 5 years and progress rapidly, whereas scoliosis in the tarda forms appears later and progresses slowly unless the curve exceeds 50 degrees.[88]

Treatment of these progressive curves is difficult. Bracing is ineffective and often harmful because it induces a thoracic cage deformity.[12,28,134] Spinal fusion is difficult because of the weak, osteoporotic bone, although successful curve stabilization has been reported.[13,28] Yong-Hing and MacEwen[134] recently conducted a worldwide survey on the treatment of scoliosis seen with osteogenesis imperfecta. Posterior fusion was primarily used with Harrington instrumentation for internal fixation in 70% of the posterior fusions. The average correction was 36% with 7% better correction in the instrumented

FIGURE 7-20
An 11-year-old girl with osteogenesis imperfecta. Severe lumbar demineralization and biconcave vertebrae ("codfish vertebrae") are seen.

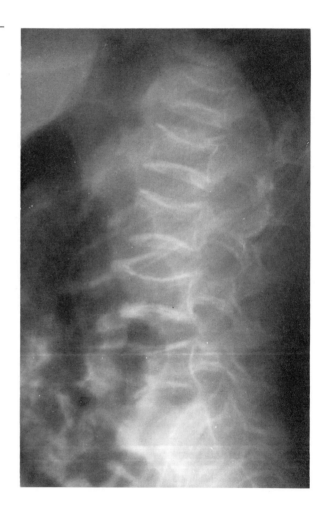

group. The incidence of pseudarthrosis was 8.3%, but the incidence of Harrington instrumentation failure was 33.3%. The incidence of complications was significantly increased in very large curves. The authors concluded that posterior spinal fusion was indicated in all patients with osteogenesis imperfecta with curves greater than 50 degrees regardless of the patient's age.[134] A recent report suggested that combined anterior and posterior fusion with fixation augmented by methylmethacrylate may reduce the arthrodesis failure rate.[44]

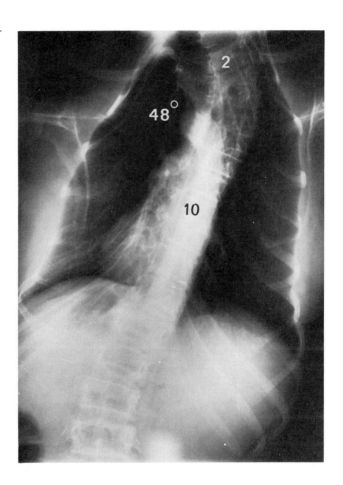

FIGURE 7-21
A 15-year-old girl with osteogenesis imperfecta and kyphoscoliosis. There is a severe secondary rib cage deformity.

SHORT-LIMBED DWARFISM

A number of the forms of dwarfism are associated with an increased incidence of scoliosis. Each of these skeletal dysplasias has characteristic clinical and radiographic findings that have been described in detail.[123] Accordingly, this discussion will focus on the incidence, patterns, and clinical significance of scoliosis in the various forms of dwarfism.

Scoliosis has been described as being frequently present in the following chondrodystrophies: (1) achondroplasia, (2) pseudoachondroplasia, (3) diastrophic dwarfism, (4) spondyloepiphyseal dysplasia, (5) metatrophic dwarfism, and (6) Morquio's syndrome.[64,87]

Achondroplasia is the most common form of short-limbed dwarfism and has an autosomal dominant pattern of inheritance.[66] The distinctive radiographic findings of achondroplasia include narrowing of the interpedicular distance in the lower lumbar spine, square ilia, narrow sacrosciatic notch, and flat acetabular roofs[66] (Fig. 7-22). Although lumbar kyphosis is a significant problem, as discussed in the next chapter, scoliosis is not a major clinical problem in these patients. One large series of 94 patients with achondroplasia found no scoliosis in 66%, scoliosis of less than 20 degrees in 26.6%, and scoliosis between 20 and 45 degrees in the remaining 7.4%.[4] The curves were relatively short and thoracolumbar or lumbar. However, another series of 71 patients did not report any patient requiring treatment of a scoliotic deformity,[87] and an even larger series of 158 patients reported only 1 patient with scoliosis (a 40 degree double structural curve).[64]

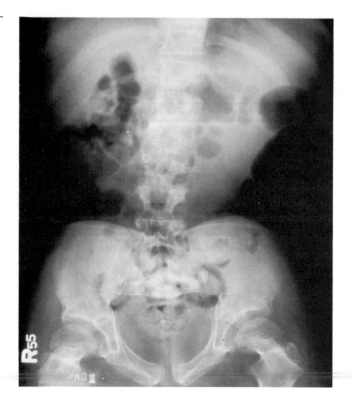

FIGURE 7-22
Achondroplasia.
Typical square ilia, flat acetabula, and progressive narrowing of interpedicular distances in lower lumbosacral spine.

Pseudoachondroplasia presents many of the same orthopedic problems as achondroplasia including hyperlordosis, hip flexion contractures, genu varum or valgum, and joint laxity.[87] The scoliosis is seen almost exclusively in patients with pelvic obliquity secondary to lower limb deformities. The curves are supple and can be managed by a Milwaukee brace or surgical alignment of the lower extremities.

Diastrophic dwarfism is a rare form of dwarfism inherited by an autosomal recessive pattern.[120] The disease is characterized radiographically by scoliosis, club feet, multiple joint dislocations, and abducted thumbs with hypoplastic first metacarpals. The interpedicular distances are frequently narrowed at multiple levels.[122] A severe, rapidly progressive scoliosis is found in most patients usually beginning about the sixth year of life.[14,64,87] The curves are most commonly double major thoracic or double major thoracic-thoracolumbar.[14] By late childhood, the curves are usually larger than 45 degrees (Fig. 7-23). Treatment with a Milwaukee brace is recommended in infancy and childhood.[14,64] Fusion of all progressive curves is recommended, although the best type of arthrodesis and instrumentation has not been defined.[14,64]

FIGURE 7-23
A 12-year-old girl with diastrophic dwarfism and severe right thoracic scoliosis. Note the uniformly narrowed interpedicular distances *(arrowheads)* in the lumbar spine.

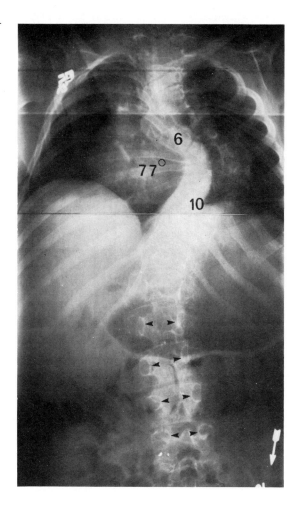

Morquio's syndrome is an autosomal recessive form of mucopolysac-charidosis characterized by corneal opacities, joint laxity, pectus carinatum, genu valgum, atlantoaxial instability, and frequent kyphoscoliosis.[64,87] The severe associated platyspondyly causes a more significant kyphosis than scoliosis, so special attention has not been paid to scoliosis in this condition. On lateral radiographs, the thoracic vertebrae are oval with a central tongue of bone extending anteriorly, and in the lumbar and thoracolumbar regions there is a large anterosuperior defect in the vertebral bodies.[15,67]

Spondyloepiphyseal dysplasia may have autosomal dominant or X-linked recessive inheritance. The radiographic findings are dominated by diffuse platyspondyly and irregular flattened epiphyses with most marked involvement of the proximal humeral and proximal femoral epiphyses.[81,118] The tarda form has a distinctive flattening of the lumbar vertebrae with a hump-shaped central protrusion of bone from the superior and inferior endplates developing in late adolescence.[65] The major spinal problem in these patients is odontoid aplasia with atlantoaxial instability.[64,87] An associated scoliosis can occur, which is usually thoracic in location and may be of a moderate to severe degree.[87]

Metatropic dwarfism is a rare chondrodystrophy for which the spinal deformity has not been described in detail. Radiographically, it is characterized by lumbar vertebral body wedging, thoracic platyspondyly, short long bones with flared metaphyses and irregular epiphyses, and a squat pelvis.[5,68,81] These patients have an early progressive kyphoscoliosis that requires treatment.[87]

Scoliosis is also present in many of the other skeletal dysplasias, but the spinal deformities have been detailed in only occasional scattered case reports.[9,11,48]

Scoliosis Secondary to Asymmetric Trunkal Growth
SURGICAL DEFORMITY

Any acquired condition that alters growth of the thorax or the abdomen during childhood has the potential to cause scoliosis. These include surgery, radiation therapy, vertebral neoplasms, and juvenile rheumatoid arthritis. Scarring from thoracic or abdominal surgery is a well documented cause of secondary scoliosis. Even if the surgery does not primarily involve the skeletal thoracic cage, such as in the repair of esophageal atresia, severe thoracic scoliosis can result requiring surgical correction.[33,43] Although these patients have their surgery in infancy, their scoliosis progresses rapidly during the adolescent growth spurt. Scoliosis most commonly develops in those patients who have had extensive pleural scarring and rib fusion from postoperative mediastinitis and empyema[43] (Fig. 7-24). The extensive adhesions in retroperitoneal fibrosis have recently been reported to cause lumbar scoliosis in two children.[71] Extensive scarring with unilateral retardation of trunkal growth is the key factor in these acquired scolioses. When the postoperative deformity is severe, scoliosis can develop even in adults. Dwork et al.[34] found a thoracic scoliosis of 20 degrees or more in 91% of 100 patients who had had a thoracoplasty as treatment for tuberculosis.

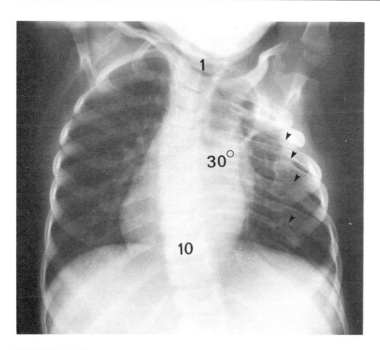

FIGURE 7-24
A 4-year-old girl who had an esophageal atresia repaired at birth but developed a postoperative fistula and empyema. Postinfectious fusion of right ribs *(arrowheads)* resulted in a progressive scoliosis.

RADIATION THERAPY

Radiation therapy of childhood thoracic or abdominal tumors is a well known cause of secondary scoliosis.[55,61,102] The most radiographically obvious cause for the induced scoliosis is the presence of retarded vertebral growth on the side of irradiation (Fig. 7-25). The wedge-shaped vertebrae presumably cause a scoliosis in a manner similar to congenital scoliosis. Older series report a 70% incidence of scoliosis after childhood irradiation for Wilms' tumor or neuroblastoma with 20% to 25% of the curves over 25 degrees.[55,102] With the current use of supervoltage rather than orthovoltage therapy and inclusion of the whole vertebrae in the treatment field, the incidence of scoliosis has decreased.[61] However, King and Stowe[61] emphasize that scoliosis can still develop due to the scarring and atrophy of the ipsilateral abdominal musculature.

Postradiation curves develop at the level of the therapy field with a concavity toward the center of the field. Because the most commonly irradiated childhood axial malignancies are Wilms' tumor and neuroblastoma, most curves are thoracolumbar or lumbar. The incidence of radiation-induced scoliosis is increased in younger children and in those receiving higher doses.[61] As in most acquired scoliosis, the curves tend to increase rapidly during the adolescent growth spurt. Since the curves are rigid, bracing is recommended only to hold the curve until growth is complete.[61,102] Because of the severe fibrosis and radiation-weakened bone, the incidence of postarthrodesis pseudarthrosis is high, and a two-stage anterior and posterior fusion is recommended.[61,102]

FIGURE 7-25
An 11-year-old boy who at age 6 years had a left paraspinal neuroblastoma irradiated and developed a left thoracic scoliosis due to hypoplasia of the left side of T10 *(arrow)*. Residual iophendylate is incidentally seen in the spinal canal.

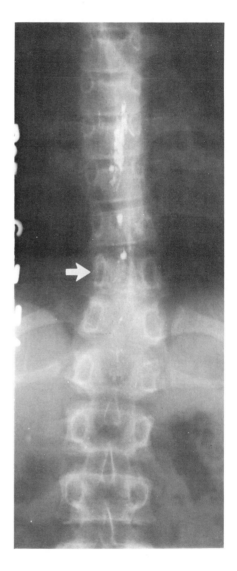

VERTEBRAL NEOPLASMS

Although osteoid osteoma and osteoblastoma of the spine are uncommon lesions, they have been the subject of multiple reports.* These benign tumors are the most frequent cause of a painful scoliosis in preadolescent and adolescent children.[83] Three fourths of the patients are between 10 and 25 years old.[1,78] Since the lesion can be difficult to locate on routine radiographs, Kirwan et al.[62] have recommended that a bone scan be obtained in all children with a painful scoliosis in whom routine radiographs are normal. In adolescent patients with true idiopathic scoliosis, the bone scan should be normal.[112]

Almost all vertebral osteoid osteomas and osteoblastomas occur in the pedicles or posterior elements. The most common spinal location for both tumors is in the lumbar vertebrae. The tumors occur on the concavity at the apex of the scoliosis except for fourth and fifth lumbar lesions, in which the apex of the curve is above the lesion.[1,56,62,98] Spinal osteoblastomas are usually expansile lytic lesions but can have significant reactive sclerosis and central calcifications (Figs. 7-26 and 7-27). Osteoid osteomas usually consist of a

*See references 1, 56, 58, 62, 78, 98.

FIGURE 7-26
Left lumbar scoliosis due to osteoblastoma of L3.
The osteoblastoma is lytic and expansile *(arrowheads)* but has central calcifications.

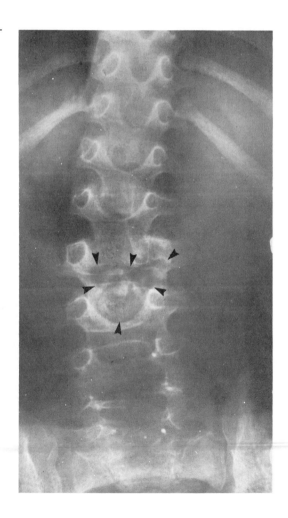

FIGURE 7-27
Osteoblastoma of the left lateral mass and
lamina of the first cervical vertebra in a
12-year-old boy. The marked expansion
and central calcifications of the lesion are
seen on the lateral cervical spine film **(A)**
and the CT scan **(B).**

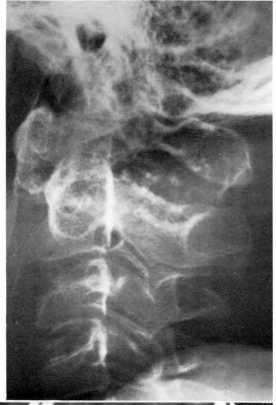

A

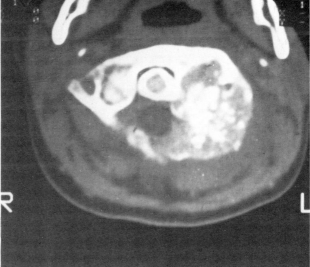

B

small, lucent nidus with central calcifications. The nidus may be difficult to detect or be obscured by dense surrounding sclerosis.

The presumed mechanism for the scoliosis is muscle spasm on the side of the tumor. In most cases, excision of the tumor eliminates the scoliosis. Recent reports have stressed the value of computed tomography for accurate preoperative localization of the nidus of an axial skeletal osteoid osteoma.[38,62] An important but little-appreciated fact is that a rigid scoliosis can develop if the lesion is present for more than 2 years.[58,98] The resultant structural scoliosis may require surgical correction.[1]

Juvenile Rheumatoid Arthritis

Patients with polyarticular juvenile rheumatoid arthritis (JRA) frequently have retarded musculoskeletal growth. Although the growth disturbances at peripheral joints are well documented, the increased incidence of scoliosis in these patients is not widely appreciated. In two large series, scoliosis of greater than 20 degrees was found in 1.7% to 2.5% of JRA patients[107,121] (Fig. 7-28). This incidence is significantly increased when compared to the well documented 0.3% to 0.4% incidence of idiopathic scoliosis of over 20 degrees in the general population. Combining the two series, the frequency of scoliosis by curve pattern and level in decreasing order was thoracic (44%), thoracolumbar (28%), double major (20%), and lumbar (8%). The cause of the scoliosis is unknown, with possible causes including muscle imbalance and asymmetrical rheumatoid involvement of apophyseal joints.[107]

FIGURE 7-28
A 17-year-old boy with long-standing juvenile
rheumatoid arthritis and right thoracolumbar scoliosis.

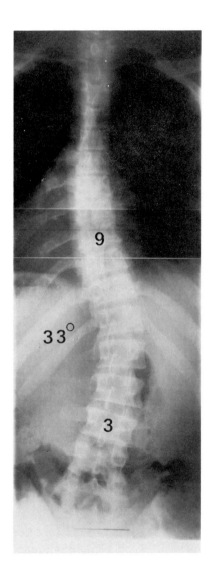

LEG-LENGTH DISCREPANCY

The scoliosis associated with leg-length discrepancy is usually described as compensatory, nonstructural, and nonprogressive. However, a recent study has shown that structural changes can develop.[94] If limb-length inequality develops prior to skeletal maturity, the scoliosis and vertebral rotation often do not disappear after correcting the limb discrepancy with a shoe lift.[94] Also, in these same patients, lateral flexion toward the short side is consistently reduced. In contrast, patients who develop limb-length inequality after skeletal maturity but before adulthood do not develop structural spinal changes.[41]

The mechanism for the development of the structural curves in the younger patient group may relate to secondary paraspinal muscle changes such as contractures. Curves related to leg-length discrepancy are predominately lumbar, although in some cases the superior end vertebra may be as high as the eighth thoracic vertebrae.[41] Scoliosis due to leg-length discrepancy is generally an infrequent and seldom significant problem.

Scoliosis and Other Inherited Diseases

Because of the well documented hereditary pattern of scoliosis (see Chapter One), it is not surprising that an increased incidence of scoliosis has also been found in patients with other inherited conditions. These diseases have no obvious reason to cause asymmetric spinal growth and include such diverse entities as cystic fibrosis, congenital heart disease, and congenital deficiencies of the upper extremity.

Scoliotic curves of greater than 10 degrees were detected in 6.9%[35] and 10%[93] of patients with cystic fibrosis in two large series. The curves were most commonly right thoracic, but 33% of the patients had left thoracic curves and 13% had double major. An equal frequency of scoliosis was found in both boys and girls with cystic fibrosis.

Similarly, scoliosis of greater than 20 degrees was found in 8.5%[99] and 4.6%[109] of patients with congenital heart disease, much greater than the expected incidence of 0.3%. These same two studies found no association between the situs of the heart or aorta and the convexity of the scoliosis. The observed curve patterns were similar to idiopathic scoliosis, with right thoracic being the most common pattern. However, unlike the female predominance in idiopathic scoliosis, the male and female incidences of scoliosis were similar in both studies.

Even more interestingly, scoliosis of greater than 10 degrees without underlying congenital spinal anomalies was found in 16% to 48% of patients with upper extremity anomalies.[79,96] No difference in the incidence of scoliosis was found in unilateral or bilateral hemimelia or bilateral phocomelia. The male and female incidences were also equal. There was no relationship between the side of a unilateral deficiency and the direction of the curve.[96] The curves (Fig. 7-29) are primarily thoracic.[79,96]

The full significance of the association between these unrelated conditions and an increased incidence of scoliosis is not known. All three conditions have curve patterns similar to idiopathic scoliosis but with a distinctive equal incidence in male and female patients. Because of these observations, it is possible that all three diseases are transmitted on particular genetic loci that are linked with at least one locus that predisposes to idiopathic scoliosis. Further genetic evaluation of these patients may be rewarding in the search for the genetic component of idiopathic scoliosis.

FIGURE 7-29
A 9-year-old boy with congenital deficiency of the left upper extremity and a left thoracic scoliosis.

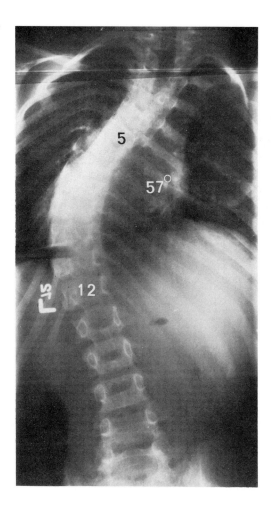

Summary

The length of this chapter reflects the complexity of the topic of secondary scoliosis. To provide a basic framework of facts, the key features of each entity are presented in this summary along with Table 7-1, which shows common radiographic patterns.

A. Congenital scoliosis
  1. Types—wedge vertebra, hemivertebra, unsegmented bar, block vertebra
  2. Related conditions
    a. Congenital heart disease (cardiac examination and chest x-ray needed)
    b. Genitourinary abnormalities (routine excretory urogram or nuclear medicine renal scan recommended)
    c. Diastematomyelia (look for spina bifida, bony midline spur, or widened pedicles about the curve apex)
  3. Patterns
    a. Short, rigid curves often relentlessly progressive
    b. Most commonly thoracic or thoracolumbar
B. Neuropathic and myopathic scoliosis
  1. General patterns
    a. Sweeping, thoracolumbar, curves—cerebral palsy, posttraumatic paralysis, poliomyelitis, spinal muscular atrophy, myelomeningocele, muscular dystrophy, arthrogryposis
    b. Associated pelvic obliquity with long thoracolumbar curves
    c. Thoracic curves resembling idiopathic scoliosis—spinocerebellar degeneration, syringomyelia, familial dysautonomia
  2. Spinal orthoses
    a. Until growth is complete or unless the curve continues to progress
    b. Not recommended in Friedrich's ataxia or familial dysautonomia
  3. Spinal fusion—progressive or large curves
    a. Posterior—Charcot-Marie-Tooth, spinal muscular atrophy, muscular dystrophy, arthrogryposis, smaller cerebral palsy, or poliomyelitis curves
    b. Two-stage anterior and posterior—cerebral palsy, poliomyelitis, myelomeningocele
C. Mesodermal scoliosis
  1. Neurofibromatosis—characteristic radiographic findings
    a. Anterior, posterior or lateral vertebral scalloping
    b. Twisted, spindled ribs or transverse processes
    c. Short (less than five vertebrae) angular thoracic scoliosis
  2. Treatment for neurofibromatosis and Marfan's syndrome
    a. Orthoses (ineffective in dystrophic scoliosis)
    b. Arthrodesis (usually posterior but two-stage if dystrophic neurofibromatosis kyphoscoliosis)
D. Skeletal dysplasia
  1. Distinctive vertebral radiographic findings

TABLE 7-1
Secondary scoliosis with key radiographic findings

Cause	Radiographic finding
Congenital	Wedge vertebra, hemivertebra, unilateral bar
Syringomyelia	Widened interpedicular distance in the cervical spine
Spinal cord tumors	Widened interpedicular distance
Myelomeningocele	Widened canal and absent posterior elements
Neurofibromatosis	Vertebral scalloping, deformed ribs, or transverse processes
Dysplasias	Distinctive for each entity
Radiation therapy	Unilateral vertebral, rib, or pelvis hypoplasia
Vertebral neoplasm	Expansile or sclerotic lesions

       a. Osteogenesis imperfecta—demineralized, compressed vertebrae
       b. Achondroplasia—narrowed interpedicular distances in lower lumbar spine
       c. Pseudachondroplasia—pelvic obliquity from lower limb deformities
       d. Diastrophic dwarfism—uniformly narrowed interpedicular distances
    2. Platyspondylic forms
       a. Morquio's syndrome—anterior beak or anterosuperior defect and pointed proximal metacarpals
       b. Spondyloepiphyseal dysplasia—tarda form with central superior and inferior humps and flattened epiphyses
       c. Metatropic dwarfism—lumbar wedging and thoracic flattening and dumbbell-shaped long bones
  E. Asymmetric trunkal growth
    1. Surgical deformity—due to soft tissue scarring or rib cage deformity
    2. Radiation therapy
       a. Typical findings wedge-shaped vertebrae at or below the thoracolumbar junction plus unilateral rib or pelvic hypoplasia
       b. Two-stage fusion recommended
    3. Vertebral neoplasms—osteoid osteoma or osteoblastoma
       a. Most common cause of painful scoliosis
       b. Usually in posterior elements
       c. Treat scoliosis by removal of lesion
    4. Juvenile rheumatoid arthritis—patterns resemble idiopathic scoliosis
  F. Scoliosis with short rigid curves
    1. Congenital
    2. Neurofibromatosis
    3. Spinal fractures
    4. Surgical scarring
    5. Radiation therapy

REFERENCES

1. Akbarnia, B.A., and Rooholamini, S.A.: Scoliosis caused by benign osteoblastoma of the thoracic or lumbar spine, J. Bone Joint Surg. (Am.) **63:**1146-1155, 1981.
2. Aprin, H., et al.: Spine fusion in patients with spinal muscular atrophy, J. Bone Joint Surg. (Am.) **64:**1179-1187, 1982.
3. Asher, M., and Olson, J.: Factors affecting the ambulatory status of patients with spina bifida cystica, J. Bone Joint Surg. (Am.) **65:**350-356, 1983.
4. Bailey, J.A., II,: Orthopaedic aspects of achondroplasia, J. Bone Joint Surg. (Am.) **52:**1285-1301, 1970.
5. Bailey, J.A., II, Dorst, J.P., and Saunderson, R.W., Jr.: Metatropic dwarfism, recognized retrospectively from the roentgenographic features, Birth Defects **5:** 376-381, 1969.
6. Baker, A.S., and Dove, J.: Progressive scoliosis as the first presenting sign of syringomyelia, J. Bone Joint Surg. (Br.) **65:**472-473, 1983.
7. Balmer, G.A., and MacEwen, G.D.: The incidence and treatment of scoliosis in cerebral palsy, J. Bone Joint Surg. (Br.) **52:**134-137, 1970.
8. Banta, J.V., et al.: Fifteen-year review of myelodysplasia, J. Bone Joint Surg. (Am.) **58:**726, 1976.
9. Bartolozzi, P., et al.: Melnick-Needles syndrome: osteodysplasty with kyphoscoliosis, J. Pediatr. Orthop. **3:**387-391, 1983.
10. Bauze, R.J., Smith, R., and Francis, M.J.O.: A new look at osteogenesis imperfecta. A clinical, radiological and biochemical study of forty-two patients, J. Bone Joint Surg. (Br.) **57:**1-12, 1975.
11. Beighton, P., et al.: Spondylo-epimetaphyseal dysplasia with joint laxity and severe, progressive kyphoscoliosis, S. Afr. Med. J. **64:**772-775, 1983.
12. Benson, D.R., Donaldson, D.H., and Millar, E.A.: The spine in osteogenesis imperfecta, J. Bone Joint Surg. (Am.) **60:**925-929, 1978.
13. Benson, D.R., and Newman, D.C.: The spine and surgical treatment in osteogenesis imperfecta, Clin. Orthop. **159:**147-153, 1981.
14. Bethem, D., Winger, R.B., and Lutter, L.: Disorders of the spine in diastrophic dwarfism, J. Bone Joint Surg. (Am.) **62:**529-536, 1980.
15. Blaw, M.E., and Langer, L.O.: Spinal cord compression in Morquio-Brailsford's disease, J. Pediatr. **74:**593-600, 1969.
16. Boldrey, E., et al.: Scoliosis as a manifestation of disease of the cervicothoracic portion of the spinal cord, Arch. Neurol. Psychiatr. **61:**528-544, 1949.
17. Bonnett, C., Brown, J.C., and Brooks, H.L.: Anterior spine fusion with Dwyer instrumentation for lumbar scoliosis in cerebral palsy—a preliminary report, J. Bone Joint Surg. (Am.) **55:**425, 1973.
18. Bonnett, C., Brown, J.C., and Grow, T.: Thoracolumbar scoliosis in cerebral palsy, J. Bone Joint Surg. (Am.) **58:**328-336, 1976.
19. Bonnett, C., et al.: Evolution of treatment of paralytic scoliosis at Rancho Los Amigos Hospital, J. Bone Joint Surg. (Am.) **57:**206-215, 1975.
20. Brown, H.P.: Management of spinal deformity in myelomeningocele, Orthop. Clin. North Am. **9:**391-402, 1978.
21. Brown, H.P., and Bonnett, C.C.: Spine deformity subsequent to spinal cord injury, J. Bone Joint Surg. (Am.) **55:**441, 1973.
22. Brown, J.C., Swank, S., and Specht, L.: Combined anterior and posterior spine fusion in cerebral palsy, Spine **7:**570-573, 1982.
23. Bunch, W.H.: The Milwaukee brace in paralytic scoliosis, Clin. Orthop. **110:**63-68, 1975.
24. Casselman, E.S., and Mandell, G.A.: Vertebral scalloping in neurofibromatosis, Radiology **131:**89-94, 1979.
25. Chaglassian, J.H., Riseborough, E.J., and Hall, J.E.: Neurofibromatous scoliosis, J. Bone Joint Surg. (Br.) **58:**695-702, 1976.
26. Colonna, P., and Vom Saal, F.: A study of paralytic scoliosis based on five hundred cases of poliomyelitis, J. Bone Joint Surg. **23:**335-353, 1941.

27. Cowell, H.R., MacEwen, G.D., and Hubben, C.: Incidence of abnormalities of the kidney and ureter in congenital scoliosis, Birth Defects 10:142-145, 1974.

28. Cristofaro, R.L., et al.: Operative treatment of spine deformity in osteogenesis imperfecta, Clin. Orthop. 139:40-48, 1979.

29. Curtiss, P.H., Jr., and Collins, W.F.: Spinal-cord tumor—a cause of progressive neurological changes in children with scoliosis, J. Bone Joint Surg. (Am.) 43:517-522, 1961.

30. Dewald, R.L., and Faut, M.M.: Anterior and posterior spinal fusion for paralytic scoliosis, Spine 4:401-409, 1979.

31. Dewald, R.L., and Ray, R.D.: Congenital kyphosis with successful treatment, J. Bone Joint Surg. (Am.) 53:587-590, 1971.

32. Drummond, D.S., and Mackenzie, D.A.: Scoliosis in arthrogryposis multiplex congenita, Spine 3:146-151, 1978.

33. Durning, R.P., Scoles, P.V., and Fox, O.D.: Scoliosis after thoracotomy in tracheoesophageal fistula patients, J. Bone Joint Surg. (Am.) 62:1156-1159, 1980.

34. Dwork, R.E., Dinken, H., and Hurst, A.: Post thoracoplasty scoliosis, Arch. Phys. Med. 32:722-729, 1951.

35. Erkkila, J.C., Warwick, W.J., and Bradford, D.S.: Spine deformities and cystic fibrosis, Clin. Orthop. 131:146-150, 1978.

36. Falvo, K.A., Root, L., and Bullough, P.G.: Osteogenesis imperfecta: clinical evaluation and management, J. Bone Joint Surg. (Am.) 56:783-793, 1974.

37. Fisk, J.R., and Bunch, W.H.: Scoliosis in neuromuscular disease, Orthop. Clin. North Am. 10:863-875, 1979.

38. Gamba, J.L., et al.: Computed tomography of axial skeletal osteoid osteomas, AJR 142:769-772, 1984.

39. Gibson, D.A., and Urs, N.D.K.: Arthrogryposis multiplex congenita, J. Bone Joint Surg. (Br.) 52:483-493, 1970.

40. Gibson, D.A., et al.: The management of spinal deformity in Duchenne's muscular dystrophy, Orthop. Clin. North Am. 9:437-450, 1978.

41. Gibson, P.H., Papaioannou, T., and Kenwright, J.: The influence on the spine of leg-length discrepancy after femoral fracture, J. Bone Joint Surg. (Br.) 65:584-587, 1983.

42. Gillespie, R., and Wedge, J.H.: The problems of scoliosis in paraplegic children, J. Bone Joint Surg. (Am.) 56:1767, 1974.

43. Gilsanz, V., et al.: Scoliosis after thoracotomy for esophageal atresia, AJR 141:457-460, 1983.

44. Gitelis, S., Whiffen, J., and DeWald, R.L.: The treatment of severe scoliosis in osteogenesis imperfecta, Clin. Orthop. 175:56-59, 1983.

45. Hall, J.E., and Bobechko, W.P.: Advances in the management of spinal deformities in myelodysplasia, Clin. Neurosurg. 20:164-173, 1973.

46. Hall, J.E., Herndon, W.A., and Levine, C.R.: Surgical treatment of congenital scoliosis with or without Harrington instrumentation, J. Bone Joint Surg. (Am.) 63:608-619, 1981.

47. Heck, A.F.: A study of neural and extraneural findings in a large family with Friedreich's ataxia, J. Neurol. Sci. 1:226-255, 1964.

48. Heilbronner, D.M., and Renshaw, T.S.: Spondylothoracic dysplasia, J. Bone Joint Surg. (Am.) 66:302-303, 1984.

49. Hensinger, R.N., and MacEwen, G.D.: Spinal deformity associated with heritable neurological conditions: spinal muscular atrophy, Friedreich's ataxia, familial dysautonomia, and Charcot-Marie-tooth disease, J. Bone Joint Surg. (Am.) 58:13-24, 1976.

50. Holt, J.F.: Neurofibromatosis in children, AJR 130:615-639, 1978.

51. Huebert, H.T., and MacKinnon, W.B.: Syringomyelia and scoliosis, J. Bone Joint Surg. (Br.) 51:338-343, 1969.

52. James, J.I.P.: Paralytic scoliosis, J. Bone Joint Surg. (Br.) 38:660-685, 1956.

53. James, J.I.P.: The management of infants with scoliosis, J. Bone Joint Surg. (Br.) 57:422-429, 1975.

54. Kahanovitz, N., Brown, J.C., and Bonnett, C.A.: The operative treatment of congenital scoliosis, Clin. Orthop. **143**:174-182, 1979.

55. Katzman, H., Waugh, T., and Berdon, W.: Skeletal changes following irradiation of childhood tumors, J. Bone Joint Surg. (Am.) **51**:825-842, 1969.

56. Kehl, D.K., Alsonso, J.E., and Lovell, W.W.: Scoliosis secondary to an osteoid-osteoma of the rib, J. Bone Joint Surg. (Am.) **65**:701-703, 1983.

57. Keim, H.A., and Greene, A.F.: Diastematomyelia and scoliosis, J. Bone Joint Surg. (Am.) **55**:1425-1435, 1973.

58. Keim, H.A., and Reina, E.G.: Osteoid-osteoma as a cause of scoliosis, J. Bone Joint Surg. (Am.) **57**:159-163, 1975.

59. Kilfoyle, R.M., Foley, J.J., and Norton, P.L.: Spine and pelvic deformity in childhood and adolescent paraplegia, J. Bone Joint Surg. (Am.) **47**:659-682, 1965.

60. King, J.D., and Bobechko, W.P.: Osteogenesis imperfecta: an orthopaedic description and surgical review, J. Bone Joint Surg. (Br.) **53**:72-89, 1971.

61. King, J., and Stowe, S.: Results of spinal fusion for radiation scoliosis, Spine **7**:574-585, 1982.

62. Kirwan, E.O'G., et al.: Osteoid osteoma and benign osteoblastoma of the spine, J. Bone Joint Surg. (Br.) **66**:21-26, 1984.

63. Klatte, E.C., Franken, E.A., and Smith, J.A.: The radiographic spectrum in neurofibromatosis, Semin. Roentgenol. **11**:17-33, 1976.

64. Kopits, S.E.: Orthopedic complications of dwarfism, Clin. Orthop. **114**:153-179, 1976.

65. Langer, L.O., Jr.: Spondyloepiphyseal dysplasia tarda, Radiology **82**:833-839, 1964.

66. Langer, L.O., Jr., Baumann, P.A., and Gorlin, R.J.: Achondroplasia, AJR **100**:12-26, 1967.

67. Langer, L.O., Jr., and Carey, L.S.: The roentgenographic features of the Ks mucopolysaccharidosis of Morquio (Morquio-Brailsford's disease), AJR **97**:1-20, 1966.

68. Larose, J.H., and Gay, B.B., Jr.: Metatrophic dwarfism, AJR **106**:156-161, 1969.

69. Leeds, N.E., and Jacobson, H.G.: Spinal neurofibromatosis, AJR **126**:617-623, 1976.

70. Leong, J.C.Y., et al: Surgical treatment of scoliosis following poliomyelitis, J. Bone Joint Surg. (Am.) **63**:726-740, 1981.

71. Letts, M.: Scoliosis in children secondary to retroperitoneal fibrosis, J. Bone Joint Surg. (Am.) **64**:1363-1368, 1982.

72. Lloyd-Roberts, G.C., and Lettin, A.W.F.: Arthrogryposis multiplex congenita, J. Bone Joint Surg. (Br.) **52**:494-508, 1970.

73. Logue, V., and Edwards, M.R.: Syringomyelia and its surgical treatment—an analysis of 75 patients, J. Neurol. Neurosurg. Psychiatry **44**:273-284, 1981.

74. Lonstein, J.E., and Akbarnia, B.A.: Operative treatment of spinal deformities in patients with cerebral palsy or mental retardation, J. Bone Joint Surg. (Am.) **65**:43-55, 1983.

75. Luque, E.R.: Paralytic scoliosis in growing children, Clin. Orthop. **163**:202-209, 1982.

76. MacEwen, G.D., Conway, J.J., and Miller, W.T.: Congenital scoliosis with a unilateral bar, Radiology **90**:711-715, 1968.

77. MacEwen, G.D., Winter, R.G., and Hardy, J.H.: Evaluation of kidney anomalies in congenital scoliosis, J. Bone Joint Surg. (Am.) **54**:1451-1454, 1972.

78. Maclellan, D.I., and Wilson, F.C., Jr.: Osteoid osteoma of the spine, J. Bone Joint Surg. (Am.) **49**:111-121, 1967.

79. Makley, J.T., and Heiple, K.G.: Scoliosis associated with congenital deficiencies of the upper extremity, J. Bone Joint Surg. (Am.) **52**:279-287, 1970.

80. Mandell, G.A.: The pedicle in neurofibromatosis, AJR **130**:675-678, 1978.

81. Maroteaux, P.: Spondyloepiphyseal dysplasias and metatropic dwarfism, Birth Defects **5**:35-44, 1969.

82. McMaster, M.J., and Ohtsuka, K.: The natural history of congenital scoliosis, J. Bone Joint Surg. (Am.) **64**:1128-1147, 1982.

83. Mehta, M.H., and Murray, R.O.: Scoliosis provoked by painful vertebral lesions, Skel. Radiol. **1**:223-230, 1977.

84. Menelaus, M.: Spinal deformity in spina bifida, J. Bone Joint Surg. (Br.) **55**:223-224, 1973.

85. Moe, J., et al.: Scoliosis and other spinal deformities, Philadelphia, 1978, W.B. Saunders Co.

86. Nasca, R.J., Stelling, F.H., and Steel, H.H.: Progression of congenital scoliosis due to hemivertebrae and hemivertebrae with bars, J. Bone Joint Surg. (Am.) **57**:456-466, 1975.

87. Nelson, M.A.: Orthopaedic aspects of the chondrodystrophies: the dwarf and his orthopaedic problems, Ann. R. Coll. Surg. Engl. **47**:185-210, 1970.

88. Norimatsu, H., Mayuzumi, T., and Takahashi, H.: The development of the spinal deformities in osteogenesis imperfecta, Clin. Orthop. **162**:20-25, 1982.

89. Norton, P.L., and Foley, J.J.: Paraplegia in children, J. Bone Joint Surg. (Am.) **41**:1291-1309, 1959.

90. O'Brien, J.P., Dwyer, A.P., and Hodgson, A.R.: Paralytic pelvic obliquity: its prognosis and management and the development of a technique for full correction of the deformity, J. Bone Joint Surg. (Am.) **57**:626-631, 1975.

91. O'Brien, J.P., and Yau, A.C.M.C.: Anterior and posterior correction and fusion for paralytic scoliosis, Clin. Orthop. **86**:151-153, 1972.

92. Osebold, W.R., et al.: Surgical treatment of paralytic scoliosis associated with myelomeningocele, J. Bone Joint Surg. (Am.) **64**:841-855, 1982.

93. Paling, M.R., and Spasovsky-Chernick, M.: Scoliosis in cystic fibrosis—an appraisal, Skel. Radiol. **8**:63-66, 1982.

94. Papaioannou, T., Stokes, I., and Kenwright, J.: Scoliosis associated with limb-length inequality, J. Bone Joint Surg. (Am.) **64**:59-62, 1982.

95. Piggott, H.: The natural history of scoliosis in myelodysplasia, J. Bone Joint Surg. (Br.) **62**:54-58, 1980.

96. Powers, T.A., et al.: Abnormalities of the spine in relation to congenital upper limb deficiencies, J. Pediatr. Orthop. **3**:471-474, 1983.

97. Poznanski, A.K., and LaRowe, P.C.: Radiographic manifestations of the arthrogryposis syndrome, Radiology **95**:353-358, 1970.

98. Ransford, A.O., et al.: The behaviour pattern of the scoliosis associated with osteoid osteoma or osteoblastoma of the spine, J. Bone Joint Surg. (Br.) **66**:16-20, 1984.

99. Reckles, L.N., et al.: The association of scoliosis and congenital heart defects, J. Bone Joint Surg. (Am.) **57**:449-455, 1975.

100. Rezaian, S.M.: The incidence of scoliosis due to neurofibromatosis, Acta Orthop. Scand. **47**:534-539, 1976.

101. Rinsky, L.A.: Perspectives on surgery for scoliosis in mentally retarded patients, Orthop. Clin. North Am. **12**:113-126, 1981.

102. Riseborough, E.J., et al.: Skeletal alterations following irradiation for Wilms' tumor, J. Bone Joint Surg. (Am.) **58**:526-536, 1976.

103. Roaf, R.: Paralytic scoliosis, J. Bone Joint Surg. (Br.) **38**:640-659, 1956.

104. Robin, G.C., and Brief, L.P.: Scoliosis in childhood muscular dystrophy, J. Bone Joint Surg. (Am.) **53**:466-476, 1971.

105. Robins, P.R., Moe, J.H., and Winter, R.B.: Scoliosis in Marfan's syndrome, J. Bone Joint Surg. (Am.) **57**:358-368, 1975.

106. Robson, P.: The prevalence of scoliosis in adolescents and young adults with cerebral palsy, Dev. Med. Child Neurol. **10**:447-452, 1968.

107. Rombouts, J.J., and Rombouts-Lindemans, C.: Scoliosis in juvenile rheumatoid arthritis, J. Bone Joint Surg. (Br.) **56**:478-483, 1974.

108. Rosenthal, R.K., Levine, D.B., and McCarver, C.L.: The occurrence of scoliosis in cerebral palsy, Dev. Med. Child Neurol. **16**:664-667, 1974.

109. Roth, A., et al.: Scoliosis and congenital heart disease, Clin. Orthop. **93**:95-102, 1973.

110. Samilson, R.L., and Bechard, R.: Scoliosis in cerebral palsy: incidence, distribu-

tion of curve patterns, natural history, and thoughts on etiology, Curr. Pract. Orthop. Surg. **5**:183-205, 1973.

111. Schwentker, E.P., and Gibson, D.A.: The orthopaedic aspects of spinal muscular atrophy, J. Bone Joint Surg. (Am.) **58**:32-38, 1976.

112. Sevastikoglou, J.A., et al.: Bone scanning of the spine and thorax in idiopathic thoracic scoliosis, Clin. Orthop. **149**:172-174, 1980.

113. Shapiro, F., and Bresnan, M.J.: Orthopaedic management of childhood neuromuscular disease, J. Bone Joint Surg. (Am.) **64**:1102-1107, 1982.

114. Shurtleff, D.B., et al.: Myelodysplasia: the natural history of kyphosis and scoliosis: a preliminary report, Dev. Med. Child Neurol. **18**:126-133, 1976.

115. Siebold, R.M., Winter, R.B., and Moe, J.H.: The treatment of scoliosis in arthrogryposis multiplex congenita, Clin. Orthop. **103**:191-198, 1974.

116. Siegel, I.M.: Scoliosis in muscular dystrophy, Clin. Orthop. **93**:235-238, 1973.

117. Spencer, G.E., Jr.: Orthopaedic considerations in the management of muscular dystrophy, Curr. Pract. Orthop. Surg. **5**:279-293, 1973.

118. Spranger, J.W., and Langer, L.O., Jr.: Spondyloepiphyseal dysplasia congenita, Radiology **94**:313-322, 1970.

119. Sriram, K., Bobechko, W.P., and Hall, J.E.: Surgical management of spinal deformities in spina bifida, J. Bone Joint Surg. (Br.) **54**:666-676, 1972.

120. Stover, C.N., Hayes, J.T., and Holt, J.F.: Diastrophic dwarfism, AJR **89**:914-922, 1963.

121. Svantesson, H., Marhaug, G., and Haeffner, F.: Scoliosis in children with juvenile rheumatoid arthritis, Scand. J. Rheumatol. **10**:65-68, 1981.

122. Taybi, H.: Diastrophic dwarfism, Radiology **80**:1-10, 1963.

123. Taybi, H.: Radiology of syndromes and metabolic disorders, ed. 2, Chicago, 1983, Year Book Medical Publishers.

124. Till, K.: Spinal dysraphism: a study of congenital malformations of the lower back, J. Bone Joint Surg. (Br.) **51**:415-422, 1969.

125. Vitko, R.J., Cass, A.S., and Winter R.B.: Anomalies of the genitourinary tract associated with congenital scoliosis and congenital kyphosis, J. Urol. **108**:655-659, 1972.

126. Wedge, J.H., and Gillespie, R.: The problems of scoliosis surgery in paraplegic children, J. Bone Joint Surg. (Br.) **57**:396, 1975.

127. Winter, R.B.: Congenital deformities of the spine, New York, 1983, Thieme-Stratton Inc.

128. Winter, R.B.: Section 26, Thoracolumbar spine: pediatric. In Orthopaedic knowledge update I: Home study syllabus, Chicago, 1984, American Academy of Orthopaedic Surgeons, pp. 217-226.

129. Winter, R.B., and Moe, J.H.: The results of spinal arthrodesis for congenital spinal deformity in patients younger than five years old, J. Bone Joint Surg. (Am.) **64**:419-432, 1982.

130. Winter, R.B., Moe, J.H., and Eilers, V.E.: Congenital scoliosis: a study of 234 patients treated and untreated. Part I: natural history, J. Bone Joint Surg. (Am.) **50**:1-15, 1968.

131. Winter, R.B., Moe, J.H., and Eilers, V.E.: Congenital scoliosis: a study of 234 patients treated and untreated. Part II: treatment, J. Bone Joint Surg. (Am.) **50**:15-47, 1968.

132. Winter, R.B., et al.: Diastematomyelia and congenital spine deformities, J. Bone Joint Surg. (Am.) **56**:27-39, 1974.

133. Winter, R.B., et al.: Spine deformity in neurofibromatosis, J. Bone Joint Surg. (Am.) **61**:677-694, 1979.

134. Yong-Hing, K., and MacEwen, G.D.: Scoliosis associated with osteogenesis imperfecta, J. Bone Joint Surg. (Br.) **64**:36-43, 1982.

135. Yoslow, W., et al.: Orthopaedic defects in familial dysautonomia, J. Bone Joint Surg. (Am.) **53**:1541-1550, 1971.

Chapter Eight

Kyphosis

General Principles

Kyphosis refers to spinal curvature in the sagittal plane of the body in which the spinal segment is convex posteriorly when viewed from the side. A kyphosis in the thoracic spine is abnormal only when the curvature exceeds the normal range. An increased thoracic kyphosis is properly termed a kyphos or hyperkyphosis. Any posteriorly convex curvature in the lumbar spine or at the thoracolumbar junction is abnormal and is indicated, respectively, by the simple terms *lumbar kyphosis* or *thoracolumbar kyphosis*.

The classification of causes of abnormal kyphosis is as extensive as that applied to scoliosis, but abnormal kyphosis is not nearly as frequent a clinical problem. A useful classification of the causes of kyphosis is presented by Moe et al.[35] in their book and includes Scheuermann's, postural, congenital, myelomeningocoele, infectious, neuromuscular, traumatic, surgical, radiation therapy, metabolic disease, and skeletal dysplasia.

RADIOGRAPHIC EVALUATION

Lateral spinal radiography for evaluation of kyphosis is as important as the routine posteroanterior radiograph in scoliosis. It serves to (1) confirm the abnormal curvature, (2) identify its etiology, (3) quantitate its severity, (4) monitor its progression or stability, and (5) evaluate the effectiveness of treatment. As described in Chapter Two, the lateral radiograph should be obtained with the patient standing, or seated if he cannot stand unassisted. The arms should be elevated to shoulder level with the hands resting on a support (Fig. 8-1, *A*). A supine cross-table lateral film obtained with the patient lying on a bolster at the curve apex evaluates the curve flexibility (Fig. 8-1, *B*).

The lateral radiograph should be evaluated carefully for the cause of the kyphos. Unlike the case for scoliosis where 85% of the curves will be idiopathic, the cause of the abnormal kyphosis will usually be radiographically identifiable. The abnormal curvature will be due to either localized or multiple vertebral abnormalities:

1. Multiple vertebral body abnormalities
   a. Scheuermann's disease
   b. Skeletal dysplasias
   c. Metabolic disease
   d. Spondyloarthropathies
2. Localized vertebral body abnormalities
   a. Congenital
   b. Traumatic
   c. Radiation therapy
   d. Infection
   e. Intraspinal mass

3. Posterior element deficiency
   a. Myelomeningocoele
   b. Postlaminectomy

In addition to the standing lateral radiograph, the initial radiographic evaluation should include a standing posteroanterior (PA) radiograph to determine if there is associated scoliosis as often occurs in kyphosis owing to Scheuermann's disease, myelomeningocoele, trauma, radiation therapy, and skeletal dysplasia. The PA radiograph also aids in identifying the cause of the kyphosis, especially in the patients with myelomeningocoele and extensive laminectomies.

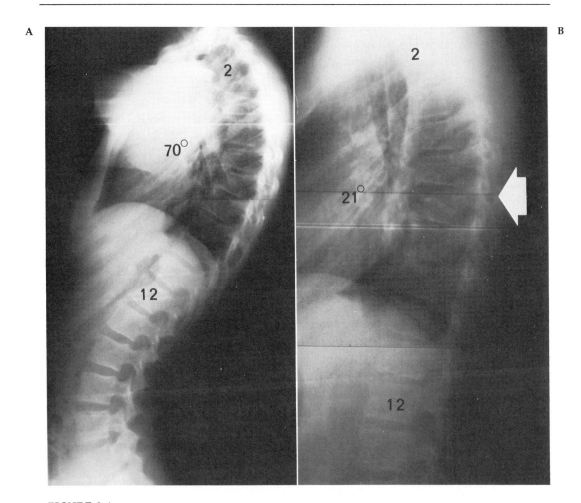

FIGURE 8-1
Adolescent girl with Scheuermann's disease.
Upright lateral film **(A)** shows flexible thoracic hyperkyphosis that significantly decreases on the supine cross-table lateral film **(B)** with arrow showing level of bolster.

TREATMENT

As a general principle, if the kyphosis warrants active therapy, treatment is begun with a spinal orthosis. For the treatment of thoracic hyperkyphosis, the only pads used are paired ones placed at the curve apex on each posterior upright. If the curve is painful and progresses during bracing or is already greater than 65 degrees, posterior fusion with internal fixation is the recommended surgical technique. Because they draw together the posterior elements and reduce kyphosis, paired Harrington compression rods are commonly used for internal fixation (Fig. 8-2). Greater control over correction of a thoracolumbar kyphosis can be achieved by bending Luque rods to the desired lumbar lordosis and thoracic kyphosis (Fig. 8-3). Anterior Dwyer or Zielke instrumentation is relatively contraindicated in the presence of abnormal kyphosis because the anterior compression increases kyphosis.

Multiple Vertebral Body Abnormalities
SCHEUERMANN'S DISEASE

Although over 60 years have passed since Scheuermann described the vertebral changes in this condition,[42] the exact etiology is still unknown. Proposed etiologies have included avascular necrosis of the vertebral ring apophysis, intravertebral disk herniation, mechanical stress, endocrine disturbances, and nutritional deficiencies.[12] Surgical evaluation of the spine in patients with Scheuermann's disease reveals a contracted anterior longitudinal ligament, normal disk space height and width, and anterior vertebral body wedging.[9] These same authors found endplate disruption with nucleus pulposus extravasation into the vertebral body spongiosa but no evidence of avascular necrosis or inflammation. A recent extensive histologic, histochemical, and electron microscopy study of vertebral tissue from six patients with Scheuermann's disease concluded that the disease was due to a defect in the matrix of the growth cartilage and vertebral endplate.[2]

Diagnostic criteria. Although in most cases the diagnosis of Scheuermann's disease is easily made on the lateral spinal radiograph, precise criteria for the condition have not been uniformly defined. In his extensive study, Sorenson suggested that the definition of Scheuermann's disease should be a hyperkyphosis that includes three central adjacent vertebrae that have wedging of 5 degrees or more.[46] Recent authorities have been less restrictive and emphasize the presence of hyperkyphosis with vertebral endplate irregularities and 5 degrees or more of wedging of one vertebral body. However, minor inconsistencies still exist. Bradford et al.[10] defined Scheuermann's disease as present whenever a patient had hyperkyphosis and at least one vertebra wedged more than 5 degrees. Although endplate irregularities were not required to establish the diagnosis of Scheuermann's disease, 95% of their patients with vertebral wedging also had these irregularities. Taylor et al.[50] diagnosed patients as having Scheuermann's disease primarily by hyperkyphosis and vertebral endplate irregularities.

A

B

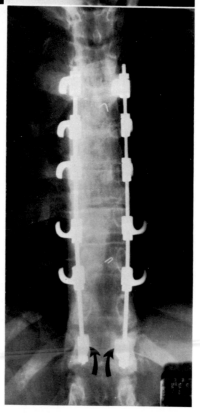

C

FIGURE 8-2
A 24-year-old man with intractable back pain.
Coned-down lateral film **(A)** shows a 75 degree Scheuermann's kyphosis with marked wedging at the curve apex. Postoperative films **(B, C)** demonstrate curve reduction to 62 degrees after posterior fusion and placement of compression rods over the lamina *(arrows)* or transverse processes (remainder of hooks).

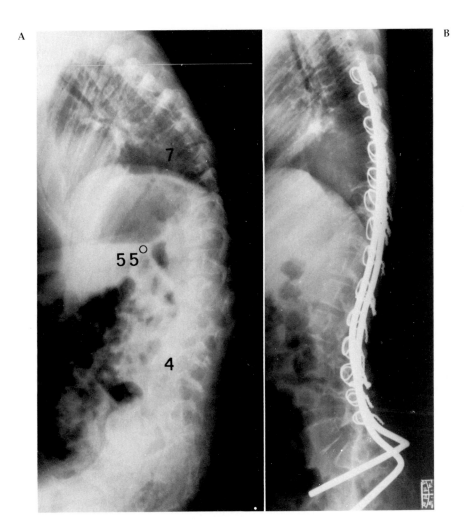

FIGURE 8-3
A, Preoperative lateral radiograph of 55 degree thoracolumbar kyphosis in an
   8-year-old boy with cerebral palsy.
B, Postoperative lateral radiograph after posterior fusion and Luque rod insertion.
   Normal thoracic kyphosis and lumbar lordosis have been restored.

The source of confusion here lies in the small set of patients with atypical radiographic findings. These patients without typical radiographic findings may have one of four radiographic patterns: (1) hyperkyphosis with vertebral wedging alone, (2) hyperkyphosis with endplate irregularities, (3) vertebral endplate irregularities without wedging or hyperkyphosis, and (4) hyperkyphosis without vertebral abnormalities. Patients with a hyperkyphosis and normal vertebrae (pattern four) should be classified as postural roundback. Their hyperkyphosis is usually modest. The curves are mobile, easily corrected, and rarely associated with muscle contractures.[35] They correct well with exercise alone or braces, if needed.

I believe that hyperkyphosis with vertebral wedging (pattern one) and hyperkyphosis with endplate irregularities (pattern two) both represent Scheuermann's disease. Since the vertebral endplate irregularities and wedging are manifestations of the same disease, it is reasonable that in mild disease some patients may show only one of the findings. The issue of vertebral endplate irregularities (frequently associated with Schmorl's nodes) without kyphosis is outside of the scope of this book, as spinal curvature is not adversely affected. The relationship of this condition to Scheuermann's disease is unknown, although the two may have similar etiologies.[21] Often these vertebral changes are detected on routine lateral chest radiographs in patients without back complaints. Further extensive discussion can be found in Schmorl's text.[43]

An important issue in the definition of Scheuermann's disease is the normal range for thoracic kyphosis. As discussed in Chapter Two, most authors have defined 20 to 40 degrees as the normal range with several recent reports giving 50 degrees as the upper limit of normal. It is significant to note that 25.3% (19/75) of Bradford's patients treated with a Milwaukee brace for hyperkyphosis had a thoracic kyphosis of 35 to 50 degrees *and* vertebral wedging of 5 degrees or more.[10] If one accepts that the upper limit for normal vertebral wedging is 5 degrees,[8,13] then these patients had one of the two key findings of Scheuermann's disease but would be normokyphotic as defined by the 20 to 50 degree normal range. Possibly the normal range is 20 to 50 degrees and these patients had early Scheuermann's disease prior to accentuation of kyphosis. However, most curves in this range are not painful, do not progress, and require no active treatment. For these reasons, I use the following two criteria for thoracic Scheuermann's disease: (1) thoracic kyphosis of greater than 50 degrees and (2) at least one vertebra wedged to 5 degrees or more with or without vertebral endplate irregularities.

Radiographic findings. Thus, there are two radiographic steps for the diagnosis of Scheuermann's disease. First, the thoracic kyphosis is measured on the standing lateral radiograph using the Cobb method from the most tilted superior and inferior end vertebrae. These are usually the third and twelfth thoracic but may be as high as the first thoracic and as low as the second lumbar[10] (Fig. 8-1).

If the kyphosis is greater than 50 degrees, then each thoracic vertebra near the apex should be checked for abnormal wedging (>5 degrees) by either visual estimation or, more accurately, by measurement (Fig. 8-4). Finally, the vertebral endplate should be evaluated for irregularities, that is, small shallow depressions with sclerotic borders (Fig. 8-4), deeper (>2 mm) localized depressions (Schmorl's nodes) (Fig. 8-4), or a persistent ring apophysis. In some cases, the routine spine film may show only vertebral wedging, while tomography reveals multiple endplate irregularities (Fig. 8-4).

The flexibility of the curve can be determined by the supine lateral film obtained with the patient lying on a bolster (Fig. 8-1, *B*). Flexibility is calculated by dividing the difference between the upright lateral Cobb and the supine lateral Cobb by the upright lateral Cobb and multiplying by 100. Flexibility does not appear to be useful in predicting effectiveness of bracing[10] or posterior fusion.[11] However, flexible curves in skeletally immature children can be managed by exercises alone.[10] Also, the supine lateral film determines the inflexible segment that needs to be fused anteriorly in the unusual case where a combined anterior and posterior fusion are indicated.[14]

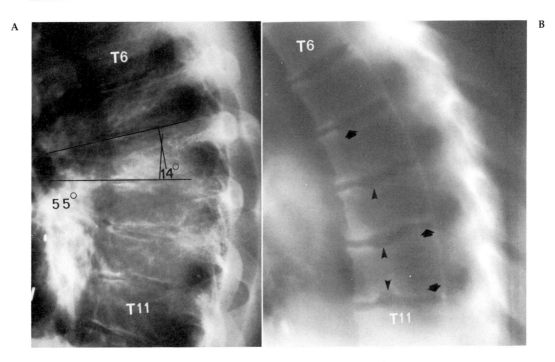

FIGURE 8-4
A 30-year-old man with 55 degree Scheuermann's kyphosis.
Routine lateral film **(A)** demonstrates vertebral wedging, but extensive endplate irregularities *(arrows)* and Schmorl's nodes *(arrowheads)* are identified confidently only on the midline lateral tomogram **(B).** Vertebral wedging is quantified **(A)** by the angle between perpendicular lines to that vertebra's endplates.

Treatment. Although some authors are skeptical,[50] others have found that Milwaukee bracing was highly effective in Scheuermann's disease.[10,33] These latter studies reported a reduction of kyphosis of 24 and 18 degrees, respectively. The vertebral wedging was also reduced an average of 41%.[10] Bradford et al. have recommended that the preadolescent child with a supple hyperkyphosis be managed with exercises alone and a Milwaukee brace be used if the curve progresses or vertebral wedging develops.[10]

Spinal fusion has been recommended in patients with a kyphosis of greater than 55 degrees and with either a progressive curve or intractable back pain.[50] Although Taylor et al.[50] reported excellent results in treating these patients with Harrington compression rods and a posterior fusion (Fig. 8-2), Bradford et al.[11] had a high rate of pseudarthrosis with this technique. These latter investigators speculated that their higher incidence of pseudarthrosis was due to longer patient follow-up and treatment of more severe cases of hyperkyphosis.[14] In fact, they have recommended that a two-stage anterior and posterior fusion be performed whenever the kyphosis is greater than 70 degrees to reduce the incidence of pseudarthrosis.[14] The anterior fusion should include the less flexible six to seven apical vertebrae and the posterior fusion should extend from the superior to the inferior end vertebrae as used for the Cobb measurement.

SKELETAL DYSPLASIAS

Many patients with dwarfism have anterior wedging deformity of one or several vertebral bodies, particularly in the upper lumbar spine. The deformed vertebral bodies have increased rotational instability. Because of the thoracic cage, most kyphoses in the skeletal dysplasias develop at the thoracolumbar junction, the point of transition between the relatively stabilized thoracic spine and more mobile lumbar spine.[19] As a consequence, thoracolumbar or lumbar kyphosis often develops. Although no official definition exists, it seems reasonable to classify a kyphosis with its apex at the twelfth thoracic vertebra (T12) or the first lumbar vertebra (L1) as thoracolumbar kyphosis and curves with lower apices as lumbar kyphoses, analogous to the definitions for curve levels in scoliosis. Most patients with dwarfism and a spinal deformity have a kyphoscoliosis in which the correction of the scoliosis is the dominant clinical concern as was discussed in Chapter Seven. However, patients with achondroplasia and Morquio's syndrome often have a dominant kyphotic deformity. Aside from the well known flame-shaped vertebral body deformity (Fig. 8-5), very little has been published on the associated kyphosis in Morquio's disease.[29]

FIGURE 8-5
An 8-year-old boy with Morquio's syndrome. Lateral upright film showing typical anterior central beaking of T11, T12, and L1 with resultant thoracolumbar kyphosis.

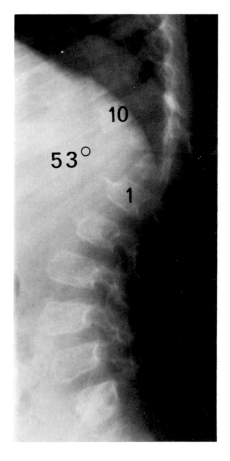

In contrast, the kyphosis of achondroplasia has been extensively studied, most likely because achondroplasia is the most common form of dwarfism, and the secondary neurologic deficits can be significant. Pure kyphotic deformities have been detected in 20% to 33.8% of patients with achondroplasia.[4,36] In infancy, the vertebral bodies are relatively normal in appearance (Fig. 8-6, *A*). As the child begins to assume an upright posture, anterior wedging of the vertebrae at the thoracolumbar junction often

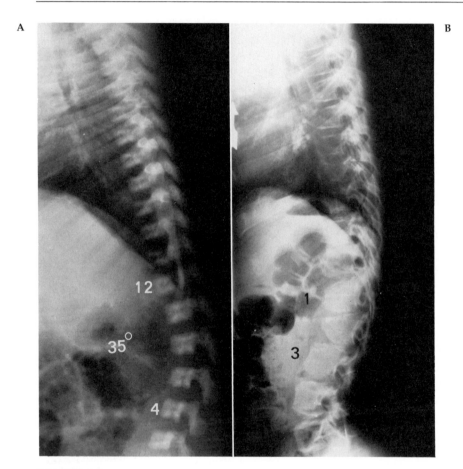

FIGURE 8-6
Kyphosis in achondroplasia.
A, Sitting lateral film of 4-week-old achondroplastic girl with proximal lumbar kyphosis with its apex at the second lumbar (L2) vertebra.
B, Standing lateral of 11-year-old boy with achondroplasia and 34 degree L1-3 lumbar kyphosis. Characteristic wedging of L1 and L2 have developed.

develops (Fig. 8-6, *B*).[32] When the curves are severe, posterior fusion and internal fixation are recommended (Fig. 8-7). Because of the small size of the spinal canal in achondroplasia, these patients often develop progressive spinal cord compression at the level of the kyphosis. Although laminectomy could theoretically increase the kyphosis, the spinal cord compression has been treated by posterior decompression without worsening of the kyphosis.[32]

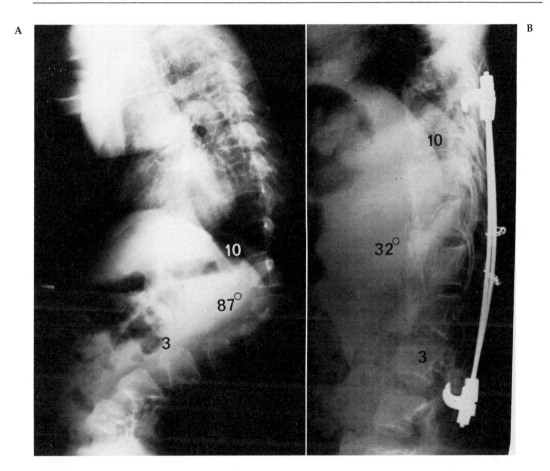

A   **B**

FIGURE 8-7
Achondroplasia in an 11-year-old boy.
A, Preoperative standing lateral radiograph with thoracolumbar kyphosis, apex at the twelfth thoracic level (T12).
B, Lateral film after two-stage anterior fusion and posterior fusion with Harrington compression rods.

METABOLIC DISEASE AND SPONDYLOARTHROPATHY

Many metabolic diseases alter osteoid formation resulting in weak bone and subsequent vertebral compression. Multiple compression fractures cause an increased kyphosis, usually in the thoracic spine. The most common cause today is osteoporosis (Fig. 8-8), but osteomalacia and renal osteodystrophy are two other frequent causes. Since these are primarily adult-onset diseases, rapid progression during the adolescent growth spurt is not of clinical concern. Rather, the diseases are chronic and slowly progressive. Treatment is directed at the underlying disease. Braces and surgery are infrequently indi-

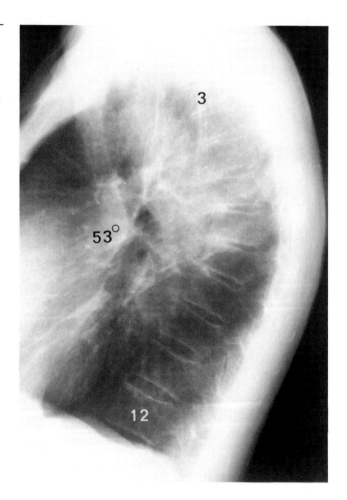

FIGURE 8-8
A 61-year-old woman with osteoporosis and thoracic hyperkyphosis owing to mild wedging of midthoracic vertebrae.

cated for curve correction. The radiographic features of these entities can be found in general radiology textbooks.[18,20]

A spondyloarthropathy is an inflammatory arthritis with predominant spinal involvement. Although ankylosing spondylitis is the prototype disease, psoriatic arthritis, Reiter's disease, and enteropathic arthritis can have similar manifestations.[40] The classic radiographic findings in ankylosing spondylitis include sacroiliitis, vertebral body squaring, and syndesmophyte formation.[39] The alteration in sagittal plane alignment may vary from mild to severe (Fig. 8-9).

FIGURE 8-9
Ankylosing spondylitis in a 47-year-old man with anterior vertebral ankylosis and hyperkyphosis.

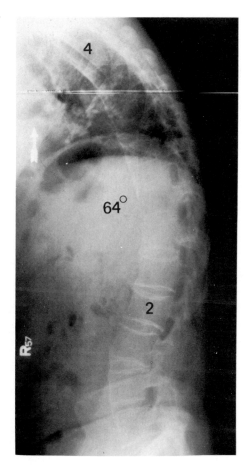

Localized Vertebral Abnormalities

The causes of abnormal kyphosis secondary to localized vertebral abnormalities include congenital anomalies, vertebral fractures, radiation-induced vertebral body wedging, and postinfectious vertebral body destruction. Because of the localized nature of the vertebral deformities, the kyphos is often severe with an acute sharp curve. The radiographic findings and treatment options vary, depending on the exact etiology.

CONGENITAL KYPHOSIS

The pathogenesis and mechanics of congenital kyphosis are similar to those for congenital scoliosis. Congenital kyphosis may be produced by failure of vertebral body formation or failure of vertebral body segmentation.[52] If the vertebral body fails to form, the posterior elements are present with only a small wedge of bone attached to the pedicles (a dorsal hemivertebra) (Fig. 8-10). Less commonly, there is failure of segmentation so that the growth plate is absent anteriorly, and two or more vertebral bodies are united by a bony bar anteriorly (Fig. 8-11). In both conditions, the kyphosis increases as the posterior elements increase in length without a corresponding increase in

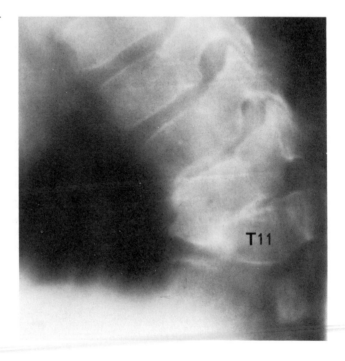

FIGURE 8-10
Lateral tomogram of dorsal T11 hemivertebra causing congenital kyphosis.

anterior vertebral height. As in most cases of abnormal spinal curvature, the deformity increases most rapidly during the adolescent growth spurt.[52] In untreated patients, the curves progress at an average of 7 degrees per year in childhood.[52] The most severe and sharply angular deformities occur in patients with dorsal hemivertebrae, while anterior bars tend to cause long, sweeping curves.[52] Paraplegia developed in 18.6% (16 of 86) of patients with untreated kyphosis owing to dorsal hemivertebrae. Bracing has not proven effective in treating congenital kyphosis, and posterior fusion of the kyphotic area prior to 3 years of age is the ideal treatment.[51] If the patient presents with a large curve (>75 degrees) already present, anterior fusion or a combined two-stage anterior and posterior fusion may be needed to prevent the high incidence of pseudarthrosis seen with posterior fusion alone.[7,13,22,45,52]

Radiographically, the lateral radiograph reveals either anterior fusion of two or more vertebrae or a dorsal hemivertebra. If a careful neurologic examination reveals any neural impairment, a myelogram is recommended to rule out spinal dysraphism. If surgery is planned, tomography is especially useful to delineate clearly the anatomical defects.[31] Both anterior bars and dorsal hemivertebrae occur most frequently at the thoracolumbar junction (62%), less commonly in the thoracic spine (30%), and infrequently in the lumbar spine.[52]

FIGURE 8-11
Congenital thoracolumbar kyphosis.
Failure of anterior segmentation resulted in an anterior bar *(arrowheads).*

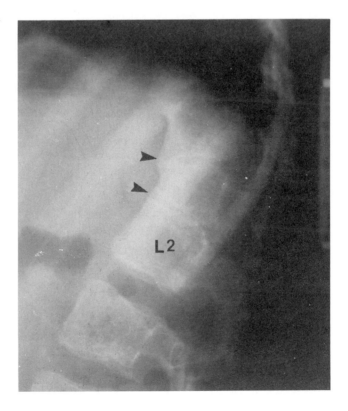

POSTTRAUMATIC KYPHOSIS

Vertebral fractures frequently involve a flexion mechanism such that the vertebral bodies are compressed and wedged anteriorly (Fig. 8-12). Although simple compression fractures are traditionally thought of as being stable spinal injuries, there are isolated reports of progressive kyphosis about these fractures. In a recent review of 105 patients with thoracic or lumbar compression fractures, progressive kyphosis was noted in two patients who had compression of two vertebrae in one case and three vertebrae in the other.[49] One patient was managed with a hyperextension cast and the other by posterior fusion.

RADIATION-INDUCED KYPHOSIS

As discussed in Chapter Seven, radiation therapy for neoplasms such as Wilms' tumor or neuroblastoma may result in vertebral body hypoplasia. The most common resultant deformity is scoliosis, but pure kyphosis is also seen.[28,41] The presence of an anteriorly wedged vertebral body may result in progressive kyphosis especially during the adolescent growth spurt. Because the kyphosis tends to distract the posterior elements, posterior fusion often results in pseudarthrosis and curve progression, so a long anterior fusion is recommended.[28]

A 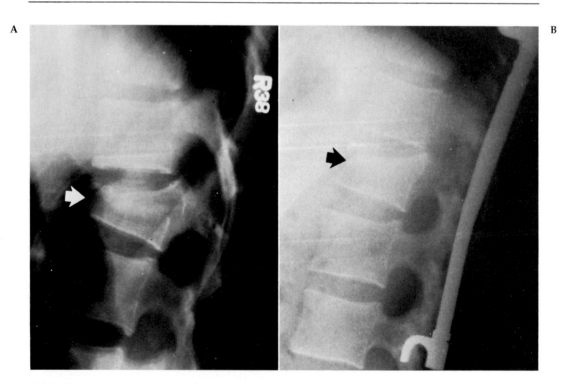 B

FIGURE 8-12
Compression fracture of L1 (arrow).
Initial lateral film (A) and lateral film (B) after fracture reduction and internal fixation with two short Harrington distraction rods.

POSTINFECTIOUS KYPHOSIS

The most frequent cause of severe kyphosis secondary to vertebral infection is spinal tuberculosis, commonly called Pott's disease. Because of the propensity of *Mycobacterium tuberculosis* to involve the spine with a low-grade, nonacutely life-threatening infection, patients with spinal tuberculosis often develop extensive vertebral destruction and paraplegia before the disease is detected.

The classic radiographic picture of spinal tuberculosis includes marked vertebral endplate destruction, relative disk space preservation, anterior vertebral body scalloping, and paraspinal abscesses (Fig. 8-13). The marked vertebral destruction has been emphasized in the reported surgical appearance of the disease.[16,24,25] These same authors emphasized that sequestra were noted more frequently at surgery than on routine radiographs. The use of tomography should aid in the detection of sequestra (Fig. 8-13).

The resistance of the intervertebral disk to destruction as seen on radiographs by disk space preservation is highlighted by the surgical observation that the disks are often intact and yet may be sequestered or sloughed within the tuberculous abscess.[3,16,24]

Anterior scalloping was noted in 41% of children with vertebral tuberculosis.[3] At surgery, the scalloped areas were found to be enveloped by the abscess which was presumed to account for the vertebral erosion. A paraspi-

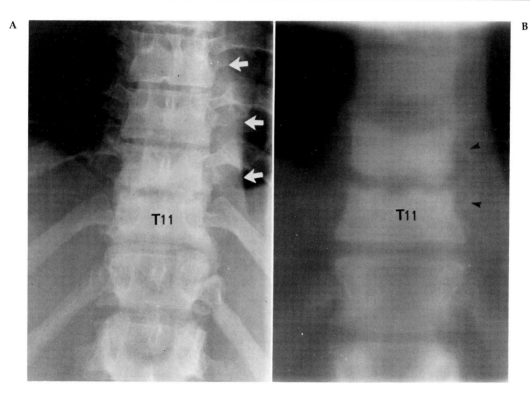

FIGURE 8-13
A 44-year-old man with tuberculosis involving T9-11.
Anteroposterior (AP) film **(A)** demonstrates the left paraspinal abscess *(arrows)*. The AP tomogram **(B)** shows extensive erosion at T9-10 and T10-11 as well as sequestra *(arrowheads)* in the paraspinal abscess.

nal abscess was noted almost universally at surgery and is manifested radiographically by displacement of the paraspinal lines about the thoracic spine (Fig. 8-13) and bulging of one or both psoas muscles in the abdomen.

Usually two to four vertebral bodies are involved with the infection, with the most common levels being between the ninth thoracic and third lumbar vertebrae.[3] Lower thoracic infection is more likely to cause paraplegia than lumbar involvement.[3]

With the advent of effective antituberculous chemotherapy in the 1950s, surgical treatment of the spinal deformity became possible. By combining surgery and chemotherapy, Hodgson and coworkers clearly proved that surgery was effective in treating the spinal deformity and reversing the associated paraplegia in most cases.[24,25] Their technique, which is still used today, consists of anterior approach to the spine with extensive debridgement of all infected soft tissue and bone followed by anterior fusion and bone grafts[25] (Fig. 8-14). Other authors have confirmed the effectiveness of this therapy.[16,34]

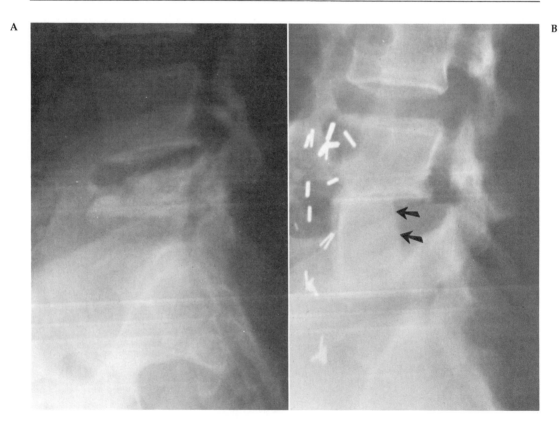

A **B**

FIGURE 8-14
A 29-year-old woman with tuberculosis involving L5 with relative preservation of the L4-5 interspace **(A)**. After sequestrectomy and anterior debridement, a large anterior bone graft *(arrows)* is placed to reduce the kyphosis **(B)**.

INTRASPINAL MASSES

Intraspinal masses presenting as spinal deformity are uncommon and usually present as scoliosis rather than kyphosis. An unusual intraspinal lesion causing kyphosis is an arachnoid cyst.[1] The cause for the associated kyphosis is unknown, although it has been speculated that the cysts interfere with vertebral body venous drainage and thus affect vertebral body growth.[1] As in the situation with spinal neoplasms causing scoliosis, these cases are diagnosed by the presence of neurologic deficits or radiographic findings of vertebral erosion such as widening of the interpedicular distance or posterior scalloping of the vertebrae[38] (Fig. 8-15).

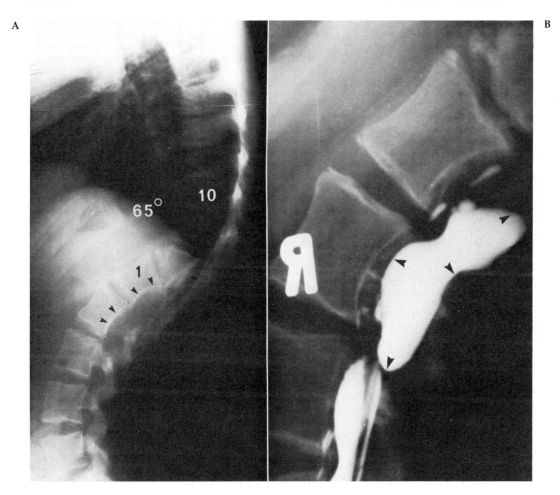

FIGURE 8-15
A 10-year-old boy with thoracolumbar kyphosis secondary to arachnoid cyst.
A, Upright lateral film shows wedging of T12 and posterior scalloping *(arrowheads)* of L1 and L2.
B, Lateral myelogram film shows iophendylate-filled arachnoid cyst *(arrowheads)*.

Posterior Element Deficiency
MYELOMENINGOCELE

The combination of muscular paralysis and absent posterior elements in patients with a myelomeningocoele often results in a lumbar kyphosis that can be more serious than their neuromuscular scoliosis.[17,47] Lumbar kyphosis was found in 27.5% of 200 infants with a myelomeningocoele.[6] The acute kyphosis may result in recurrent, overlying skin ulceration, respiratory insufficiency owing to upward pressure on the diaphragm, and lumbar spine pain. The deformity may prevent the child from ambulating with leg braces and crutches because they are markedly out of balance with the upper torso displaced forward.[27] Finally, the anterior abdominal wall surface may be so reduced by the kyphosis that a urinary diversion for a neurogenic bladder cannot be performed.

The radiographic appearance is fairly typical on the lateral sitting film showing a lumbar kyphosis. In early infancy, there is a long lumbar kyphosis (Fig. 8-16). In older children, the vertebral bodies at and near the apex, which is usually one of the upper lumbar vertebrae, are often secondarily wedged

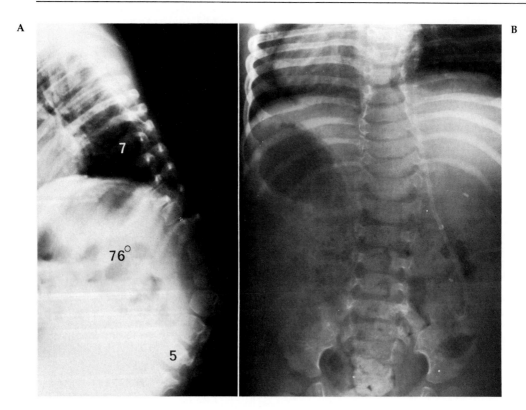

FIGURE 8-16

Thoracolumbar myelomeningocele and lumbar kyphosis **(A).** The AP film **(B)** reveals absent posterior spinal elements and widened interpedicular distances from T7 through the sacrum. Owing to the lumbar kyphosis, the lower thoracic ribs are elevated superiorly from their normal inferior course.

anteriorly with gibbus formation (Fig. 8-17).[6,23,44] On the anteroposterior film, in addition to widened interpedicular distances and absent posterior elements, the intervertebral disk spaces appear narrowed at the level of the kyphosis, and the lower ribs are elevated compared to their normal downward angulation[26] (Fig. 8-16).

If the curves are not surgically corrected, they tend to progress[44] at an average rate of 3 degrees per year.[5] As the children begin to assume an upright posture with sitting, a secondary lordosis develops at the thoracolumbar junction.[44] The lordosis is initially nonstructural but frequently becomes rigid. Because of the rigidity of the kyphosis, most authors[15,17,26,44,47] have recommended treatment by anterior fusion after resection of one or more lumbar vertebrae. This should be followed by posterior fusion and Luque instrumentation to the pelvis. Park and Watt[37] found that preoperative aortography was useful to locate the aorta and its major branches to prevent operative arterial injury. Stephen and Bodel[48] recently reported that Luque rod fixation may be useful in recurrent kyphosis if a prior fusion is unsuccessful.

FIGURE 8-17
A 7-year-old girl with myelomeningocele and severe thoracolumbar kyphosis requiring vertebral body resection and posterior fusion for treatment.

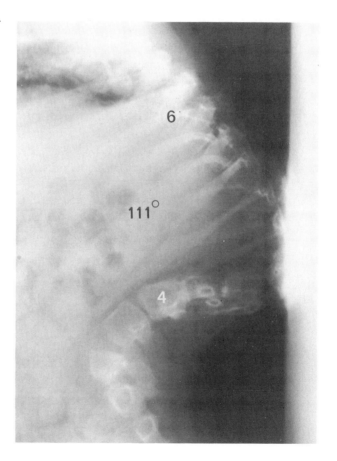

POSTLAMINECTOMY KYPHOSIS

In a manner similar to the myelomeningocoele patients, children who have had extensive laminectomies may also develop kyphosis. Because these patients are not paralyzed, the deformity is not as rapidly progressive but can still be severe. In a series of 32 children who had laminectomies for spinal tumors, Lonstein et al.[30] found an average kyphosis at the laminectomy site of 82 degrees. Anterior fusion was recommended as the appropriate treatment.

Summary

A. General principles
   1. Evaluate with upright lateral and supine cross-table lateral radiographs
   2. Determine if posterior element defects or localized or diffuse vertebral abnormalities exist
   3. Treat with Milwaukee brace or posterior internal fixation
B. Multiple vertebral abnormalities
   1. Scheuermann's disease
      a. Thoracic kyphosis over 50 degrees and at least one vertebra wedged 5 degrees or more
      b. Often associated endplate irregularities and Schmorl's nodes
      c. Milwaukee bracing as primary treatment
      d. Posterior or two-stage fusion in larger or progressive curves
   2. Skeletal dysplasia
      a. Predominant kyphosis—achondroplasia, Morquio's syndrome
      b. About thoracolumbar junction most commonly
   3. Metabolic disease and spondyloarthropathy
      a. Affect primarily adults
      b. Treatment directed toward underlying disease
C. Localized vertebral abnormalities, key radiographic findings
   1. Congenital—anterior bar or dorsal hemivertebra
   2. Traumatic—anterior compression fractures
   3. Radiation therapy—anterior hypoplasia
   4. Tuberculosis—vertebral destruction with relative disk preservation, anterior scalloping, and paraspinal abscess
   5. Intraspinal masses—posterior vertebral body scalloping
D. Posterior element deficiency
   1. Myelomeningocele
      a. Initial long lumbar kyphosis with subsequent secondary vertebral wedging and an apical gibbus
      b. Secondary thoracic structural lordosis may develop
   2. Postlaminectomy—less severe kyphosis than in myelomeningocele

REFERENCES

1. Adelstein, L.J.: Spinal extradural cyst associated with kyphosis dorsalis juvenilis, J. Bone Joint Surg. **23**:93-101, 1941.
2. Ascani, E., Montanaro, A., and Ippolito, E.: Scheuermann's kyphosis: histological, histochemical and ultrastructural studies, Orthop. Trans. **7**:28, 1983.
3. Bailey, H.L., et al.: Tuberculosis of the spine in children, J. Bone Joint Surg. (Am.) **54**:1633-1657, 1972.
4. Bailey, J.A., II: Orthopaedic aspects of achondroplasia, J. Bone Joint Surg. (Am.) **52**:1285-1301, 1970.
5. Banta, J.V., and Hamada, J.S.: Natural history of the kyphotic deformity in myelomeningocele, J. Bone Joint Surg. (Am.) **58**:279, 1976.
6. Barson, A.J.: Radiological studies of spina bifida cystica. The phenomenon of congenital lumbar kyphosis, Br. J. Radiol. **38**:294-300, 1965.
7. Bjerkreim, I., Magnaes, B., and Semb, G.: Surgical treatment of severe angular kyphosis, Acta Orthop. Scand. **53**:913-917, 1982.
8. Bradford, D.S.: Kyphosis, Clin. Orthop. **128**:2-4, 1977.
9. Bradford, D.S., and Moe, J.H.: Scheuermann's juvenile kyphosis, Clin. Orthop. **110**:45-53, 1975.
10. Bradford, D.S., et al.: Scheuermann's kyphosis and roundback deformity, J. Bone Joint Surg. (Am.) **56**:740-758, 1974.
11. Bradford, D.S., et al.: Scheuermann's kyphosis: results of surgical treatment by posterior spine arthrodesis in twenty-two patients, J. Bone Joint Surg. (Am.) **57**: 439-448, 1975.
12. Bradford, D.S., et al.: Scheuermann's kyphosis: a form of osteoporosis? Clin. Orthop. **118**:10-15, 1976.
13. Bradford, D.S., et al.: Techniques of anterior spinal surgery for the management of kyphosis, Clin. Orthop. **128**:129-139, 1977.
14. Bradford, D.S., et al.: The surgical management of patients with Scheuermann's disease, J. Bone Joint Surg. (Am.) **62**:705-712, 1980.
15. Brown, H.P.: Management of spinal deformity in myelomeningocele, Orthop. Clin. North Am. **9**:391-402, 1978.
16. Chu, C.-B.: Treatment of spinal tuberculosis in Korea using focal debridement and interbody fusion, Clin. Orthop. **50**:235-253, 1967.
17. Eckstein, H.B., and Vora, R.M.: Spinal osteotomy for severe kyphosis in children with myelomeningocele, J. Bone Joint Surg. (Br.) **54**:328-333, 1972.
18. Edeiken, J.: Roentgen diagnosis of diseases of bone, ed. 3, Baltimore, 1981, The Williams & Wilkins Co.
19. Eulert, J.: Scoliosis and kyphosis in dwarfing conditions, Arch. Orthop. Trauma Surg. **102**:45-47, 1983.
20. Greenfield, G.B.: Radiology of bone diseases, ed. 3, Philadelphia, 1980, J.B. Lippincott Co.
21. Hafner, R.H.V.: Localised osteochondritis (Scheuermann's disease), J. Bone Joint Surg. (Br.) **34**:38-40, 1952.
22. Hall, J.E.: The anterior approach to spinal deformities, Orthop. Clin. North Am. **3**:81-98, 1972.
23. Hall, J.E., and Bobechko, W.P.: Advances in the management of spinal deformities in myelodysplasia, Clin. Neurosurg. **20**:164-173, 1973.
24. Hodgson, A.R., and Stock, F.E.: Anterior spinal fusion. A preliminary communication on the radical treatment of Pott's disease and Pott's paraplegia, Br. J. Surg. **44**:266-275, 1956.
25. Hodgson, A.R., et al.: Anterior spinal fusion. The operative approach and pathological findings in 412 patients with Pott's disease of the spine, Br. J. Surg. **48**:172-178, 1960.
26. Hoppenfeld, S.: Congenital kyphosis in myelomeningocele, J. Bone Joint Surg. (Br.) **49**:276-280, 1967.

27. Kilfoyle, R.M., Foley, J.J., and Norton, P.L.: Spine and pelvic deformity in child-hood and adolescent paraplegia, J. Bone Joint Surg. (Am.) **47**:659-682, 1965.

28. King, J., and Stowe, S.: Results of spinal fusion for radiation scoliosis, Spine **7**:574-585, 1982.

29. Kopits, S.E.: Orthopedic complications of dwarfism, Clin. Orthop. **114**:153-179, 1976.

30. Lonstein, J.E., et al.: Post-laminectomy spine deformity, J. Bone Joint Surg. (Am.) **58**:727, 1976.

31. Lorenzo, R.L., et al.: Congenital kyphosis and subluxation of the thoraco-lumbar spine due to vertebral aplasia, Skeletal Radiol. **10**:255-257, 1983.

32. Lutter, L.D., and Langer, L.O.: Neurological symptoms in achondroplastic dwarfs —surgical treatment, J. Bone Joint Surg. (Am.) **59**:87-92, 1977.

33. McAllister, D.T., and Hardy, J.H.: Juvenile kyphosis: a statistical survey and comparison of methods of treatment, J. Bone Joint Surg. (Am.) **55**:1323, 1973.

34. Medical Research Council Working Party on Tuberculosis of the Spine: A controlled trial of anterior spinal fusion and debridement in the surgical management of tuberculosis of the spine in patients on standard chemotherapy: a study in Hong Kong, Br. J. Surg. **61**:853-866, 1974.

35. Moe, J., et al.: Scoliosis and other spinal deformities, Philadelphia, 1978, W.B. Saunders Co.

36. Nelson, M.A.: Orthopaedic aspects of the chondrodystrophies: the dwarf and his orthopaedic problems, Ann. R. Coll. Surg. **47**:185-210, 1970.

37. Park, W.M., and Watt, I.: The pre-operative aortographic assessment of children with spina bifida cystica and severe kyphos, J. Bone Joint Surg. (Br.) **57**:112, 1975.

38. Price, H.I., et al.: The computed tomographic findings in benign disease of the vertebral column, RadioGraphics **4**:283-313, 1984.

39. Resnick, D.: Radiology of seronegative spondyloarthropathies, Clin. Orthop. **143**:38-45, 1979.

40. Resnick, D., and Niwayama, G.: Diagnosis of bone and joint disorders with emphasis on articular abnormalities, Philadelphia, 1981, W.B. Saunders Co.

41. Riseborough, E.J., et al.: Skeletal alterations following irradiation for Wilms' Tumor, J. Bone Joint Surg. (Am.) **58**:526-536, 1976.

42. Scheuermann, H.W.: Kyfosis dorsalis juvenilis, Ugeskr. Laeger **82**:385, 1920.

43. Schmorl, G.: The human spine in health and disease, New York, 1971, Grune & Stratton, Inc.

44. Sharrard, W.J.W., and Drennan, J.C.: Osteotomy-excision of the spine for lumbar kyphosis in older children with myelomeningocele, J. Bone Joint Surg. (Br.) **54**:50-60, 1972.

45. Simmons, E.H.: Congenital kyphosis, J. Bone Joint Surg. (Br.) **55**:233, 1973.

46. Sorenson, K.H.: Scheuermann's juvenile kyphosis, Copenhagen, 1964, Munksgaard.

47. Sriram, K., Bobechko, W.P., and Hall, J.E.: Surgical management of spinal deformities in spina bifida, J. Bone Joint Surg. (Br.) **54**:666-676, 1972.

48. Stephen, J.P.H., and Bodel, J.G.: Luque rod fixation in meningomyelocele kyphosis: a preliminary report, Aust. N.Z. J. Surg. **53**:473-477, 1983.

49. Sutherland, C.J., Miller, F., and Wang, G.-J.: Early progressive kyphosis following compression fractures, Clin. Orthop. **173**:216-220, 1983.

50. Taylor, T.C., et al.: Surgical management of thoracic kyphosis in adolescents, J. Bone Joint Surg. (Am.) **61**:496-503, 1979.

51. Winter, R.B., and Moe, J.H.: The results of spinal arthrodesis for congenital spinal deformity in patients younger than five years old, J. Bone Joint Surg. (Am.) **64**:419-432, 1982.

52. Winter, R.B., Moe, J.H., and Wang, J.F.: Congenital kyphosis, J. Bone Joint Surg. (Am.) **55**:223-256, 1973.

Chapter Nine

Lordosis and Spondylolisthesis

*L*ordosis or spinal curvature convex anteriorly is abnormal whenever it occurs in the thoracic spine and is abnormal in the lumbar spine when it exceeds the upper limits of normal (probably 60 degrees, see Chapter Two). Abnormal lordosis has many potential causes including congenital anomalies, skeletal dysplasia, postsurgical deformity, and neuromuscular disease. Active medical management of the lordosis is seldom needed in most of these conditions, so only a limited discussion of these entities will be presented. Although these conditions are relatively uncommon, a related problem, spondylolisthesis, is common. Spondylolisthesis is actually a kyphosis at the lumbosacral junction, but it often causes secondary hyperlordosis in the lumbar spine.

Abnormal lordosis is evaluated radiographically in a manner similar to that used for abnormal kyphosis. The standing lateral film is the primary diagnostic radiograph. After carefully reviewing the radiograph for vertebral abnormalities, the sagittal plane curvature in the lumbar spine is quantified using the Cobb method. Wiltse and Winter have recommended that the superior endplate of the fifth lumbar vertebrae be used as the distal line for the Cobb angle because the inferior endplate is often deformed, especially in patients with spondylolisthesis[31] (Fig. 9-1).

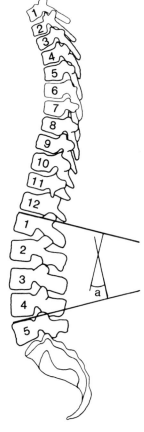

FIGURE 9-1
Cobb measurement of lumbar lordosis.
In the presence of spondylolisthesis, the distal tangential line is across the superior endplate of the fifth lumbar *(L5)* vertebra rather than the traditional inferior endplate. Perpendicular lines to the tangential lines form the lordosis angle *(a)*.

Spondylolysis and Spondylolisthesis
ETIOLOGY

Spondylolysis refers to a defect in the bony integrity of the pars interarticularis. This region of the posterior vertebral elements represents the junction of the transverse process, pedicle, lamina, and articular facets. The defect is now considered to be acquired rather than congenital because it has not been discovered in the fetus or the newborn but is present in 5% to 6% of young adults.[9] Spondylolysis appears to be caused by an acute fracture, a fatigue fracture related to abnormal stress, or an underlying dysplasia of the pars interarticularis.[9] Support for this traumatic etiology comes from mechanical in vitro studies of cadaver spines in which loading of the spine, similar to walking while carrying a heavy load, resulted in mechanical fatigue fractures almost exclusively through the pars interarticularis.[5] In addition, analysis of 485 skeletons revealed that unilateral spondylolysis is often associated with surrounding callus suggesting that these are healing fractures.[8]

FIGURE 9-2
Spondylolisthesis classes.
Dysplastic type has hypoplasia of superior sacrum *(curved arrow)* allowing slippage. Isthmic class has either pars fracture *(arrow)* or elongated pars *(arrowheads).*

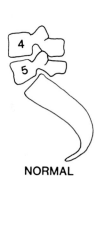

NORMAL

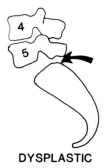

DYSPLASTIC

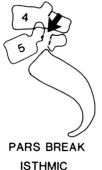

PARS BREAK
ISTHMIC

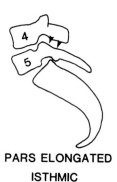

PARS ELONGATED
ISTHMIC

SPONDYLOLISTHESIS PATTERNS

Spondylolisthesis is defined as forward slippage of one vertebral body on another. Wiltse et al.[30] have divided spondylolisthesis into five basic classes: (1) dysplastic, (2) isthmic, (3) degenerative, (4) traumatic, and (5) pathologic. Dysplastic spondylolisthesis is due to congenital anomalies at the lumbosacral junction with hypoplasia of the superior facets of the sacrum (Figs. 9-2 and 9-3). The isthmic variety may be due to either fracture (Figs. 9-2 and 9-4) or elongation of the pars interarticularis (Figs. 9-2 and 9-5). Degenerative spondylolisthesis or spondylolisthesis with an intact pars interarticularis is due to degenerative disease of the apophyseal joints[23] (Fig. 9-6). Traumatic spondylolisthesis refers to anterior displacement from posterior element fractures (Fig. 9-7) at sites other than the pars. Pathologic spondylolisthesis describes the condition when posterior element fractures develop in diseased bone.

Text continued on p. 272.

FIGURE 9-3
Dysplastic spondylolisthesis.
The L5 pars *(straight arrow)* is intact but attenuated. The superior sacral facets *(curved arrow)* are hypoplastic (confirmed at surgery).

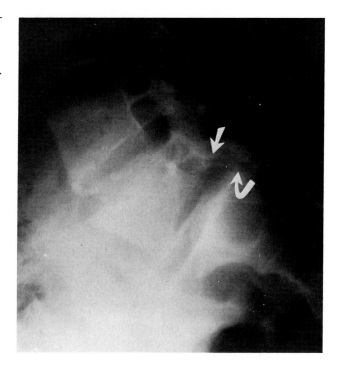

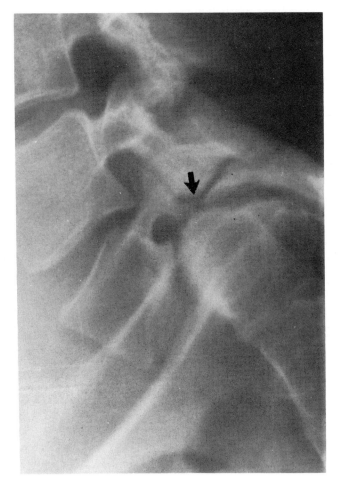

FIGURE 9-4
Severe isthmic spondylolisthesis with fracture of the L5 pars
interarticularis *(arrow)*.

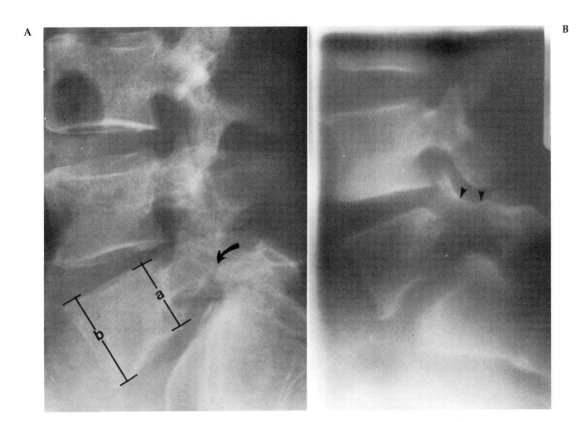

FIGURE 9-5
Isthmic spondylolisthesis with elongated pars.
L5 pars shows questionable fracture *(arrow)* on routine lateral film **(A)** but lateral
tomogram **(B)** reveals an intact but elongated L5 pars *(arrowheads)*. Opposite pars
had identical tomographic appearance. The percentage of wedging of the body of
L5 is defined as 100 × a/b.

FIGURE 9-6
Degenerative spondylolisthesis of
L4-5 owing to facet joint
osteoarthritis indicated by facet
joint sclerosis *(arrow)*.

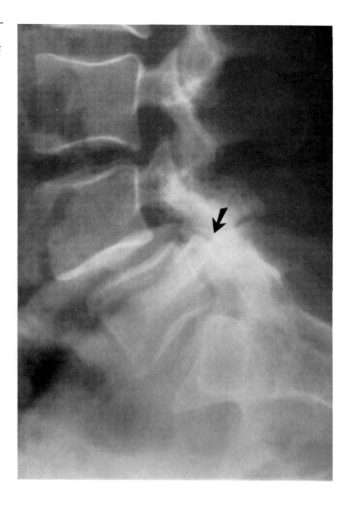

FIGURE 9-7
Combined isthmic spondylolysis and pedicle fracture in a 19-year-old football
player with chronic midlumbar pain.

A, AP radiograph of L2-4. Typical AP appearance of isthmic spondylolysis *(arrows)*
at L3. The right L3 pedicle *(curved arrow)* is sclerotic.

B, Right posterior oblique radiograph reveals an intact pars *(arrowheads)*. The
opposite oblique film (not shown) confirmed a typical isthmic left spondylolysis.

C, Lateral tomogram. Vertical fracture *(arrowheads)* through sclerotic right pedicle of
L3.

D, CT scan of L3. Right nonisthmic pedicle fracture *(arrowheads)* and left isthmic
spondylolysis *(curved arrow)*.

A

B

C

D

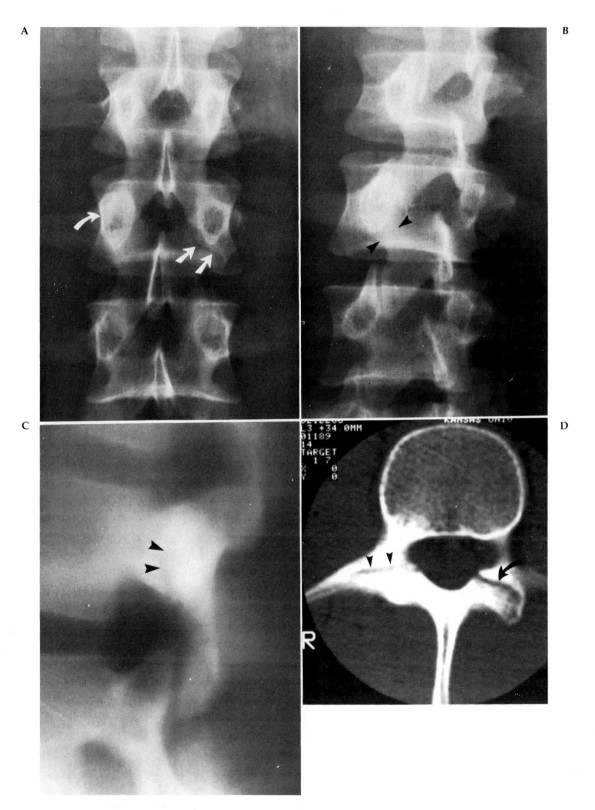

FIGURE 9-7
For legend see opposite page.

Patients with dysplastic spondylolisthesis have a 33% incidence of spondylolisthesis among their first-degree relatives.[35] They also have a 94% incidence of segmentation defects or spina bifida occulta at the fifth lumbar or first sacral level but no evidence of neural tube defects. Thus it appears that the dysplastic form of spondylolysis has a genetic predisposition related to mild bony anomalies of the lumbosacral junction. Dysplastic spondylolysis occurs in 1% of the population and is less common than isthmic spondylolysis, which is present in 5% of the population.[35]

Spondylolysis occurs almost exclusively in the lumbar spine, most commonly at the fifth lumbar level (L5) with a decreasing incidence from L4 to L3 to L2 to L1. Spondylolysis has also been reported rarely in the cervical spine.[15,25] Like spondylolysis, spondylolisthesis occurs most commonly at L5 with a decreasing incidence proximally up the lumbar spine. In the presence of spondylolisthesis, the pars defect is usually easily seen on a lateral radiograph, and oblique films are not necessary.

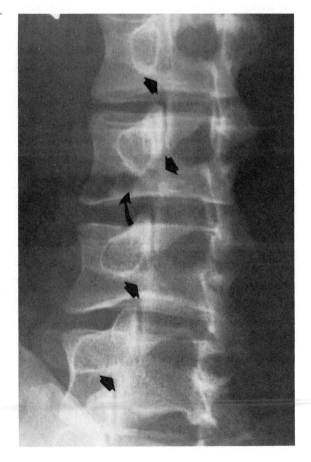

FIGURE 9-8
Normal right posterior oblique
radiograph of L2-5.
The pars interarticularis *(arrows)* is intact at all levels. Bowel gas *(curved arrow)* overlies one pars simulating spondylolysis.

RADIOGRAPHIC APPEARANCE

Spondylolysis is most easily diagnosed on oblique radiographs of the lumbar spine. The outlines of the posterior elements on the oblique view have been likened to a Scotch terrier or a "Scotty dog."[4] The region of the neck of the Scotty dog represents the pars interarticularis (Fig. 9-8). Any defect in this region indicates spondylolysis (Fig. 9-9). Bilateral spondylolysis can almost always be diagnosed on the lateral film alone (Fig. 9-10), but in two large studies of lumbar spine examinations comparing lateral and oblique views approximately 80% of the cases of unilateral spondylolysis could be recognized only on the oblique views.[17,24] Occasionally, spondylolysis can be detected using anteroposterior (AP) radiographs alone, such as abdominal or excretory urogram films by the presence of horizontal lucencies projected over the pedicles (Fig. 9-10). With marked spondylolisthesis of L5 on S1, the body of L5 may be viewed en face. This appearance has been termed the "inverted Napoleon hat sign"[7] (see Fig. 9-19, *A*). In the presence of unilateral spondylolysis, the contralateral pedicle may hypertrophy or become sclerotic, and the spinous process at that level may shift out of the midline away from the defect[18,22,28] (Fig. 9-11). This sclerotic pedicle might be mistaken for infection or neoplasm.[28] A recently described helpful sign for recognizing spondylolysis on the AP film (Fig. 9-11) is a bony fragment at the superior edge of the lamina near the spondylolysis.[1]

FIGURE 9-9
Large left L4 spondylolysis defect *(arrow)* easily seen on left posterior oblique radiograph.

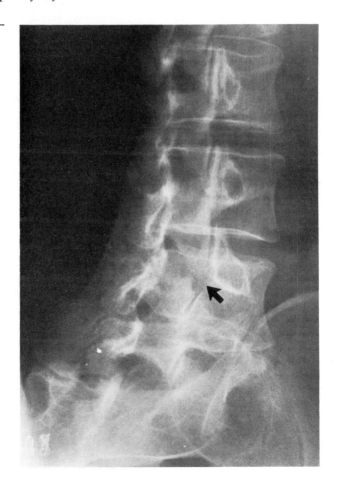

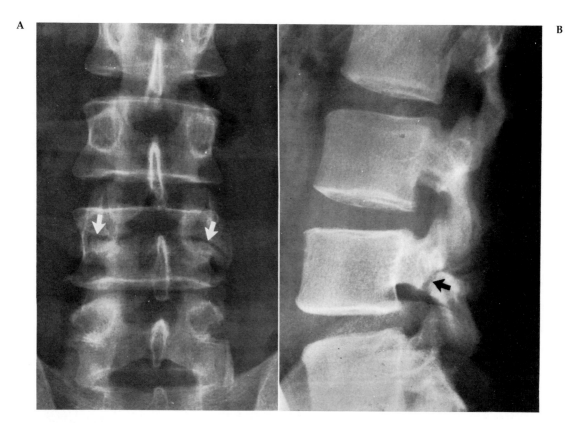

FIGURE 9-10
Bilateral L4 spondylolysis *(arrows)* well visualized on AP **(A)** and lateral **(B)** films.

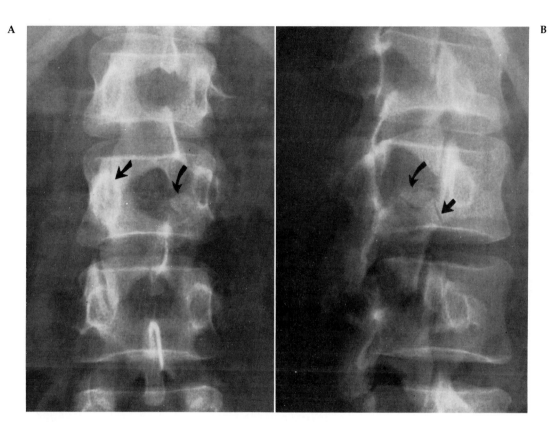

FIGURE 9-11
Left L3 spondylolysis.

A, AP film reveals bony fragment *(curved arrow)* near the site of the nonvisualized
  spondylolysis. The opposite pedicle *(arrow)* is sclerotic.

B, The left posterior oblique film demonstrates the spondylolysis *(arrow)* and the
  laminar fragment *(curved arrow)*.

SPECIAL STUDIES

Occasionally, if there is lumbar hyperlordosis, the pars interarticularis is not well seen on the routine oblique radiographs. If spondylolysis is suspected, the oblique films can be obtained with 15 degrees of cephalad tube tilt. If there is still uncertainty as to the presence of spondylolysis, tomograms represent the gold standard. Thin section tomograms at 5 mm intervals through the posterior elements are required. These may be either the routine antero-posterior (AP) and lateral or both posterior oblique projections. The oblique tomograms provide the clearest evaluation of the pars interarticularis if that is the major clinical consideration (Fig. 9-12). If the clinical problem is unexplained back pain, routine AP and lateral tomograms are recommended to exclude other disease processes as well as spondylolysis (Fig. 9-13).

FIGURE 9-12
Normal oblique hypocycloidal tomogram of the lumbar spine. Each pars interarticularis *(arrows)* is intact.

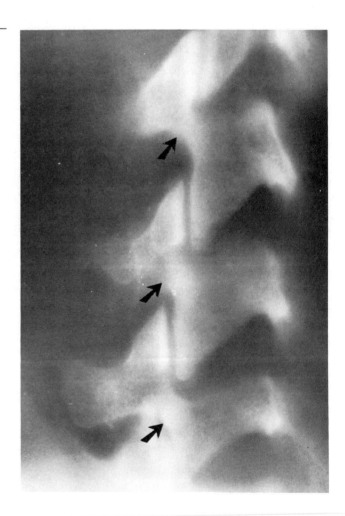

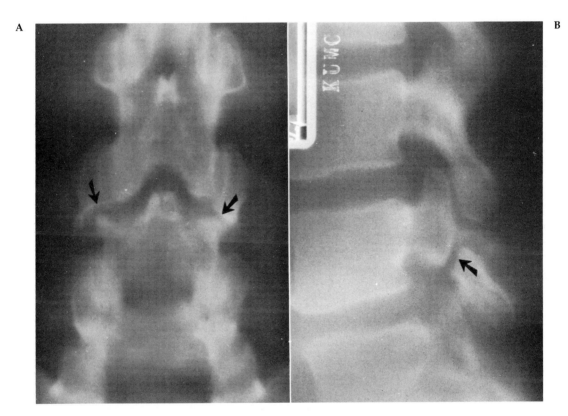

FIGURE 9-13
AP **(A)** and lateral **(B)** hypocycloidal tomograms from L3 to L5 showing bilateral L4
spondylolysis *(arrows)*.

Radionuclide bone scanning has been used to evaluate the activity of spondylolytic lesions.[10] The sensitivity of bone scanning for detecting spondylolysis has not been determined. One study found that out of ten defects, there was increased uptake at the defect in six cases (Fig. 9-14), at the opposite pars in one, and at a higher level in one while there was no area of increased uptake in two patients.[10] Some of these defects may not have been acute because two authorities have recently stated that bone scanning is useful to detect acute spondylolysis even before plain films show the defect.[29,32] Other imaging procedures can also be used to study patients with spondylolysis. Contrast medium injection of a facet above or below a spondylolysis often fills the adjacent facet joint across the pars defect.[11,19] Although the passage of contrast material across the defect does exclude a fibrous union, the clinical significance is undetermined.

A   B

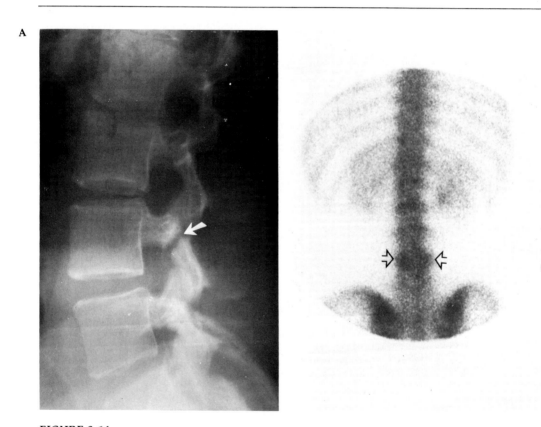

FIGURE 9-14
A 13-year-old girl with bilateral L4 spondylolysis (*arrow,* **A**) with increased uptake at both sites on a radionuclide bone scan (*arrows,* **B**).

The appearance of spondylolysis on computed tomography (CT) of the spine (Fig. 9-7, *D*) has been thoroughly described.[12] Optimal visualization was found to require thin 5 mm sections through the pedicles at a level 10 to 15 mm above the disk. A wide bone window (1000 H) was required. In view of the expense of CT scanning, routine AP, lateral, and oblique radiographs are recommended as the primary method for evaluation. In rare cases, CT may provide additional useful information.

SPONDYLOLISTHESIS MEASUREMENT

The grading and description of spondylolisthesis can be either brief or extensive. The simplest and most commonly used classification is that of Meyerding in which the superior aspect of the lower vertebral segment is divided into quarters (Fig. 9-15). The slip is then graded from I to IV, depending on which quartile the posterior edge of the upper vertebral body is displaced into.[21] A grade V spondylolisthesis occurs when the upper vertebral body has slipped completely off the lower vertebra.

More precise quantitation of the spondylolisthesis and associated deformity has recently been standardized by Wiltse and Winter.[31] The *anterior displacement* or extent of anterior slippage is measured as a percentage of the AP diameter of the first sacral vertebral body (Fig. 9-16). The *sacral inclination* (also called sacral tilt) refers to the tilt of the sacrum from the vertical (Fig. 9-17). A related measurement, the *sacrohorizontal angle,* is the angle between the superior endplate of the sacrum and the horizontal (Fig. 9-17). *Sagittal rotation* is the angular relationship between the fifth lumbar and first sacral segments as measured by lines drawn along the front of L5 and back of the

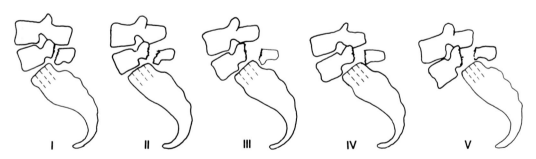

FIGURE 9-15
Meyerding grading of the degree of spondylolisthesis.
Grades I to IV represent the posterior edge of the upper vertebral body as it moves across the quartile divisions of the endplate of the inferior vertebra. Complete displacement is grade V.

FIGURE 9-16
Quantitation of anterior
displacement.
L4-5 isthmic spondylolysis with
spondylolisthesis. The percentage
anterior displacement equals
(a/b) × 100.

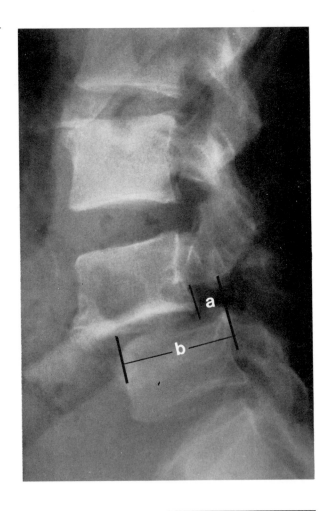

FIGURE 9-17
The sacral inclination angle (a) lies between a vertical line
and a line across the back of the sacrum. The
sacrohorizontal angle (b) is between a horizontal line and
the superior surface of the sacrum.

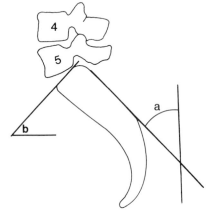

upper sacrum (Fig. 9-18). The *percent of wedging* of the slipped vertebra is obtained by dividing the height of the posterior border of the vertebra by the height of its anterior border and multiplying by 100 (Fig. 9-5, *A*). *Lumbar lordosis* is quantified using the Cobb angle from the superior endplate of L1 to the superior end plate of L5 (Fig. 9-1). The inferior endplate of L5 should not be used owing to the frequent rounding off which occurs with spondylolisthesis. In a recent study of spondylolisthesis, Boxall et al.[2] found that the percentage of anterior displacement and the sagittal rotation were the most important measurements in defining instability and progression.

In evaluating spondylolisthesis, one must remember that there is a 42% incidence of associated scoliosis.[20] However, these same authors found that the curves are often insignificant, with 50% of the curves measuring less than 10 degrees, 43% measuring from 10 to 15 degrees, 7% measuring from 25 to 35 degrees. Upon follow-up, only one of the curves in this study progressed, and many of the smaller curves disappeared.

FIGURE 9-18
The sagittal rotation angle (*a*) reflects the lumbosacral kyphosis. If rotation is severe, lines across the front surface of L5 and the back of the sacrum determine the angle (*a*). If the rotation is small, the lines will not intersect but perpendicular lines (*arrows*) create an equal angle.

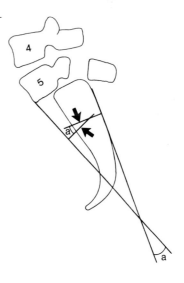

TREATMENT

Grades I and II spondylolisthesis (<50% anterior displacement) are usually treated conservatively with orthotic back supports, back strengthening exercises, and a weight reduction program if the patient is obese.

For higher grades of symptomatic spondylolisthesis, surgery is usually necessary.[13] The more traditional approach has been in situ posterolateral fusion without reduction of the anterior displacement.[14,16] Lateral column fusion has also been effective.[13] Reduction of the slippage and internal fixation with Harrington distraction rods has been used in selected cases,[26] although the reduction has not always been maintained.[2] The indications for reduction have not been defined, but it is generally used where there is significant lumbosacral kyphosis (Fig. 9-19).[32] A decompression laminectomy may also be necessary if there are signs of nerve root impingement.[6]

A   B

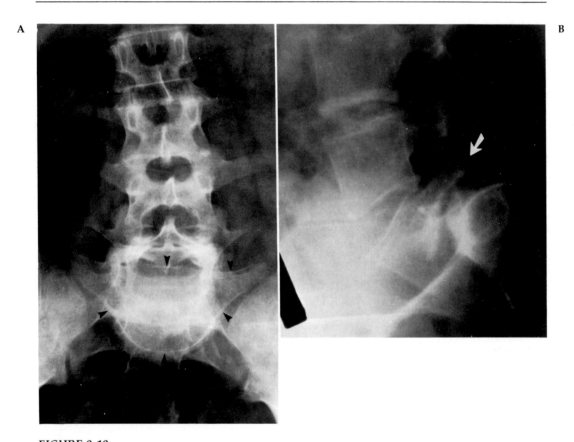

FIGURE 9-19
Painful L5-S1 spondylolisthesis in a 14-year-old boy.
AP film **(A)** shows "inverted Napoleon hat sign" *(arrowheads)* owing to severe slippage of L5 resulting in its almost en face visualization. Lateral film **(B)** reveals grade 4 spondylolisthesis with marked erosion and sclerosis of opposite L5 and S1 borders. Spondylolysis is faintly seen *(arrow)*.

C   D

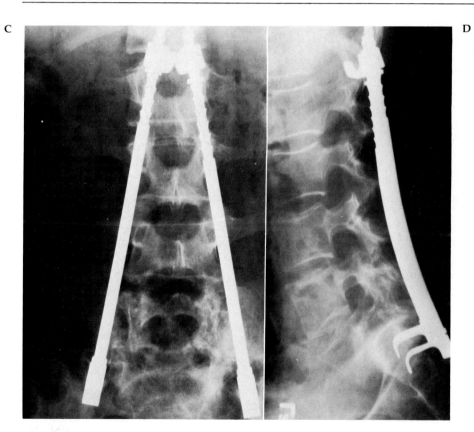

FIGURE 9-19, cont'd
AP **(C)** and lateral **(D)** films 8 months after reduction and internal fixation with
Harrington rods and posterolateral L4-S1 fusion which is now solid.

Abnormal Lordosis
IDIOPATHIC LORDOSCOLIOSIS

Significant thoracic lordosis is a rare clinical problem, most commonly being associated with idiopathic scoliosis when it does occur. Thoracic lordoscoliosis fortunately is uncommon (Fig. 9-20). Winter et al.[33] have emphasized that idiopathic thoracic lordoscoliosis compromises respiratory function even more severely than kyphoscoliosis. They stressed that the Milwaukee brace should be avoided in this situation as it increases the lordosis. Posterior fusion and Harrington distraction rods stabilize the curve, but normal thoracic kyphosis cannot be restored with this technique.[33] A new operative procedure has been described that allows restoration of the normal thoracic kyphosis in these patients. The technique consists of initial anterior fusion and multiple rib osteotomies followed by a posterior fusion using square-end contoured Harrington distraction rods secured by sublaminar wires at multiple levels.[3]

A 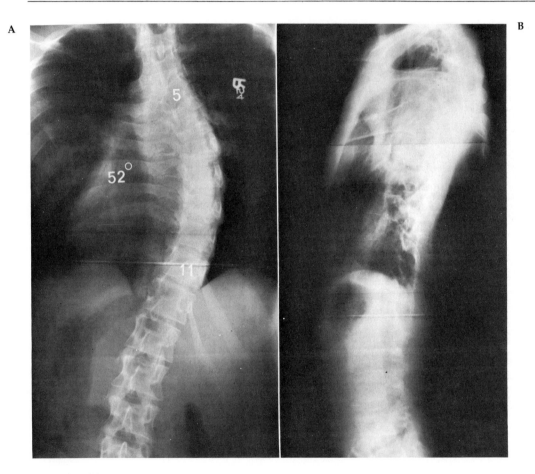 B

FIGURE 9-20
Adolescent lordoscoliosis.
The degree of scoliosis **(A)** is only moderate but the lateral view **(B)** shows marked anterior convexity of the thoracic spine and narrowing of the anteroposterior (AP) diameter of the chest.

CONGENITAL LORDOSIS

This rare entity has been described only sporadically in the literature with the largest series being the five patients described by Winter et al.[34] These patients have synostosis of the posterior elements alone so that with progressive enlargement of the anterior elements, there is a relentless increase in the thoracic lordosis (Fig. 9-21). The resultant decrease in the thoracic cage anteroposterior diameter results in restrictive lung disease and cor pulmonale. Early anterior fusion has been recommended as the optimal method of treatment.[34]

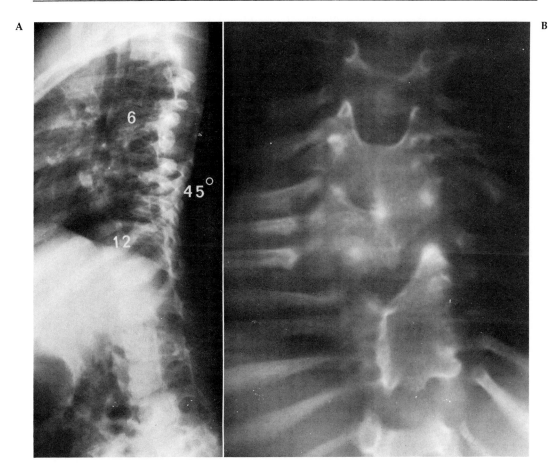

FIGURE 9-21
A 3-year-old girl with congenital lordosis subsequently treated by anterior fusion.
Lateral film **(A)** shows marked thoracic lordosis owing to posterior laminar fusion evident on the AP tomogram **(B)**.

POSTSURGICAL LUMBAR HYPERLORDOSIS

If extensive scarring develops eccentrically along any region of the growing spine, there is a potential for asymmetric spinal growth and resultant abnormal curvature. Previously, children with hydrocephalus were treated with lumboperitoneal shunts. In rare cases, the surgical insertion of the tube resulted in lumbar laminar fusion and hyperlordosis.[27] Although lumboperitoneal shunts are no longer used, these cases emphasize that any child having spinal or paraspinal surgery should be monitored clinically for the development of an abnormal spinal curvature.

Summary

A. Spondylolysis
  1. Etiology—acquired acute or stress fractures
  2. Diagnosis
     a. Oblique lumbar spine films usually adequate
     b. AP and lateral or oblique tomograms, if necessary
     c. Radionuclide bone scans and CT in special circumstances only
B. Spondylolisthesis
  1. Types: dysplastic, isthmic with fractured pars, isthmic with elongated pars, degenerative, traumatic, and pathologic
  2. Measurement
     a. Meyerding—grades I to V by quartile displacement
     b. Anterior displacement—percentage of AP diameter of S1
     c. Sacral inclination—tilt of sacrum from the vertical
     d. Sacrohorizontal angle—tilt of sacral superior endplate from the horizontal
     e. Sagittal rotation—rotation of L5 relative to posterior border of sacrum
     f. Percent of wedging = 100 × posterior height/anterior height
  3. Treatment
     a. Posterior fusion in situ or fusion after reduction with Harrington instrumentation
     b. Laminectomy added if neurologic deficit present
C. Thoracic lordosis
  1. Idiopathic lordoscoliosis
     a. Associated with respiratory insufficiency
     b. Two-stage anterior and posterior fusion after osteotomy restores normal thoracic kyphosis
  2. Congenital
     a. Owing to synostosis of posterior elements
     b. Early anterior fusion recommended
D. Lumbar hyperlordosis: may be secondary to lumboperitoneal shunts or other causes of posterior spinal fusion

REFERENCES

1. Amato, M.E., Gilula, L.A., and Totty, W.G.: Laminal fragmentation: a valuable sign of lumbar isthmic defect. Presented at the Radiological Society of North America, Chicago, 1983.
 2. Boxall, D., et al.: Management of severe spondylolisthesis in children and adolescents, J. Bone Joint Surg. (Am.) **61**:479-495, 1979.
 3. Bradford, D.S., Blatt, J.M., and Rasp, F.L.: Surgical management of severe thoracic lordosis: a new technique to restore normal kyphosis, Spine **8**:420-428, 1983.
 4. Brown, R.C., and Evans, E.T.: What causes the "eye in the Scotty dog" in the oblique projection of the lumbar spine? AJR **118**:435-437, 1973.
 5. Cyron, M., and Hutton, W.C.: The fatigue strength of the lumbar neural arch in spondylolysis, J. Bone Joint Surg. (Br.) **60**:234-238, 1978.
 6. Davis, I.S., and Bailey, R.W.: Spondylolisthesis: indications for lumbar nerve root decompression and operative technique, Clin. Orthop. **117**:129-134, 1976.
 7. Eisenberg, R.L.: Atlas of signs in radiology, Philadelphia, 1984, J.B. Lippincott Co.
 8. Eisenstein, S.: Spondylolysis, J. Bone Joint Surg. (Br.) **60**:488-494, 1978.
 9. Fullenlove, T.M., and Wilson, J.G.: Traumatic defects of the pars interarticularis of the lumbar vertebrae, AJR **122**:634-638, 1974.
10. Gelfand, M.J., Strife, J.L., and Kereiakes, J.G.: Radionuclide bone imaging in spondylolysis of the lumbar spine in children, Radiology **140**:191-195, 1981.
11. Ghelman, B., and Doherty, J.H.: Demonstration of spondylolysis by arthrography of the apophyseal joint, AJR **130**:986-987, 1978.
12. Grogan, J.P., et al.: Spondylolysis studied with computed tomography, Radiology **145**:737-742, 1982.
13. Hensinger, R.N., Lang, J.R., and MacEwen, G.D.: Surgical management of spondylolisthesis in children and adolescents, Spine **1**:207-216, 1976.
14. Johnson, J.R., and Kirwan, E.O'B.: The long-term results of fusion in situ for severe spondylolisthesis, J. Bone Joint Surg. (Br.) **65**:43-46, 1983.
15. Karasick, S., Karasick, D., and Wechsler, R.J.: Unilateral spondylolysis of the cervical spine, Skeletal Radiol. **9**:259-261, 1983.
16. Laurent, L.E., and Osterman, K.: Operative treatment of spondylolisthesis in young patients, Clin. Orthop. **117**:85-91, 1976.
17. Libson, E., et al.: Oblique lumbar spine radiographs: importance in young patients, Radiology **151**:89-90, 1984.
18. Maldague, B.E., and Malghem, J.J.: Unilateral arch hypertrophy with spinous process tilt: a sign of arch deficiency, Radiology **121**:567-574, 1976.
19. Maldague, B., Mathurin, P., and Malghem, J.: Facet joint arthrography in lumbar spondylolysis, Radiology **140**:29-36, 1981.
20. McPhee, I.B., and O'Brien, J.P.: Scoliosis in symptomatic spondylolisthesis, J. Bone Joint Surg. (Br.) **62**:155-157, 1980.
21. Meyerding, H.W.: Spondylolisthesis, Surg. Gynecol. Obstet. **54**:371-377, 1932.
22. Ravichandran, G.: A radiologic sign in spondylolisthesis, AJR **134**:113-117, 1980.
23. Rosenberg, N.J.: Degenerative spondylolisthesis, Clin. Orthop. **117**:112-120, 1976.
24. Scavone, J.G., Latshaw, R.F., and Weidner, W.A.: Anteroposterior and lateral radiographs: an adequate lumbar spine examination, AJR **136**:715-717, 1981.
25. Schwartz, A.M., et al.: Posterior arch defects of the cervical spine, Skeletal Radiol. **8**:135-139, 1982.
26. Sijbrandij, S.: Reduction and stabilisation of severe spondylolisthesis, J. Bone Joint Surg. (Br.) **65**:40-42, 1983.
27. Steel, H.H., and Adams, D.J.: Hyperlordosis caused by the lumboperitoneal shunt procedure for hydrocephalus, J. Bone Joint Surg. (Am.) **54**:1537-1542, 1972.
28. Wilkinson, R.H., and Hall, J.E.: The sclerotic pedicle: tumor or pseudotumor? Radiology **111**:683-688, 1974.

29. Wiltse, L.L.: Section 29, Lumbosacral spine: reconstruction. In Orthopaedic knowledge update I: Home study syllabus, Chicago, 1984, American Academy of Orthopaedic Surgeons, pp. 254-255.

30. Wiltse, L.L., Newman, P.H., and Macnab, I.: Classification of spondylolisis and spondylolisthesis, Clin. Orthop. **117:**23-29, 1976.

31. Wiltse, L.L., and Winter, R.G.: Terminology and measurement of spondylolisthesis, J. Bone Joint Surg. (Am.) **65:**768-772, 1983.

32. Winter, R.B.: Section 26, Thoracolumbar spine: pediatric. In Orthopaedic knowledge update I: Home study syllabus, Chicago, 1984, American Academy of Orthopaedic Surgeons, p. 223.

33. Winter, R.B., Lovell, W.W., and Moe, J.H.: Excessive thoracic lordosis and loss of pulmonary function in patients with idiopathic scoliosis, J. Bone Joint Surg. (Am.) **57:**972-977, 1975.

34. Winter, R.B., Moe, J.H., and Bradford, D.S.: Congenital thoracic lordosis, J. Bone Joint Surg. (Am.) **60:**806-809, 1978.

35. Wynne-Davies R., and Scott, J.H.S.: Inheritance and spondylolisthesis, J. Bone Joint Surg. (Br.) **61:**301-305, 1979.

Chapter Ten
Three-Dimensional Analysis of Spinal Curvature

Larry T. Cook

ANATOMIC LANDMARKS

DEVICE CONSTRUCTION

SYSTEM VALIDATION

MATHEMATICS OF THREE-DIMENSIONAL LOCALIZATION

ACQUISITION OF DATA

DATA DISPLAY

CLINICAL IMPLICATIONS

*T*he key to the assessment and treatment of spinal deformities is found in the ability to perceive changes in the spinal geometry of the patient. Standard plane projections of the spine involve geometric distortion of curved structures, cannot reliably document rotation, and cannot explicitly describe the true three-dimensional extent of spinal deformities. Furthermore, the accurate data that are available (angles) are strictly limited to that particular projection. Consequently, there has been a strong impetus to develop the means to obtain accurate three-dimensional radiographic data describing spinal geometry. Analogous needs have elicited the development of a family of related radiographic devices for accurately determining the geometry of various anatomic structures, including spines, knees, elbows, and hips.*

All of these devices are based fundamentally on the principle of triangulation as used in surveying for localization of a structure. By obtaining two or more radiographic projections without moving the patient, any object seen on several projections can be located in three-dimensional space if the accurate positions of the x-ray tube and film are known. The resultant calculations are also very complex, so the use of a computer is required if many examinations are to be performed. Our investigations into these problems and the details of our system will be presented.

A concomitant problem is that of presenting spinal coordinate data to the physician. Coordinates of points in space alone provide little insight into curve shape. Hence, the construction of this device requires that the calculated data be presented in a quickly understandable form. Presentation of the data in an integrated form is most easily accomplished through the use of a computer graphics system. We have explored several display systems, which will be discussed.

Anatomic Landmarks

In order to obtain meaningful and reasonably precise geometric information about the spine through radiographic means, either radiopaque markers can be implanted in the spine[14] or natural anatomic landmarks must be found. The localization procedure for our technique is analogous with the triangulation technique that is used for locating an unknown geographic position by observing azimuths to known landmarks. We modify the procedure by observing an anatomic feature from several fixed, separated positions and then triangulating on the unknown position of the feature. Consequently, we must observe a selected feature on several radiographic projections. Since it is difficult to implant markers in precisely standard places in each subject,

---

*See references 1-5, 9-11, 13-26.

markers can be used to document change precisely in a single patient, but they are not good for establishing standard guides to different classes of geometrically defined pathologies. Furthermore, the scoliosis patient population is not appropriate for the implanting of markers, so this technique is out of the question.

Certain anatomic structures such as the tips of the spinous processes,[1,11,13] the transverse processes,[13] and the articular facets[14,18] have been used as anatomic landmarks. However, the spinous processes may not follow the center line in a normal person but instead might bend away on either side of the sagittal plane, and the transverse processes and facets in the thoracic spine can be very difficult to locate on radiographs. Hence, these potential landmarks are not recommended.

It is believed that there are two types of reasonably reliable landmarks: the pedicles and the center of the vertebral body (Fig. 10-1). We are in agreement with other investigators that the inferior surface of the pedicle is a useful landmark.[1,11,13] However, we have found that these points may be difficult to locate when the spine is rotated because of overlapping ribs and marked vertebral tilting in some spinal deformities. It has been found experimentally that although the pedicles in nonrotated vertebrae can be seen in at least two of three projections separated by 45 degrees, these landmarks are not consistently seen when the vertebrae are rotated.[6] Thus the pedicles are reliable landmarks, but, unfortunately, in many patients with moderate spinal deformities, they cannot be located to use as landmarks.

The second and more reliable landmark is not an explicit anatomic point. It is the "center" of the vertebral body (Fig. 10-1). The "waist" of the vertebral body as seen on a radiograph is used to locate the center in the vertical direction. Two points on either side of the pinched-in waist of the vertebral body as seen in each projection are specified. The "center" lies halfway between them (Fig. 10-2). Location of this landmark is based on the assumption that a cross section of a vertebral body is an ellipse and on the second as-

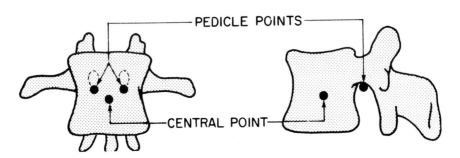

FIGURE 10-1
Reliable spinal landmarks that are detectable in multiple radiographic projections include the pedicle points and the vertebral body center.
From Cook, L.T., et al.: IEEE Trans. Biomed. Engin. **28**:366-371, 1981. © 1981 IEEE.

sumption that the lines from the x-ray source are essentially parallel. However, the cross section of a vertebral body is modified in its posterior aspect where the body is concave to accommodate the spinal canal. The consequence of this fact is that "center" is not a unique point, but its location may be shifted depending on which border of the vertebral body is visualized (Fig. 10-2). Rather than obtaining just the center of the vertebral body, the center for each endplate can similarly be obtained by identifying the outer points of the superior and inferior edges of each vertebral body.[1]

We evaluated six vertebrae to determine how close the cross-sectional shape of a vertebral body is to an ellipse.[8] Axial radiographs of six vertebral specimens from the thoracic and lumbar spine were used. Data were obtained from each projection corresponding to the central vertebral cross section excluding the spinal canal region. Each of these contours was fitted to the equation of an ellipse using a standard least–squares procedure. The fits obtained were good to very good.[6] We concluded that the outline of a vertebral body was a truncated ellipse. Using these data, we then calculated the variability that is introduced with different techniques of finding the "center" of a vertebral body because the shape is not a true ellipse but a truncated ellipse. We found less variation using three views at 45 degree angles than when two views at 90 degrees were used.[6] High thoracic vertebral bodies demonstrated more variability than lumbar or low thoracic vertebrae because their cross section forms less of an ellipse.[6] Using the 45 degree projections, the interexamination error from a 20 degree rotation was 0.6 mm for T3 and 0.7 mm for L5. Using the two 90 degree views, the errors were 2.6 mm and 3.0 mm, respectively. Our investigation demonstrated that we can fix the magnitude of the variation in position that can be expected when anatomic landmarks are used. This is an important aspect of an evaluation of the accuracy and repeatability of the measurements made by the device we describe. In practice, variations such as these are limited by the need to position the patient consistently in the device.

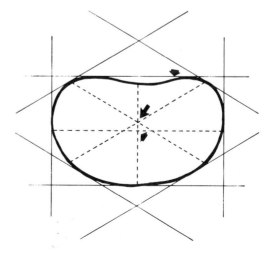

FIGURE 10-2
Cross section of the midportion of a vertebral body.
The dotted lines halfway between parallel tangents intersect at a constant point *(long arrow)* except when the tangent is across the spinal canal region *(upper short arrow)*. For the spinal canal tangent, the midway dotted line intersection is shifted anteriorly *(lower short arrow)*.

From De Smet, A.A., et al.: Radiology **137**:343-348, 1980.

Device Construction

The general layout of our device is seen in Fig. 10-3. Three whole-spine radiographs, separated by 45 degrees, are taken of each patient. The triangulation method is used first to calculate the positions of the x-ray tubes using reference points that are held fixed by the metal framework of the device (Fig. 10-4). By using a framework in front of and in back of the patient, the x-ray tube does not have to be positioned at a precise point for each exposure. After this calculation, triangulation is again used to calculate the coordinates of spinal landmarks (Fig. 10-5).

The device evolved through several stages during which we corrected problems that had arisen. Despite the use of a steel backframe and steel undersurface in our prototype model, the framework wobbled when a patient stood in the device. Braces were added between the backsurface and the undersurface to hold the framework rigid. The fixed reference points initially were formed by tensioned horizontal and vertical wires in an open framework. Technicians had to handle the framework, since it was detached when the device was not in use. The handling of the framework caused the wires to be displaced or disturbed. Consequently, we developed the current system, described below, in which the reference points are protected from inadvertent displacement. Finally, it was difficult to position the x-ray tube since the arrangement of the reference point, the patient, and the cassette holder was

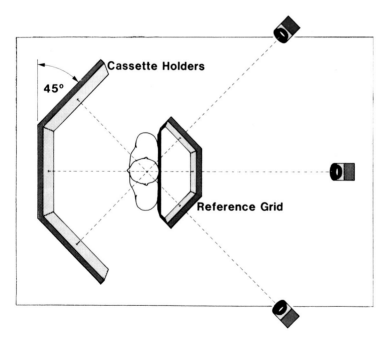

FIGURE 10-3
Plan view of the three-dimensional scoliosis apparatus.
The x-ray tube is moved to three separate positions to produce three radiographs.
From De Smet, A.A., et al.: Automedica **4**:25-36, 1981.

FIGURE 10-4
Reference points from the wire frame are projected onto a film. The x-ray tube coordinates (x, y) can be calculated by knowing the location of both the projected points on the film and the points on the reference frame.

From De Smet, A.A., et al.: Radiology **137**:343-348, 1980.

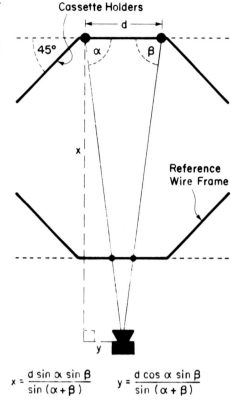

$$x = \frac{d \sin \alpha \sin \beta}{\sin (\alpha + \beta)} \qquad y = \frac{d \cos \alpha \sin \beta}{\sin (\alpha + \beta)}$$

FIGURE 10-5
If the locations of two x-ray tubes, *B1* and *B2*, (see Fig. 10-4) and the projected images, *A1* and *A2*, are known, then the x and y coordinates of the object A can be calculated as indicated.

From De Smet, A.A., et al.: Radiology **137**:343-348, 1980.

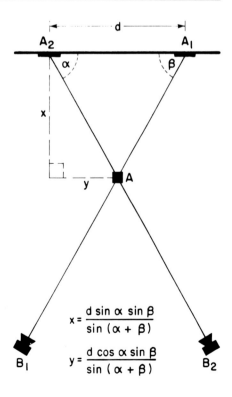

$$x = \frac{d \sin \alpha \sin \beta}{\sin (\alpha + \beta)}$$

$$y = \frac{d \cos \alpha \sin \beta}{\sin (\alpha + \beta)}$$

critical, as can be seen in Fig. 10-3. Positioning holes were drilled in the floor so that the device was always in the same position in the room. Tape markers were placed on the overhead x-ray tube rails indicating the location for each of the three tube positions. The result was that the tube could be moved quickly from position to position, and we reliably obtain radiographs that demonstrate the entire spine.

In summary, the physical device is designed to support fixed-wire reference points, hold film cassettes, and position a patient (Fig. 10-6). The fixed-wire reference points are formed by the intersections of horizontal and vertical wires of 0.010 inch diameter. The wires are embedded in plexiglas plates which, in turn, are fastened to the main framework. The film cassette holders are height adjustable and each has two markers called film reference points that define the center line on each film. The coordinates of the source and film reference points were established by surveying the completed apparatus with a theodolite of 1 second accuracy. This accuracy at the surveying distance translated into an accuracy of ±0.001 inch at the apparatus.

The theodolite was set up in several distinct positions. From each position sights were taken on known reference points not on the device and the unknown points on the device. Each set of observations consisted of two

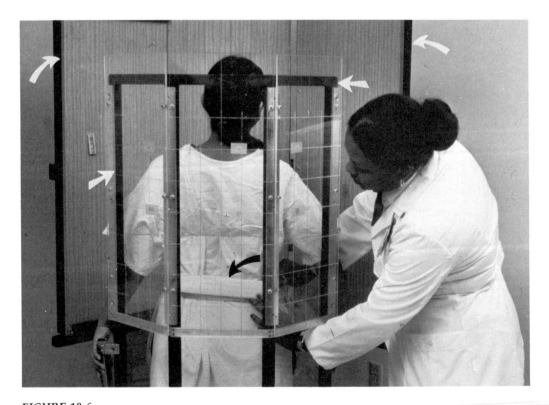

FIGURE 10-6
A photograph of the device showing cassette holders *(white curved arrows)* and wire reference frame *(white arrows)*. The Velcro pelvic band is being adjusted on the patient *(black curved arrow)*.

angles for each unknown reference point. The angles were the azimuthal angle and the angle of inclination from the horizontal. Then a triangulation procedure was used to calculate the coordinates of the unknown points. The mathematics used are the same as those used to locate spinal landmarks as described in detail later in this chapter. The algorithm was programmed into a hand calculator to determine the coordinates of the fixed reference points on the framework.

The patient is positioned in the device by means of a band that holds the pelvis against a plexiglas sheet (Fig. 10-6). The patient stands naturally with relaxed arms hanging down. This position does not induce any extraneous forces or curves in the spine. Referring to the plan view of this set-up in Fig. 10-3, we observe that the patient must occupy that place in the device that is covered by all three x-ray beams. When films are exposed, the information recorded on each film includes the wire reference points, the film reference points, and the spinal landmarks of the patient.

Since there is an air gap between the patient and the film, which reduces scattered radiation, no grids are used. Our measurements indicate that the total radiation dose to a patient from the three projections we use is about the same as the total dose received from an anteroposterior and a lateral radiograph.[3]

System Validation

We validated the system using a phantom constructed from 5.08 cm diameter rods.[3] Three sections were cut, measuring 2.58 cm in height, and two ball bearings were embedded posteriorly to simulate pedicles. Flat disks with central pivot pins were used to simulate the intervertebral disks and also to allow rotation. Spacers with 10 degree wedge angles were used to simulate curvature. Three sets of radiographs were exposed with rotations of 0, 15, and 30 degrees and lateral curvature of 10 degrees. The resulting coordinate data obtained indicated that the system provided spatial resolution within 1.0 mm and measured rotation within 2 degrees.

An important consideration in any three-dimensional localization device used clinically is the potential for patient movement. Experimental determinations of accuracy may be irrelevant if patient movement can produce errors that are a magnitude larger than the system error. To address this problem, several approaches have been used. Biplane simultaneous exposures have been used to eliminate totally patient motion,[1] but they significantly increase patient exposure due to the need for high-ratio crisscross grids to reduce scatter radiation. As discussed above, biplanar (90 degree) exposures also result in less consistent determination of the vertebral body center. Alternatively, an automatic, vertically shifted x-ray tube and film changer have been devised to reduce the time between two anteroposterior exposures to 5 seconds.[11] The problem with this system is that the angle between the two projections is very small. As a result, small errors in marking the landmarks result in large errors in the calculated spatial location. All of the current systems thus have limitations in the degree of precision attainable.

The three 45 degree views we have selected have the advantage of minimizing the error in locating vertebral centers due to rotation and are widely separated to minimize the deleterious effects of slightly mislocating a vertebral landmark. However, an average of 5 minutes is required for the film sequence, so the potential for patient movement is great. Because of concern over this issue, we have analyzed the potential magnitude of error due to patient motion with our system assuming that a patient, when asked to stand normally, always stands so that each vertebral center is within a distance, e, of some ideal point. Since the patient is constrained by a back support and an anterior band, this error should be from side to side in a horizontal line. Then, if two orthogonal views are used to establish vertebral landmarks, the maximal interexamination variation is 2e. Surprisingly, the same assumption leads us to conclude that the maximal interexamination variation using our apparatus is also 2e. Fig. 10-7 illustrates this point. The shaded area shows where our method will calculate the position of a landmark, given that the true position of the landmark was somewhere on the dark line segment. The distance, d, represents the incremental increase in variability due to the shape of the region shaded in Fig. 10-7. The maximum distance between any two points in this region is 2e + d, where d is much smaller than e and d depends on e. For our apparatus, $d = 2e^3/[(144)^2 - e^2]$ cm. If e = 2 cm, then d = 0.008 mm. Given that the design goal for accuracy was ±1 mm, the number d is insignificant. Even if e (or patient side to side movement) is large, for instance e = 10 cm, then d is only 1 mm.

We concluded that if a patient can assume a stance repeatedly within a horizontal error of e, then our apparatus will find landmarks within e of the ideal or true position, and, furthermore, the interexamination error due to stance is 2e. These figures match the performance of systems in which patient movement is minimized by simultaneous biplane exposures.

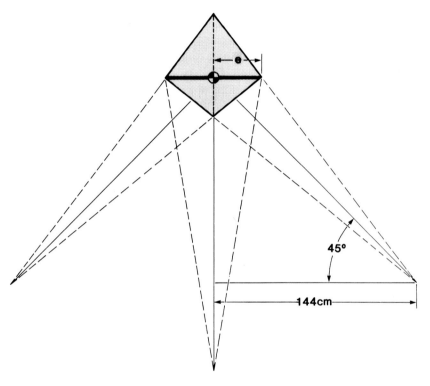

FIGURE 10-7
The theoretical position of a landmark is indicated at the center of the heavy line segment. If the actual position moves along the heavy line segment, the three-view method will calculate the position of the landmark to be inside the shaded region.

Mathematics of Three-Dimensional Localization

As discussed above, the scoliosis device uses the principle of triangulation to locate anatomic landmarks in space. Simply stated, an anatomic landmark lies on the ray drawn from the focal spot of the x-ray tube to the projection of the landmark on the film. If two distinct lines are constructed by using different tube and film locations, then the lines intersect at the immobile anatomic landmark. This situation is shown in Fig. 10-5.

For a formal mathematical description, we assume that all points are taken relative to a fixed coordinate system. Suppose line i passes through the points P_i and Q_i. Define

$$A_i = P_i - Q_i$$
$$i = 1,2$$

where P_i and Q_i are considered as vectors. Let

$$B = P_2 - P_1$$

then the intersection point, X, satisfies both

$$Y = sA_1 + P_1$$

and

$$Y = tA_2 + P_2$$

for an appropriate pair s,t. Unfortunately, in three-dimensional space, these lines may not actually intersect. To allow for that situation, suppose that X_1 and X_2 are the points on lines one and two that are closest to the other line. Then

$$s = [(A_1 \circ A_2)(B \circ A_2) - (A_2 \circ A_2)(B \circ A_1)]/C$$

and

$$t = [(A_1 \circ A_1)(B \circ A_2) - (A_1 \circ A_2)(B \circ A_1)]/C$$

where

$$C = (A_1 \circ A_2)^2 - A_1^2 A_2^2$$

(The symbol "$\circ$" refers to scalar product.)

An estimate of the intersection point is given by

$$X = (X_1 + X_2)/2.$$

The error due to this algorithm has been investigated by Sherlock and Aitken.[20] Their results demonstrate that the error is least when the angle between views is 90 degrees. The error remains low until the angle between views is less than 45 degrees. Consequently, we do not expect this algorithm to introduce a significant error into our calculations. Furthermore, the algorithm is easily implemented on any computer or programmable calculator.

Acquisition of Data

The anatomic landmarks, wire reference points, and film reference points are entered into a computer using a digitizing stylus and tablet. On each radiograph, there are two film registration points and between 2 and 12 wire frame reference points (Fig. 10-8). Each vertebral body has four points to be digitized, namely the two pedicles and the left and right sides of the vertebral body (Fig. 10-8). Three radiographs must be digitized. In practice, the landmarks are marked by the radiologist and the actual digitization is carried out by a technician. Digitization accuracy is ±0.1 mm for the digitizer itself. A larger error is undoubtedly introduced when the observers locate the landmarks and place the digitizer.

FIGURE 10-8
Digitized points for computer data entry.
The film reference points *(arrows)* and several of the wire reference points *(curved arrows)* and vertebral landmarks *(arrowheads)* are shown. The thick white line *(short white arrow)* is produced by the joint between two intensifying screens in the cassette.

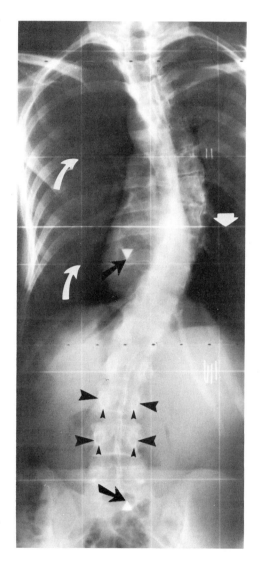

Data Display

Subsequent to the digitization of coordinate data, the three-dimensional coordinates of the vertebral centers and pedicles are calculated. Using these data, the spine can be displayed on a computer graphics display from any desired viewing angle. We have investigated multiple methods of display and currently utilize three modes: (1) static display, (2) rotating display, and (3) the top view. Because of the ability of a computer to manipulate mathematical data rapidly, more numbers describing spinal geometry can be generated than reasonably comprehended. We had hoped that using color bars to show relative magnitude of a particular variable would allow rapid detection of significant abnormal values. However, since the importance of a particular variable and specific values is as yet undetermined, the color bars have not proven useful. At this point, we would not recommend that other investigators include them in their display systems.

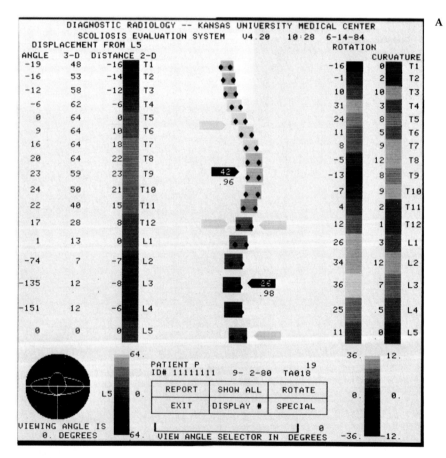

FIGURE 10-9

A 13-year-old girl with idiopathic scoliosis. Her 42 degree right thoracic and 26 degree left lumbar scoliosis is seen from five computer-generated perspectives.

A, Posterior view at 0 degrees (angle of view indicated by drawing in lower left-hand corner).

The basic and most important display is the static display of the spine from a desired viewing angle. The standard posteroanterior and left lateral views are routinely generated and hard copies are made of these images (Fig. 10-9, *A* and *B*). The computer automatically determines the end vertebrae, apical vertebra, and Cobb angle more accurately and reproducibly than is manually possible.[12] The ability to view the spine from other projections is occasionally useful to find the plane of largest curvature (the "Stagnara" view, Fig. 10-9, *C*) and to view the spine along the axis of the curve (a true, nonrotated posterior view, Fig. 10-9, *D*). Each vertebral body is shown as a rectangle and the pedicles are projected as circles in various positions on the rectangle depending on whether they can be seen in the selected projection. The plain arrows pointing at the vertebrae indicate the end vertebrae. The darker arrows point at the apical vertebrae and give the Cobb angle within the

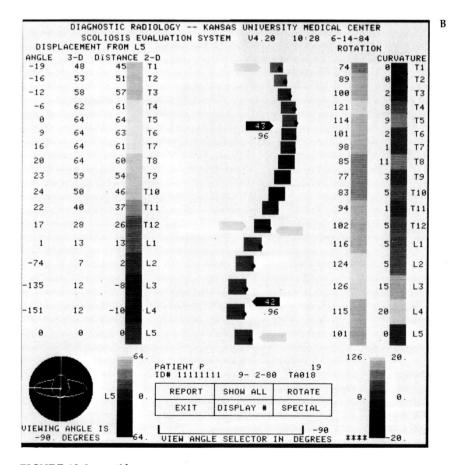

FIGURE 10-9, cont'd
B, Left lateral view at −90 degrees. The thoracic kyphosis and lumbar lordosis are normal at 43 and 42 degrees respectively.

Continued.

arrow. The fraction beneath the Cobb angle arrow is the arc of curvature where 1.00 is a straight line and decreasing fractions indicate progressive curvature.

The mathematical information is arranged in vertical columns on the television screen. In Fig. 10-9, *A*, the left-most column gives the direction of axial displacement of each vertebra on a polar coordinate system relative to L5. A posterior view would be 0 degrees (Fig. 10-9, *A*), a left lateral view would be −90 degrees (Fig. 10-9, *B*), a right lateral view would be +90 degrees, and so on. The figure in the lower left shows the viewing plane and direction. The viewing angle is selected by moving a cursor along the scale in the lower part of the middle of the screen.

The second column contains the magnitude in millimeters of the axial displacement of each vertebra in the direction specified by the corresponding

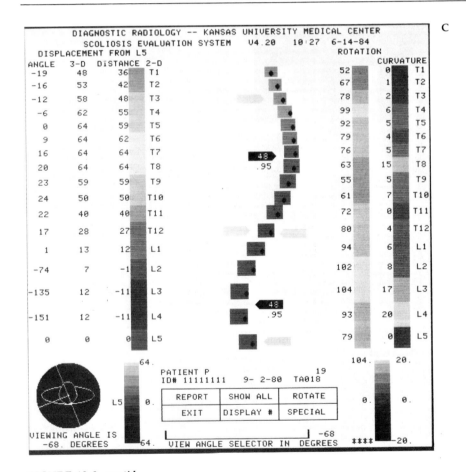

FIGURE 10-9, cont'd

C, Left posterior oblique view at −68 degrees demonstrates maximum size of the thoracic curve.

angle in the first (left-most) column. For example, in Fig. 10-9, *A*, the body of T1 is displaced 48 mm (column 2) along the −19 degree vector (column 1).

The third column contains the magnitudes of the displacement to the left or right of a vertical line through L5 for the chosen viewing angle. This measurement allows determination of the relative balance of each vertebral body and trunkal balance relative to the midline, which is arbitrarily determined at L5. In Fig. 10-9, *A*, T1 is displaced 16 mm (column 3) to the left of the midline so the patient is out of balance to the left.

The column immediately to the right of the spinal display gives the axial rotation of each vertebral body relative to the localizing framework. Relative rotations of one vertebra to another are determined by subtraction. In Fig. 10-9, *A* the lumbar apex (L3) is rotated 36 degrees to the right.

The last column contains curvature values (Ferguson angle) for each ver-

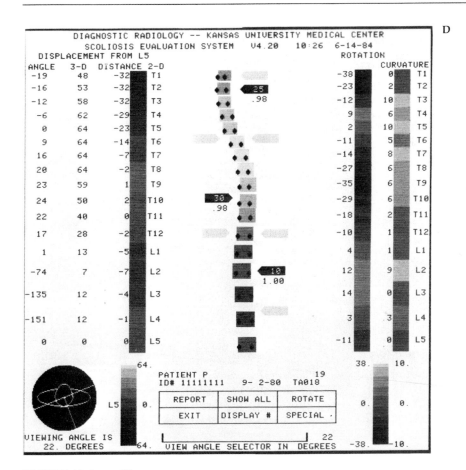

FIGURE 10-9, cont'd

D, View at right angle to maximum thoracic curvature view shows straightening of the segment of the thoracic scoliosis but increased curvature in the upper thoracic segment.

Continued.

tebral body relative to the vertebra above and the vertebra below. This is a measure of the local curvature and represents the degree of angular deformity at each segment of the spine.

The second major display is the rotating line display, which dynamically changes a line drawing in 1 degree increments. This display allows a viewer to appreciate the shape of a spine by seeing it rotate in real time. Although this is difficult to quantitate, it provides a visual approximation of a true three-dimensional or holographic-type image.

The most potentially useful value of the three-dimensional technique is the top view (Fig. 10-9, *E*), a cephalocaudad view of the spine. Each vertebral body is represented by a rectangle, and the data are presented in a stylized drawing. This view is used as another visual summary and can be of great utility in expanding the physician's ability to integrate the data produced by a three-dimensional scoliosis system.[6]

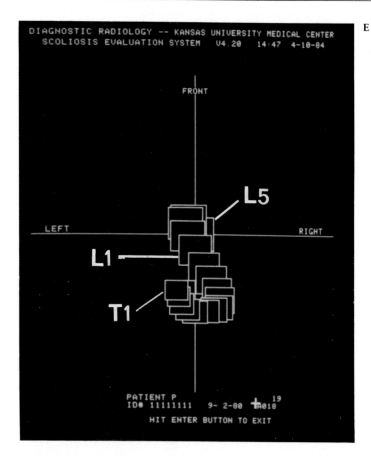

FIGURE 10-9, cont'd

E, Top view as if the spine is viewed from above with overlapping of the rectangles representing vertebrae from T1 above to L5 on the bottom. The spine is seen not to deform in one plane but to curve like a helix. The lumbar spine has mostly lordosis without much side-to-side swing. The thoracic spine sweeps far to the right before ending out of balance to the left at T1.

The final display technique available to us but not an integral part of the scoliosis system is demonstrated in Fig. 10-10. The raw data consist of the coordinates of vertebral body centroids and pedicles. An idealized three-dimensional vertebral body is placed at each centroid and it is rotated in space to match the rotation inferred from the pedicle locations. Its size is specified by its locations (T1, T2, and so on). Geometrically, each idealized vertebral body is a polyhedron with its lateral surfaces defined by triangular faces. Using advanced computer graphics display techniques, a reconstructed spine can be viewed from any angle, or stereoscopic pairs can be created, as can be observed in Fig. 10-10.

FIGURE 10-10
Stylized three-dimensional stereo pair depicting the lateral aspect of a right lower thoracic scoliosis.

From De Smet, A.A., et al.: Radiology **136:**343-348, 1980.

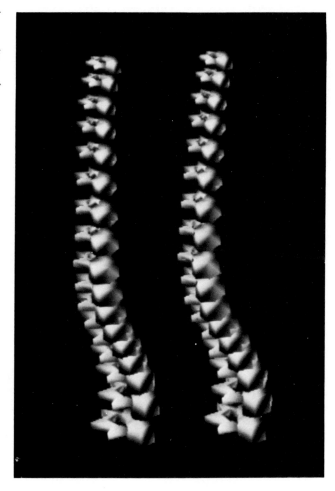

Clinical Implications

A three-dimensional scoliosis device offers some definite advantages over routine two-dimensional radiographs. Cobb angles are computed with better reproducibility and a lower standard deviation using our mathematical model.[12] With the restrictions noted earlier, vertebral rotation is obtained with excellent precision.[4]

Through the use of computer graphics techniques, any desired view of the spine can be constructed. These views help to understand the three-dimensional shape of each patient's spine. In particular, the top view graphically demonstrates that two spines with the same frontal plane curves can have dramatically different three-dimensional morphologies. A collapse of a curve, over time, as seen in the top view accompanies scoliotic curve progression, suggesting a common mechanism of curve progression.[7] Proper placement of pads in a brace may be suggested by an analysis of the top view, for instance, to determine if a pad should exert a purely lateral force or a composite lateral and anterior force.[7]

The potential uses of this device include the collection of data for the calculation of the mechanical properties of the spine and the resolution of the forces acting on the spine. Other avenues of research are also available; for example, when sufficient data have been collected we might be able to identify shape descriptors that will help to predict those curves most likely to progress.

REFERENCES

1. Brown, R.H., et al.: Spinal analysis using a three-dimensional radiographic technique, J. Biomech. **9:**355-365, 1976.
2. Chao, E.Y., and Morrey, B.F.: Three-dimensional rotation of the elbow, J. Biomech. **11:**57-73, 1978.
3. Cook, L.T., et al.: Assessment of scoliosis using three-dimensional analysis, IEEE Trans. Biomed. Engin. **28:**366-371, 1981.
4. DeSmet, A.A., et al.: A radiographic method for three-dimensional analysis of spinal configuration, Radiology **137:**343-348, 1980.
5. DeSmet, A.A., et al.: Assessment of scoliosis using three-dimensional radiographic measurements, Automedica **4:**25-36, 1981.
6. DeSmet, A.A., et al.: Evaluation of radiographic landmarks for three-dimensional spinal analysis. Proceedings International Conference on the Pathogenesis of Scoliosis, Denver, Colorado, 1982.
7. DeSmet, A.A., et al.: The top view for analysis of scoliosis progression, Radiology **147:**369-372, 1983.
8. DeSmet, A.A., et al.: Evaluation of radiographic landmarks for three-dimensional spinal analysis. In Jacobs, R.R., editor: Pathogenesis of idiopathic scoliosis, Chicago, 1984, Scoliosis Research Society.
9. Frymoyer, J.W., et al.: The mechanical and kinematic analysis of the lumbar spine in normal living human subjects in vivo, J. Biomech. **12:**165-172, 1979.
10. Hierholzer, E.: The display-stereocomparator, a new device for biostereometric measurements, Appl. Hum. Biostereometr. (NATO) SPIE Proc. **166:**31-35, 1978.
11. Hindmarsh, J., Larsson, J., and Mattsson, O.: Analysis of changes in the scoliotic spine using a three-dimensional radiographic technique, J. Biomech. **13:**279-290, 1980.
12. Jeffries, B.F., et al.: Computerized measurement and analysis of scoliosis, Radiology **134:**381-385, 1980.
13. Kratky, V.: Analytical x-ray photogrammetry in scoliosis, Photogrammetria **31:** 195-210, 1975.
14. Matteri, R.E., Pope, M.H., and Frymoyer, J.W.: A biplane radiographic method of determining vertebral rotation in postmortem specimens, Clin. Orthop. **116:**95-98, 1976.

15. Olsson, T.H., Selvik, G., and Willner, S.: Kinematic analysis of spinal fusions, Invest. Radiol. **11**:202-209, 1976.
16. Panjabi, M., and White, A.A.: A mathematical approach for three-dimensional analysis of the mechanics of the spine, J. Biomech. **4**:203-211, 1971.
17. Pearcy, M., and Burrough, S.: Assessment of bony union after interbody fusion of the lumbar spine using a biplanar radiographic technique, J. Bone Joint Surg. (Br.) **64**:228-232, 1982.
18. Pope, M.H., et al.: Experimental measurements of vertebral motion under load, Orthop. Clin. North Am. **8**:155-167, 1977.
19. Reuben, J.D., et al.: In vivo effects of axial loading on healthy, adolescent spines, Clin. Orthop. **139**:17-27, 1979.
20. Reuben, J.D., et al.: In vivo effects of axial loading on double-curve scoliotic spines, Spine **7**:440-447, 1982.
21. Sherlock, R.A., and Aitken, W.M.: A method of precision position determination using x-ray stereography, Phys. Med. Biol. **25**:349-355, 1980.
22. Suh, C.H.: The fundamentals of computer aided x-ray analysis of the spine, J. Biomech. **7**:161-169, 1974.
23. van Dijk, R., Huiskes, R., and Selvik, G.: Roentgen stereophotogrammetric methods for the evaluation of the three dimensional kinematic behavior and cruciate ligament length patterns of the human knee joint, J. Biomech. **12**:727-731, 1979.
24. Veress, S.A., et al.: Patellar tracking patterns measurement by analytical x-ray photogrammetry, J. Biomech. **12**:639-650, 1979.
25. White, A.A.: Kinematics of the normal spine as related to scoliosis, J. Biomech. **4**:405-411, 1971.
26. Wientroub, S., et al.: The use of stereophotogrammetry to measure acetabular and femoral anteversion, J. Bone Joint Surg. (Br.) **63**:209-213, 1981.

Appendix

Approved Glossary of the Scoliosis Research Society (1981)

Adolescent scoliosis

Scoliosis appearing at or about the onset of puberty and before maturity.

Adult scoliosis

Scoliosis of any etiology present after skeletal maturity.

Angle of thoracic inclination

With the trunk flexed 90 degrees at the hips, the angle between the horizontal and a plane across the posterior rib cage at the greatest prominence of a rib hump.

Apical vertebra

The most rotated vertebra in a curve; the most deviated from the vertical axis of the patient.

Cafe-au-lait spots

Light brown irregular areas of skin pigmentation with smooth margins. If six or more measuring 1.5 cm or more in diameter are present, neurofibromatosis is suggested.

Cervical scoliosis

Scoliosis having its apex at or between C1 and C6.

Cervicothoracic scoliosis

Scoliosis having its apex at C7, T1, or the intervening disk space.

Compensation

The alignment of the inion with the midpoint of the sacrum. (In patients without cervical scoliosis, the midpoint of C7 may be used in place of the inion.)

Compensatory curve

A curve above or below a structural curve that tends to maintain compensation.

Congenital scoliosis

Scoliosis owing to congenitally anomalous vertebral development.

Curve measurement

>   (1) Select the most caudal vertebrae whose inferior endplate tilts to the concavity of the curve and erect a perpendicular from this endplate.
>   (2) Select the most cephalad vertebra whose superior endplate tilts to the concavity of the curve and erect a perpendicular from this endplate.
>   (3) The curve value is the number of degrees formed by the angle of intersection of these perpendiculars.

Double structural scoliosis

>   When two structural scolioses occur in the same spine.

Double thoracic

>   A double structural scoliosis with the apex of each curve located in the thoracic spine.

End vertebra

>   The most cephalad vertebra of a curve whose superior surface, or transverse axis or the most caudal one, whose inferior surface or transverse axis tilts maximally toward the concavity of the curve.

Fractional curve

>   A compensatory curve that is incomplete because it returns to the erect. Its only horizontal vertebra is its caudad or cephalad one.

Gibbus

>   A sharply angular kyphosis.

Hyperkyphosis

>   A kyphosis greater than the normal range, that is, a kyphos.

Hyperlordosis

>   A lordosis of greater than the normal range.

Hypokyphosis

>   A kyphosis of the thoracic spine of less than the normal range.

Hypolordosis

>   A lordosis of the cervical or lumbar spine of less than the normal range.

Hysterical scoliosis

>   A nonstructural scoliosis owing to a conversion reaction.

Idiopathic scoliosis

>   A scoliosis of unknown etiology.

Iliac epiphysis

>   The epiphysis along the crest of the ilium.

Iliac epiphysis (apophysis) sign

> In the anteroposterior roentgenogram of the pelvis, the state of ossification of the iliac epiphysis (apophysis) is used to denote the degree of skeletal maturity:
> (0) Equals no presence of the epiphysis.
> (1) Equals 25% excursion.
> (2) Equals 50% excursion.
> (3) Equals 75% excursion.
> (4) Equals 100% excursion.
> (5) Equals fusion of the epiphysis to the iliac crest.

Infantile idiopathic scoliosis

> An idiopathic scoliosis appearing before the skeletal age of 3 years.

Infantile scoliosis

> Scoliosis developing during the first 3 years of life.

Juvenile scoliosis

> Scoliosis developing between skeletal age 3 years and the onset of puberty.

Kyphos

> An abnormally increased kyphosis.

Kyphoscoliosis

> A structural scoliosis associated with a kyphos in the same area.

Kyphosis

> A posterior convex angulation of the spine.

Lordoscoliosis

> A structural scoliosis associated with an abnormal lordosis in the same area.

Lordosis

> An anterior convex angulation of the spine.

Lumbar scoliosis

> A scoliosis that has its apex from the L1-2 disk space to the L4-5 disk space.

Lumbosacral scoliosis

> A scoliosis with its apex at L5, S1, or the intervening disk space.

Major curve

> Term used to designate the larger(est) curve(s), usually structural.

Minor curve

> Term used to refer to smaller(est) curve(s).

Myopathic scoliosis

> Scoliosis owing to a muscular disorder.

Neuropathic scoliosis
> Scoliosis owing to a neurologic disorder.

Nonstructural (functional) curve
> A curve that has no structural component.

Pelvic inclination
> Deviation of the pelvis from the vertical in the sagittal plane.

Pelvic obliquity
> Deviation of the pelvis from the horizontal in the frontal plane.

Pelvic rotation
> Deviation of the pelvis from normal around the longitudinal axis of the body.

Primary curve
> The first structural curve to appear.

Skeletal age
> The age obtained by comparing posteroanterior roentgenogram of the left wrist and hand with the standards of the Gruelich and Pyle Atlas.

Structural scoliosis
> A lateral curvature of the spine that does not demonstrate normal segmental mobility on lateral bending or distraction.

Thoracic scoliosis
> Scoliosis in which the apex of the curvature is between T2 and T11.

Thoracogenic scoliosis
> Spinal curvature attributable to disease or operative trauma in or on the thoracic cage.

Thoracolumbar scoliosis
> A scoliosis with its apex at T12, L1, or the intervening disk space.

Index